Learning Disabilities Sourcebook, 3rd Edition

Leukemia Sourcebook

Liver Disorders Sourcebook

Lung Disorders Sourcebook

Medical Tests Sourcebook, 3rd Edition

Men's Health Concerns Sourcebook, 2nd Edition

Mental Health Disorders Sourcebook, 4th Edition

Mental Retardation Sourcebook

Movement Disorders Sourcebook, 2nd Edition

Multiple Sclerosis Sourcebook

Muscular Dystrophy Sourcebook

Obesity Sourcebook

Osteoporosis Sourcebook

Pain Sourcebook, 3rd Edition

Pediatric Cancer Sourcebook

Physical & Mental Issues in Aging Sourcebook

Podiatry Sourcebook, 2nd Edition

Pregnancy & Birth Sourcebook, 2nd Edition

Prostate & Urological Disorders Sourcebook

Prostate Cancer Sourcebook

Reconstructive & Cosmetic Surgery Sourcebook

Rehabilitation Sourcebook

Respiratory Disorders Sourcebook, 2nd Edition

Sexually Transmitted Diseases Sourcebook, 3rd Edition

Sleep Disorders Sourcebook, 3rd Edition

Smoking Concerns Sourcebook

Sports Injuries Sourcebook, 3rd Edition

Stress-Related Disorders Sourcebook, 2nd Edition

Stroke Sourcebook, 2nd Edition

Surgery Sourcebook, 2nd Edition

Thyroid Disorders Sourcebook

Transplantation Sourcebook

Traveler's Health Sourcebook

Urinary Tract & Kidney Diseases & Disorders Sourcebook, 2nd Edition

Vegetarian Sourcebook

Women's Health Concerns Sourcebook, 3rd Edition

Workplace Health & Safety Sourcebook

Worldwide Health Sourcebook

Teen Health Series

Abuse & Violence Information for Teens

Accident & Safety Information for Teens

Alcohol Information for Teens, 2nd Edition

Allergy Information for Teens

Asthma Information for Teens, 2nd Edition

Body Information for Teens

Cancer Information for Teens

Complementary & Alternative Medicine Information for Teens

Diabetes Information for Teens

Diet Information for Teens, 2nd Edition

Drug Information for Teens, 3rd Edition

Eating Disorders Information for Teens, 2nd Edition

Fitness Information for Teens, 2nd Edition

Learning Disabilities Information for Teens

Mental Health Information for Teens, 3rd Edition

Pregnancy Information for Teens

Sexual Health Information for Teens, 2nd Edition

Skin Health Information for Teens, 2nd Edition

Sleep Information for Teens

Sports Injuries Information for Teens, 2nd Edition

Stress Information for Teens

Suicide Information for Teens, 2nd Edition

Tobacco Information for Teens, 2nd Edition

Allergies
SOURCEBOOK

Fourth Edition

Health Reference Series

Fourth Edition

Allergies
SOURCEBOOK

*Basic Consumer Health Information about the
Immune System and Allergic Disorders, Including
Rhinitis (Hay Fever), Sinusitis, Conjunctivitis, Asthma,
Atopic Dermatitis, and Anaphylaxis, and Allergy Triggers
Such As Pollen, Mold, Dust Mites, Animal Dander,
Chemicals, Foods and Additives, and Medications*

*Along with Facts about Allergy Diagnosis and
Treatment, Tips on Avoiding Triggers and Preventing
Symptoms, a Glossary of Related Terms, and
Directories of Resources for Additional
Help and Information*

Edited by
Amy L. Sutton

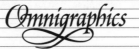

P.O. Box 31-1640, Detroit, MI 48231

Bibliographic Note
Because this page cannot legibly accommodate all the copyright notices, the Bibliographic Note portion of the Preface constitutes an extension of the copyright notice.

Edited by Amy L. Sutton

Health Reference Series

Karen Bellenir, *Managing Editor*
David A. Cooke, MD, FACP, *Medical Consultant*
Elizabeth Collins, *Research and Permissions Coordinator*
Cherry Edwards, *Permissions Assistant*
EdIndex, Services for Publishers, *Indexers*

* * *

Omnigraphics, Inc.
Matthew P. Barbour, *Senior Vice President*
Kevin M. Hayes, *Operations Manager*

* * *

Peter E. Ruffner, *Publisher*

Copyright © 2011 Omnigraphics, Inc.

ISBN 978-0-7808-1144-7

Library of Congress Cataloging-in-Publication Data

Allergies sourcebook : basic consumer health information about the immune system and allergic disorders, including rhinitis (hay fever), sinusitis, conjunctivitis, asthma, atopic dermatitis, and anaphylaxis, and allergy triggers such as pollen, mold, dust mites, animal dander, chemicals, foods and additives, and medications ; along with facts about allergy diagnosis and treatment, tips on avoiding triggers and preventing symptoms, a glossary of related terms, and directories of resources for additional help and information / edited by Amy L. Sutton. -- 4th ed.
     p. cm.
  Includes bibliographical references and index.
  Summary: "Provides basic consumer health information about causes, triggers, and treatment of allergic disorders, along with coping strategies and prevention tips. Includes index, glossary of related terms, and other resources"--Provided by publisher.
   ISBN 978-0-7808-1144-7 (hardcover : alk. paper) 1. Allergy--Popular works. I. Sutton, Amy L. II. Title.

  RC584.A3443 2011
  616.97--dc22

                                                                            2010048879

Table of Contents

Visit www.healthreferenceseries.com to view *A Contents Guide to the Health Reference Series*, a listing of more than 15,000 topics and the volumes in which they are covered.

vi

Part III: Foods and Food Additives That Trigger Allergic Reactions

Part IV: Airborne, Chemical, and Other Environmental Allergy Triggers

Part V: Diagnosing and Treating Allergies

Part VI: Avoiding Allergy Triggers, Preventing Symptoms, and Getting Support

Part VII: Additional Help and Information

Preface

About This Book

Allergies are the sixth leading cause of chronic disease in the United States, and according to the National Institute of Allergy and Infectious Diseases, "About half of all Americans test positive for at least one of the ten most common allergens: ragweed, Bermuda grass, rye grass, white oak, Russian thistle, Alternaria mold, cat, house dust mite, German cockroach, and peanut." Symptoms associated with allergic reactions can range from mild annoyances to anaphylaxis, a life-threatening emergency. Combined, allergies cost the U.S. healthcare system an estimated $18 billion annually.

Despite their widespread occurrence, however, many people do not understand the basic biological processes involved in allergic reactions and the role the immune system plays in causing common symptoms. Furthermore, medical science has yet to identify the specific genetic and environmental interactions that lead to the development of allergies or to fully understand why the prevalence of allergic diseases is increasing.

Allergies Sourcebook, Fourth Edition provides updated information about the causes, triggers, treatments, and prevalence of common allergic disorders, including rhinitis, sinusitis, conjunctivitis, allergic asthma, dermatitis, eczema, hives, and anaphylaxis. It discusses the immune system and its role in the development of allergic disorders and describes such commonly encountered allergens as pollen, mold, dust mites, and animal dander. Facts about allergies to foods and food additives, insect stings, medications, and chemicals are also included, along with information about allergy diagnosis, treatments, coping strategies, and prevention efforts. The book concludes with a glossary of related terms and directories of resources, including one to help people with food allergies find allergen-free foods and recipes.

How to Use This Book

This book is divided into parts and chapters. Parts focus on broad areas of interest. Chapters are devoted to single topics within a part.

Part I: Introduction to Allergies and the Immune System discusses the components and function of the immune system and explains the link between genes, environment, and allergy development. Facts about how allergies impair aspects of daily life, including sleep and cognitive function, and the impact of allergies on children are also included, along with current information about economic costs and trends in allergic disease.

Part II: Types of Allergic Reactions identifies the signs and symptoms of common allergic reactions, including rhinitis (hay fever), sinusitis, conjunctivitis (eye allergies), asthma, atopic dermatitis (eczema), rashes, hives, and life-threatening anaphylaxis.

Part III: Foods and Food Additives That Trigger Allergic Reactions provides information about the most common food allergens, including milk, egg, fish and shellfish, peanut and tree nut, wheat, and soy. Information about food additives and ingredients that trigger reactions, food intolerances, and tips on living with a food allergy are also included.

Part IV: Airborne, Chemical, and Other Environmental Allergy Triggers discusses symptoms of allergies to pollen and ragweed, mold, dust mites, cockroaches, animal dander, insect stings, medications, and components used to manufacture medical products. People whose allergies flare when exposed to tobacco smoke, fragrance, or building materials will also find suggestions on coping at home and in the workplace.

Part V: Diagnosing and Treating Allergies identifies tests, therapies, and medications that alleviate allergy symptoms, including antihistamines, decongestants, nasal sprays, and allergy shots. It also provides tips on choosing an allergist and updated information about how recent health care reform laws affect health insurance coverage for people with allergies and asthma.

Part VI: Avoiding Allergy Triggers, Preventing Symptoms, and Getting Support provides information about reducing indoor allergy triggers and improving air quality. This part also offers strategies for preventing allergy symptoms during travel, exercise, and pregnancy, finding an allergy support group, and remaining free of symptoms at school.

Part VII: Additional Help and Information provides a glossary of important terms related to allergies and the immune system. A directory of organizations that provide health information about allergies and asthma is also included, along with a list of cookbooks, websites, and companies that market allergy-free products for people with food allergies.

Bibliographic Note

This volume contains documents and excerpts from publications issued by the following U.S. government agencies: Agency for Healthcare Research and Quality (AHRQ); Centers for Disease Control and Prevention (CDC); Environmental Protection Agency (EPA); National Center for Complementary and Alternative Medicine (NCCAM); National Heart, Lung, and Blood Institute (NHLBI); National Human Genome Research Institute (NHGRI); National Institute of Allergy and Infectious Diseases (NIAID); National Institute of Arthritis and Musculoskeletal and Skin Diseases (NIAMS); National Institute of Environmental Health Sciences (NIEHS); National Institutes of Health (NIH); Office on Women's Health (OWH); U.S. Department of Health and Human Services (HHS); and the U.S. Food and Drug Administration (FDA).

In addition, this volume contains copyrighted documents from the following organizations and individuals: A.D.A.M., Inc.; Access Media Group, LLC; Allergy and Asthma Network Mothers of Asthmatics; Allergy/Asthma Information Association; American Celiac Disease Alliance; American College of Allergy, Asthma and Immunology; American Medical ID; American Rhinologic Society; Asthma and Allergy Foundation of America; Canadian Centre for Occupational Health and Safety; Children's Hospital of Philadelphia–Vaccine Education Center; Children's Hospital of Wisconsin; Children's Hospitals and Clinics of Minnesota; Cleveland Clinic Foundation; Linda Marienhoff Coss; Duke University Health System; EatingWithFoodAllergies.com; Florida Cooperative Extension Service–University of Florida; Food Allergy Initiative; Humane Society of the United States; International Food Information Council Foundation; Job Accommodation Network;

Kids With Food Allergies, Inc.; Joe Kraynak; National Eczema Association; Nemours Foundation; New Zealand Dermatological Society; Northwestern Nasal and Sinus; Oregon Alliance Working for Antibiotic Resistance Education–Oregon Department of Human Services; Leonard P. Perry, PhD; University of Michigan Health System; University of Texas Health Science Center at Houston; Vickerstaff Health Services, Inc.; and Robert A. Wood, MD.

Full citation information is provided on the first page of each chapter or section. Every effort has been made to secure all necessary rights to reprint the copyrighted material. If any omissions have been made, please contact Omnigraphics to make corrections for future editions.

Acknowledgements

Thanks go to the many organizations, agencies, and individuals who have contributed materials for this *Sourcebook* and to medical consultant Dr. David Cooke and prepress service provider WhimsyInk. Special thanks go to managing editor Karen Bellenir and research and permissions coordinator Liz Collins for their help and support.

About the Health Reference Series

The *Health Reference Series* is designed to provide basic medical information for patients, families, caregivers, and the general public. Each volume takes a particular topic and provides comprehensive coverage. This is especially important for people who may be dealing with a newly diagnosed disease or a chronic disorder in themselves or in a family member. People looking for preventive guidance, information about disease warning signs, medical statistics, and risk factors for health problems will also find answers to their questions in the *Health Reference Series*. The *Series*, however, is not intended to serve as a tool for diagnosing illness, in prescribing treatments, or as a substitute for the physician/patient relationship. All people concerned about medical symptoms or the possibility of disease are encouraged to seek professional care from an appropriate health care provider.

A Note about Spelling and Style

Health Reference Series editors use *Stedman's Medical Dictionary* as an authority for questions related to the spelling of medical terms and the *Chicago Manual of Style* for questions related to grammatical structures, punctuation, and other editorial concerns. Consistent adherence is not always possible, however, because the individual volumes within the *Series* include many documents from a wide variety of different producers and copyright holders, and the editor's primary goal is to present material from each source as accurately as is possible following the terms specified by each document's producer. This sometimes means that information in different chapters or sections may follow other guidelines and alternate spelling authorities. For example, occasionally a copyright holder may require that eponymous terms be shown in possessive forms (Crohn's disease vs. Crohn disease) or that British spelling norms be retained (leukaemia vs. leukemia).

Locating Information within the Health Reference Series

The *Health Reference Series* contains a wealth of information about a wide variety of medical topics. Ensuring easy access to all the fact sheets, research reports, in-depth discussions, and other material contained within the individual books of the *Series* remains one of our highest priorities. As the *Series* continues to grow in size and scope, however, locating the precise information needed by a reader may become more challenging.

A *Contents Guide to the Health Reference Series* was developed to direct readers to the specific volumes that address their concerns. It presents an extensive list of diseases, treatments, and other topics of general interest compiled from the Tables of Contents and major index headings. To access *A Contents Guide to the Health Reference Series*, visit www.healthreferenceseries.com.

Medical Consultant

Medical consultation services are provided to the *Health Reference Series* editors by David A. Cooke, MD, FACP. Dr. Cooke is a graduate of Brandeis University, and he received his M.D. degree from the University of Michigan. He completed residency training at the University of Wisconsin Hospital and Clinics. He is board-certified in Internal Medicine. Dr. Cooke currently works as part of the University of Michigan Health System and practices in Ann Arbor, MI. In his free time, he enjoys writing, science fiction, and spending time with his family.

Our Advisory Board

We would like to thank the following board members for providing guidance to the development of this *Series*:

- Dr. Lynda Baker, Associate Professor of Library and Information Science, Wayne State University, Detroit, MI

- Nancy Bulgarelli, William Beaumont Hospital Library, Royal Oak, MI

- Karen Imarisio, Bloomfield Township Public Library, Bloomfield Township, MI

- Karen Morgan, Mardigian Library, University of Michigan-Dearborn, Dearborn, MI

- Rosemary Orlando, St. Clair Shores Public Library, St. Clair Shores, MI

Health Reference Series *Update Policy*

The inaugural book in the *Health Reference Series* was the first edition of *Cancer Sourcebook* published in 1989. Since then, the *Series* has been enthusiastically received by librarians and in the medical community. In order to maintain the standard of providing high-quality health information for the layperson the editorial staff at Omnigraphics felt it was necessary to implement a policy of updating volumes when warranted.

Medical researchers have been making tremendous strides, and it is the purpose of the *Health Reference Series* to stay current with the most recent advances. Each decision to update a volume is made on an individual basis. Some of the considerations include how much new information is available and the feedback we receive from people who use the books. If there is a topic you would like to see added to the update list, or an area of medical concern you feel has not been adequately addressed, please write to:

Editor
Health Reference Series
Omnigraphics, Inc.
P.O. Box 31-1640
Detroit, MI 48231
E-mail: editorial@omnigraphics.com

Part One

Introduction to Allergies and the Immune System

Chapter 1

Understanding the Immune System and Allergic Reactions

The immune system is a network of cells, tissues, and organs that work together to defend the body against attacks by "foreign" invaders. These are primarily microbes—tiny organisms such as bacteria, parasites, and fungi that can cause infections. Viruses also cause infections, but are too primitive to be classified as living organisms. The human body provides an ideal environment for many microbes. It is the immune system's job to keep them out or, failing that, to seek out and destroy them.

When the immune system hits the wrong target, however, it can unleash a torrent of disorders, including allergic diseases, arthritis, and a form of diabetes. If the immune system is crippled, other kinds of diseases result.

The immune system is amazingly complex. It can recognize and remember millions of different enemies, and it can produce secretions (release of fluids) and cells to match up with and wipe out nearly all of them.

The secret to its success is an elaborate and dynamic communications network. Millions and millions of cells, organized into sets and subsets, gather like clouds of bees swarming around a hive and pass information back and forth in response to an infection. Once immune cells receive the alarm, they become activated and begin to produce

Excerpted from "Understanding the Immune System: How It Works," by the National Institute of Allergy and Infectious Diseases (NIAID, www.niaid.nih.gov), part of the National Institutes of Health, September 2007. Table 1.1, "Is It a Cold or Allergy?" is from the NIAID, November 2008.

powerful chemicals. These substances allow the cells to regulate their own growth and behavior, enlist other immune cells, and direct the new recruits to trouble spots.

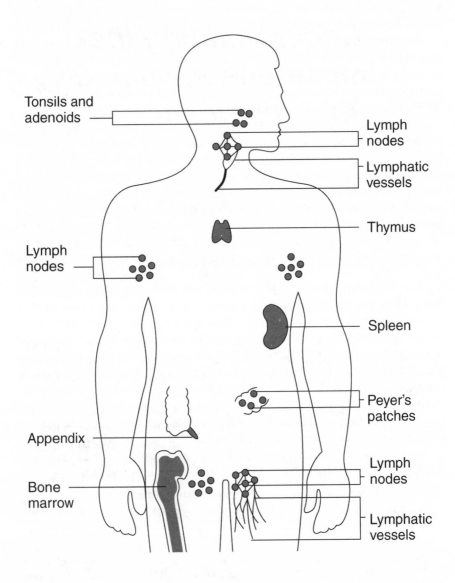

Figure 1.1. *The lymphoid organs.*

Self and Nonself

The key to a healthy immune system is its remarkable ability to distinguish between the body's own cells, recognized as "self," and foreign cells, or "nonself." The body's immune defenses normally coexist peacefully with cells that carry distinctive "self" marker molecules. But when immune defenders encounter foreign cells or organisms carrying markers that say "nonself," they quickly launch an attack.

Anything that can trigger this immune response is called an antigen. An antigen can be a microbe such as a virus, or a part of a microbe such as a molecule. Tissues or cells from another person (except an identical twin) also carry nonself markers and act as foreign antigens. This explains why tissue transplants may be rejected.

In abnormal situations, the immune system can mistake self for nonself and launch an attack against the body's own cells or tissues. The result is called an autoimmune disease. Some forms of arthritis and diabetes are autoimmune diseases. In other cases, the immune system responds to a seemingly harmless foreign substance such as ragweed pollen. The result is allergy, and this kind of antigen is called an allergen.

The Structure of the Immune System

The organs of the immune system are positioned throughout the body. They are called lymphoid organs because they are home to lymphocytes, small white blood cells that are the key players in the immune system. Bone marrow, the soft tissue in the hollow center of bones, is the ultimate source of all blood cells, including lymphocytes. The thymus is a lymphoid organ that lies behind the breastbone. Lymphocytes known as T lymphocytes or T cells ("T" stands for "thymus") mature in the thymus and then migrate to other tissues. B lymphocytes, also known as B cells, become activated and mature into plasma cells, which make and release antibodies.

Lymph nodes, which are located in many parts of the body, are lymphoid tissues that contain numerous specialized structures:

- T cells from the thymus concentrate in the paracortex.
- B cells develop in and around the germinal centers.
- Plasma cells occur in the medulla.

Lymphocytes can travel throughout the body using the blood vessels. The cells can also travel through a system of lymphatic vessels that closely parallels the body's veins and arteries.

Cells and fluids are exchanged between blood and lymphatic vessels, enabling the lymphatic system to monitor the body for invading microbes. The lymphatic vessels carry lymph, a clear fluid that bathes the body's tissues.

Small, bean-shaped lymph nodes are laced along the lymphatic vessels, with clusters in the neck, armpits, abdomen, and groin. Each lymph node contains specialized compartments where immune cells congregate, and where they can encounter antigens.

Immune cells, microbes, and foreign antigens enter the lymph nodes via incoming lymphatic vessels or the lymph nodes' tiny blood vessels. All lymphocytes exit lymph nodes through outgoing lymphatic vessels. Once in the bloodstream, lymphocytes are transported to tissues throughout the body. They patrol everywhere for foreign antigens, then gradually drift back into the lymphatic system to begin the cycle all over again.

The spleen is a flattened organ at the upper left of the abdomen. Like the lymph nodes, the spleen contains specialized compartments where immune cells gather and work. The spleen serves as a meeting ground where immune defenses confront antigens.

Other clumps of lymphoid tissue are found in many parts of the body, especially in the linings of the digestive tract, airways, and lungs—territories that serve as gateways to the body. These tissues include the tonsils, adenoids, and appendix.

Immune Cells and Their Products

The immune system stockpiles a huge arsenal of cells, not only lymphocytes but also cell-devouring phagocytes and their relatives. Some immune cells take on all intruders, whereas others are trained on highly specific targets. To work effectively, most immune cells need the cooperation of their comrades. Sometimes immune cells communicate by direct physical contact, and sometimes they communicate releasing chemical messengers.

The immune system stores just a few of each kind of the different cells needed to recognize millions of possible enemies. When an antigen first appears, the few immune cells that can respond to it multiply into a full-scale army of cells. After their job is done, the immune cells fade away, leaving sentries behind to watch for future attacks.

All immune cells begin as immature stem cells in the bone marrow. They respond to different cytokines and other chemical signals to grow into specific immune cell types, such as T cells, B cells, or phagocytes. Because stem cells have not yet committed to a particular future, their use presents an interesting possibility for treating some immune system disorders. Researchers currently are investigating if a person's own stem cells can be used to regenerate damaged immune responses in autoimmune diseases and in immune deficiency disorders, such as HIV [human immunodeficiency virus] infection.

B Cells

B cells and T cells are the main types of lymphocytes. B cells work chiefly by secreting substances called antibodies into the body's fluids. Antibodies ambush foreign antigens circulating in the bloodstream. They are powerless, however, to penetrate cells. The job of attacking target cells—either cells that have been infected by viruses or cells that have been distorted by cancer—is left to T cells or other immune cells.

Each B cell is programmed to make one specific antibody. For example, one B cell will make an antibody that blocks a virus that causes the common cold, while another produces an antibody that attacks a bacterium that causes pneumonia. When a B cell encounters the kind of antigen that triggers it to become active, it gives rise to many large cells known as plasma cells, which produce antibodies.

- Immunoglobulin G, or IgG, is a kind of antibody that works efficiently to coat microbes, speeding their uptake by other cells in the immune system.

- IgM is very effective at killing bacteria.

- IgA concentrates in body fluids—tears, saliva, and the secretions of the respiratory and digestive tracts—guarding the entrances to the body.

- IgE, whose natural job probably is to protect against parasitic infections, is responsible for the symptoms of allergy.

- IgD remains attached to B cells and plays a key role in initiating early B cell responses.

T Cells

Unlike B cells, T cells do not recognize free-floating antigens. Rather, their surfaces contain specialized antibody-like receptors that see fragments of antigens on the surfaces of infected or cancerous cells. T cells contribute to immune defenses in two major ways: Some direct and regulate immune responses, whereas others directly attack infected or cancerous cells.

Table 1.1. Is It a Cold or an Allergy?

Symptoms	Cold	Airborne allergy
Cough	Common	Sometimes
General aches, pains	Slight	Never
Fatigue, weakness	Sometimes	Sometimes
Itchy eyes	Rare or never	Common
Sneezing	Usual	Usual
Sore throat	Common	Sometimes
Runny nose	Common	Common
Stuffy nose	Common	Common
Fever	Rare	Never
Duration	3 to 14 days	Weeks (for example, six weeks for ragweed or grass pollen seasons)
Treatment	Antihistamines; decongestants; nonsteroidal anti-inflammatory medicines	Antihistamines; nasal steroids; decongestants
Prevention	Wash your hands often with soap and water; Avoid close contact with anyone with a cold	Avoid those things that you are allergic to such as pollen, house dust mites, mold, pet dander, cockroaches
Complications	Sinus infection; middle ear infection; asthma	Sinus infection; asthma

Helper T cells, or Th cells, coordinate immune responses by communicating with other cells. Some stimulate nearby B cells to produce antibodies, others call in microbe-gobbling cells called phagocytes, and still others activate other T cells.

Cytotoxic T lymphocytes (CTLs)—also called killer T cells—perform a different function. These cells directly attack other cells carrying certain foreign or abnormal molecules on their surfaces. CTLs are especially useful for attacking viruses because viruses often hide from other parts of the immune system while they grow inside infected cells. CTLs recognize small fragments of these viruses peeking out from the cell membrane and launch an attack to kill the infected cell.

In most cases, T cells only recognize an antigen if it is carried on the surface of a cell by one of the body's own major histocompatibility complex, or

MHC, molecules. MHC molecules are proteins recognized by T cells when they distinguish between self and nonself. A self-MHC molecule provides a recognizable scaffolding to present a foreign antigen to the T cell. In humans, MHC antigens are called human leukocyte antigens, or HLA.

Although MHC molecules are required for T cell responses against foreign invaders, they also create problems during organ transplantations. Virtually every cell in the body is covered with MHC proteins, but each person has a different set of these proteins on his or her cells. If a T cell recognizes a nonself-MHC molecule on another cell, it will destroy the cell. Therefore, doctors must match organ recipients with donors who have the closest MHC makeup. Otherwise the recipient's T cells will likely attack the transplanted organ, leading to graft rejection.

Natural killer (NK) cells are another kind of lethal white cell, or lymphocyte. Like CTLs, NK cells are armed with granules filled with potent chemicals. But CTLs look for antigen fragments bound to self-MHC molecules, whereas NK cells recognize cells lacking self-MHC molecules. Thus, NK cells have the potential to attack many types of foreign cells.

Both kinds of killer cells slay on contact. The deadly assassins bind to their targets, aim their weapons, and then deliver a lethal burst of chemicals.

T cells aid the normal processes of the immune system. If NK T cells fail to function properly, asthma, certain autoimmune diseases—including type 1 diabetes—or the growth of cancers may result. NK T cells get their name because they are a kind of T lymphocyte that carries some of the surface proteins, called "markers," typical of NK T cells. But these T cells differ from other kinds of T cells. They do not recognize pieces of antigen bound to self-MHC molecules. Instead, they recognize fatty substances (lipids and glycolipids) that are bound to a different class of molecules called CD1d. Scientists are trying to discover methods to control the timing and release of chemical factors by NK T cells, with the hope they can modify immune responses in ways that benefit patients.

Phagocytes and Their Relatives

Phagocytes are large white cells that can swallow and digest microbes and other foreign particles. Monocytes are phagocytes that circulate in the blood. When monocytes migrate into tissues, they develop into macrophages. Specialized types of macrophages can be found in many organs, including the lungs, kidneys, brain, and liver.

Macrophages play many roles. As scavengers, they rid the body of worn-out cells and other debris. They display bits of foreign antigen in a way that draws the attention of matching lymphocytes and, in that respect, resemble dendritic cells. And they churn out an amazing variety of powerful chemical signals, known as monokines, which are vital to the immune response.

Granulocytes are another kind of immune cell. They contain granules filled with potent chemicals, which allow the granulocytes to destroy microorganisms. Some of these chemicals, such as histamine, also contribute to inflammation and allergy.

One type of granulocyte, the neutrophil, is also a phagocyte. Neutrophils use their prepackaged chemicals to break down the microbes they ingest. Eosinophils and basophils are granulocytes that "degranulate" by spraying their chemicals onto harmful cells or microbes nearby.

Mast cells function much like basophils, except they are not blood cells. Rather, they are found in the lungs, skin, tongue, and linings of the nose and intestinal tract, where they contribute to the symptoms of allergy. Related structures, called blood platelets, are cell fragments. Platelets also contain granules. In addition to promoting blood clotting and wound repair, platelets activate some immune defenses.

Dendritic cells are found in the parts of lymphoid organs where T cells also exist. Like macrophages, dendritic cells in lymphoid tissues display antigens to T cells and help stimulate T cells during an immune response. They are called dendritic cells because they have branch-like extensions that can interlace to form a network.

T Cell Receptors

T cell receptors are complex protein molecules that peek through the surface membranes of T cells. The exterior part of a T cell receptor recognizes short pieces of foreign antigens that are bound to self-MHC molecules on other cells of the body. It is because of their T cell receptors that T cells can recognize disease-causing microorganisms and rally other immune cells to attack the invaders, or kill the invaders themselves.

Toll-like receptors (TLRs), which occur on cells throughout the immune system, are a family of proteins the body uses as a first line of defense against invading microbes. Like T cell receptors, some TLRs peek through the surface membranes of immune cells, allowing them to respond to microbes in the cells' environment.

Some TLRs are activated by molecules that make up viruses, whereas other TLRs respond to molecules that make up the cell walls of bacteria. Once activated, TLRs relay the alarm to other actors in the immune system. For example, some TLRs play important roles in the all-purpose "first-responder" arm of the immune system, also called the innate immune system. In short order, the innate immune system responds with a surge of chemical signals that together cause inflammation, fever, and other responses to infection or injury. Other TLRs help initiate responses from genetically identical groups of lymphocytes, called clones, that are already programmed to recognize specific antigens. Such responses are called adaptive immunity.

Overall, the cellular receptors important for the first-line responses of innate immunity are encoded by genes people inherit from their parents. In contrast, adaptive immune responses rely on antigen receptors that are pieced together in the genomes of lymphocytes during their development in various tissues of the body. In addition to TLRs, other kinds of innate immune receptors can stimulate phagocytosis by macrophages, trigger the inflammatory responses that help control local infections, and play a range of crucial roles in defending the body against invading microbes.

Cytokines

Cells of the immune system communicate with one another by releasing and responding to chemical messengers called cytokines. These proteins are secreted by immune cells and act on other cells to coordinate appropriate immune responses. Cytokines include a diverse assortment of interleukins, interferons, and growth factors.

Some cytokines are chemical switches that turn certain immune cell types on and off. One cytokine, interleukin 2 (IL-2), triggers the immune system to produce T cells. IL-2's immunity-boosting properties have traditionally made it a promising treatment for several illnesses. Clinical studies are underway to test its benefits in diseases such as cancer, hepatitis C, and HIV infection and AIDS [acquired immunodeficiency syndrome]. Scientists are studying other cytokines to see whether they can also be used to treat diseases.

One group of cytokines chemically attracts specific cell types. These so-called chemokines are released by cells at a site of injury or infection and call other immune cells to the region to help repair the damage or fight off the invader. Chemokines often play a key role in inflammation and are a promising target for new drugs to help regulate immune responses.

Complement

The complement system is made up of about 25 proteins that work together to assist, or "complement," the action of antibodies in destroying bacteria. Complement also helps to rid the body of antibody-coated antigens (antigen-antibody complexes). Complement proteins, which cause blood vessels to become dilated and then leaky, contribute to the redness, warmth, swelling, pain, and loss of function that characterize an inflammatory response.

Complement proteins circulate in the blood in an inactive form. When the first protein in the complement series is activated—typically by antibody that has locked onto an antigen—it sets in motion a domino effect. Each component takes its turn in a precise chain of steps known as the complement cascade. The end products are molecular cylinders that are inserted into—and that puncture holes in—the cell walls that surround the invading bacteria. With fluids and molecules flowing in and out, the bacterial cells swell, burst, and die. Other components of the complement system make bacteria more susceptible to phagocytosis or beckon other immune cells to the area.

Mounting an Immune Response

Infections are the most common cause of human disease. They range from the common cold to debilitating conditions like chronic hepatitis to life-threatening diseases such as AIDS. Disease-causing microbes (pathogens) attempting to get into the body must first move past the body's external armor, usually the skin or cells lining the body's internal passageways.

The skin provides an imposing barrier to invading microbes. It is generally penetrable only through cuts or tiny abrasions. The digestive and respiratory tracts—both portals of entry for a number of microbes—also have their own levels of protection. Microbes entering the nose often cause the nasal surfaces to secrete more protective mucus, and attempts to enter the nose or lungs can trigger a sneeze or cough reflex to force microbial invaders out of the respiratory passageways. The stomach contains a strong acid that destroys many pathogens that are swallowed with food.

If microbes survive the body's front-line defenses, they still have to find a way through the walls of the digestive, respiratory, or urogenital passageways to the underlying cells. These passageways are lined with tightly packed epithelial cells covered in a layer of mucus, effectively blocking the transport of many pathogens into deeper cell layers.

Mucosal surfaces also secrete a special class of antibody called IgA, which in many cases is the first type of antibody to encounter an invading microbe. Underneath the epithelial layer a variety of immune cells, including macrophages, B cells, and T cells, lie in wait for any microbe that might bypass the barriers at the surface.

Next, invaders must escape a series of general defenses of the innate immune system, which are ready to attack without regard for specific antigen markers. These include patrolling phagocytes, NK T cells, and complement.

Microbes cross the general barriers then confront specific weapons of the adaptive immune system tailored just for them. These specific weapons, which include both antibodies and T cells, are equipped with singular receptor structures that allow them to recognize and interact with their designated targets.

Allergic Reactions

The most common types of allergic diseases occur when the immune system responds to a false alarm. In an allergic person, a normally harmless material such as grass pollen, food particles, mold, or house dust mites is mistaken for a threat and attacked.

Allergies such as pollen allergy are related to the antibody known as IgE. Like other antibodies, each IgE antibody is specific; one acts against oak pollen and another against ragweed, for example.

Chapter 2

How Allergies Develop

Chapter Contents

Section 2.1

Genetic Connections

From "Genetic Finding Suggests Alternative Treatment Strategy for Common, Complex Skin Disorders and Asthma," by the National Human Genome Research Institute (NHGRI, www.genome.gov), part of the National Institutes of Health, April 25, 2006.

A genetic finding by researchers at the National Institutes of Health provides new insight into the cause of a series of related, common, and complex illnesses—including hay fever and asthma as well as the skin disorders eczema and psoriasis—and suggests a novel therapeutic approach. All of these illnesses are essentially inflammatory disorders of the tissues that separate the inside of the body from the outside world, such as the skin and the linings of the throat and lungs.

Researchers from the National Human Genome Research Institute, the National Eye Institute, and the National Institute of Child Health and Human Development, all part of the National Institutes of Health, report that excessive production of a specific protein disrupts the protective properties of the skin barrier. Once the skin barrier is compromised, immune-system-stimulating chemicals—allergens—can enter the body and cause an inflammatory reaction that, in turn, stimulates skin cells to grow rapidly, further diminishing the protective function of the skin. The compromised barrier, in turn, becomes more porous to allergens that then stimulate more inflammation in a cycle that eventually produces common skin conditions such as psoriasis and eczema.

It may, however, be possible to break the cycle by creating a temporary, artificial barrier on the skin that blocks incoming allergens. The solution could be as simple as developing a lotion that effectively blocks allergens from getting through damaged skin. Keeping allergens out of the skin would keep the immune system from overstimulating cell growth, giving the skin time to recreate a normal barrier. Current therapies for these skin conditions principally focus on suppressing the immune system, but the medicines used can produce undesired side effects.

"The human body is an incredibly complex system," said Elias A. Zerhouni, MD, director of the National Institutes of Health. "Only by conducting this kind of basic research can we hope to understand the causes of complex diseases. And only by understanding disease can we produce a future in which we can predict who is at risk, pre-empt the illness from ever occurring, and personalize the treatment when it does."

Several recent studies have suggested that defects in the skin barrier may be as important to eczema and psoriasis as the hyperactive response of the immune system. In addition, doctors have observed that individuals with eczema are also likely to develop hay fever and asthma, suggesting a common mechanism for both disorders. The other risk factor for these conditions is having a relative with the disorder, suggesting a genetic connection.

To test whether a defective skin barrier can produce these diseases, a team of NIH researchers focused on a specific gene called connexin 26, which makes a protein that forms connections between skin cells that create the normal barrier. When the skin is intact, the production of connexin 26 is turned off once there is enough to hook all the skin cells together. When skin is damaged by a cut or a scrape, connexin 26 is produced while new skin cells reproduce and heal the wound. Researchers have shown that connexin 26 production is turned on in the sore skin of people with psoriasis, but it wasn't clear what role connexin 26 played in the disorder.

To determine connexin 26's role in psoriasis, NIH researchers created a line of transgenic mice that overproduce connexin 26. The resulting mice develop psoriatic-type skin sores, just like humans with psoriasis.

"This discovery demonstrates the power of animal models to unravel complex conditions of medical importance," said Eric D. Green, MD, PhD, NHGRI's scientific director and the director of the institute's Division of Intramural Research, where the research was conducted. "Our current abilities to rapidly create new genetically altered animal models allow researchers to move from conception of an idea to its implementation at an incredible pace." The discovery broadens the basic understanding of the causes of skin disorders such as psoriasis and eczema, and may well contribute to the basic understanding of asthma and hay fever, conditions that arise when allergens penetrate the tissue barrier in the lungs and nose, respectively.

"Hopefully, this will help us understand the complex genetics of psoriasis," said Julie A. Segre, PhD, an investigator in NHGRI's Genetics and Molecular Branch. "Previous genetic studies have focused on the genes that regulate immune response. We are now examining the effect of genes that are involved in both regulating the growth of skin cells and signaling to the immune cells."

The problem causing these related disorders may simply be the body over-reacting to an allergen getting through the barrier that is supposed to block it. "The skin goes into a stress response and overcompensates by trying to rebuild the barrier too fast, actually becoming less effective," Dr. Segre said. "The skin cells grow so fast that they fail to make a normal barrier, and the body is stimulating the immune response because of material (chemicals and allergens) coming through the barrier."

Understanding the genetics of skin disorders may well have important implications for other serious illnesses, such as asthma. It is not uncommon for a family doctor to face the dilemma of a child who has eczema and then having to decide how aggressively to treat the disease. Eczema is not particularly dangerous, but children presenting with eczema commonly go on to develop asthma, which severely compromises quality of life and in rare cases can be lethal. Treating eczema with immune-suppressing drugs, which may also prevent asthma from developing, may cause undesirable side effects.

The genetic studies suggest that researchers now need to focus on both turning down the immune response, as well as restoring a normal skin barrier to keep the outside world out of the body.

"The barrier function of epithelial surfaces is important in all tissues that have contact with the outside world. In addition to the skin and respiratory tract, it includes the gastrointestinal tract, and the ocular surface," said Ali Djalilian, MD, formerly a research fellow and medical officer at the National Eye Institute but now at the University of Illinois in Chicago. "These findings underline the importance of this barrier function and suggests a new strategy for restoring it in human diseases."

Additional Information

- Among the most serious, common chronic conditions in the United States, asthma affects more than 20 million people. Some 5 million asthmatics are U.S. children younger than 18 and approximately 3.6 million children have had an asthma attack within the last year. Nearly half a million attacks resulted in a trip to the emergency room each year and more than 5,000 asthmatics died from their illness.

- An estimated 4.5 million U.S. adults suffer from psoriasis, up to a third suffer moderate to a severe form of the disorder, including 1 million who have psoriatic arthritis.

- More than 15 million Americans suffer from the symptoms of eczema, according to the National Institute of Arthritis and Musculoskeletal and Skin Diseases, a part of the National Institutes of Health.

• Approximately 50 million Americans suffer some form of allergy or hay fever, experiencing sneezing, runny nose, or watery eyes, though the symptoms can range from mild to life-threatening.

Section 2.2

Breastfeeding and Allergic Disease Development

"Prevention of Allergy in 2008," by Edmond S. Chan, MD, FRCPC, *Allergy & Asthma News*, Issue 4, 2008. © 2008 Allergy/Asthma Information Association (www.aaia.ca/en). Reprinted with permission.

The purpose of this editorial by Sicherer and Burks [*Editorial Note: See Source at the end of this section*] is to describe how the American Academy of Pediatrics (AAP) has changed its recommendations for prevention of allergy in infants at high risk of developing allergies, based on updated evidence. In addition, the authors speculate on future directions in this area, and provide some practical advice on how decisions may need to be individualized in certain scenarios (e.g., having an older sibling with peanut allergy).

In 2000, the AAP defined high risk infants as those who have two parents (or one parent plus one sibling) with allergy. It suggested that there may be benefit from avoidance of peanut during pregnancy, as well as avoidance of peanut and tree nuts in the mother's diet while breastfeeding. For the young child, it suggested delay of dairy until 12 months of age, egg until 2 years, and peanuts, nuts, fish until 3 years.

In early 2008, the AAP published an updated set of recommendations, which are very similar to European recommendations that have been available for years. The AAP changed their definition of high risk to describe an infant with either one parent or one sibling with allergy, making the definition less strict. Most significantly, it has stated that there is a lack of evidence for doing anything beyond exclusive breastfeeding for 4 to 6 months (or use of a hypoallergenic formula if one cannot exclusively breastfeed). In other words, there is no good reason from an allergy point of view for mothers to avoid any foods during pregnancy or while breastfeeding. Similarly, there is no good reason for young infants to delay any specific foods beyond 6 months of age (including egg, peanut, etc.) from an allergy perspective.

What has not changed is that both the 2000 and 2008 AAP recommendations have supported use of exclusive breastfeeding for at least 4 to 6 months in high risk infants, which has been shown to have a preventive effect against eczema and cow's milk allergy. This would also mean avoiding any solids until 4 to 6 months of age. If not breastfeeding or if supplementing during the first 4 to 6 months, use of an extensively hydrolyzed casein formula (or a partially hydrolyzed whey formula, although it may be less effective) instead of cow's milk or soy formula is recommended.

In the last section of their editorial, Sicherer and Burks recognize that the 2008 AAP recommendations are a reflection of the limitations of currently available data on prevention, since they focus on explaining what doesn't appear to work rather than giving a lengthy "to-do list." They comment on current thoughts that delay of foods such as peanut by mouth may be increasing the chance of developing peanut allergy due to a missed opportunity for oral tolerance when young. Furthermore, delay of peanut by mouth may be increasing the odds of early skin contact with peanut, a route of exposure which is suspected to increase the risk of developing peanut allergy. Although these are intriguing thoughts, Sicherer and Burks do make it clear that they are not ready to advise parents to start peanut butter by mouth for their infant at 6 months of age, since the whole situation is still so unclear. It is hoped that studies such as the "Learning Early About Peanut allergy" study in the United Kingdom will provide us with further direction. In the meantime, Sicherer and Burks advise individualizing decisions about when to introduce specific foods such as peanut in the young child, through a discussion of the evidence available and consideration of unique factors for the family of concern. An example would be having an older sibling with peanut allergy, which may cause some to prefer either avoiding peanut for the entire family including the younger sibling (for simplicity), or waiting until an allergy assessment for the younger sibling has taken place. It has been shown that a young sibling's risk of peanut allergy is increased by having an older sibling with peanut allergy. To conclude, the authors identify that much more research on prevention is needed.

Source: Sicherer SH and Burks AW. Maternal and infant diets for prevention of allergic diseases: Understanding menu changes in 2008. *J Allergy Clin Immunol:* 2008;122:29–33.

Section 2.3

The Hygiene Hypothesis

From "Asthma: The Hygiene Hypothesis," by the U.S. Food
and Drug Administration (FDA, www.fda.gov), June 18, 2009.

One of the many explanations for asthma being the most common chronic disease in the developed world is the hygiene hypothesis. This hypothesis suggests that the critical postnatal period of immune response is derailed by the extremely clean household environments often found in the developed world. In other words, the young child's environment can be too clean to pose an effective challenge to a maturing immune system.

According to the hygiene hypothesis, the problem with extremely clean environments is that they fail to provide the necessary exposure to germs required to educate the immune system so it can learn to launch its defense responses to infectious organisms. Instead, its defense responses end up being so inadequate that they actually contribute to the development of asthma.

Scientists based this hypothesis in part on the observation that, before birth, the fetal immune system's default setting is suppressed to prevent it from rejecting maternal tissue. Such a low default setting is necessary before birth—when the mother is providing the fetus with her own antibodies. But in the period immediately after birth the child's own immune system must take over and learn how to fend for itself.

The hygiene hypothesis is supported by epidemiologic studies demonstrating that allergic diseases and asthma are more likely to occur when the incidence and levels of endotoxin (bacterial lipopolysaccharide, or LPS) in the home are low. LPS is a bacterial molecule that stimulates and educates the immune system by triggering signals through a molecular switch called TLR4, which is found on certain immune system cells.

The Science behind the Hygiene Hypothesis

The Inflammatory Mechanisms Section of the Laboratory of Immunobiochemistry is working to better understand the hygiene hypothesis,

21

by looking at the relationship between respiratory viruses and allergic diseases and asthma, and by studying the respiratory syncytial virus (RSV) in particular.

What Does RSV Have to Do with the Hygiene Hypothesis?

- RSV is often the first viral pathogen encountered by infants.

- RSV pneumonia puts infants at higher risk for developing childhood asthma. (Although children may outgrow this type of asthma, it can account for clinic visits and missed school days.)

- RSV carries a molecule on its surface called the F protein, which flips the same immune system switch (TLR4) as do bacterial endotoxins.

It may seem obvious that, since both the RSV F protein and LPS signal through the same TLR4 switch, they both would educate the infant's immune system in the same beneficial way. But that may not be the case.

The large population of bacteria that normally lives inside humans educates the growing immune system to respond using the TLR4 switch. When this education is lacking or weak, the response to RSV by some critical cells in the immune system's defense against infections—called T-cells—might inadvertently trigger asthma instead of protecting the infant and clearing the infection. How this happens is a mystery that we are trying to solve.

In order to determine RSV's role in triggering asthma, the laboratory studied how RSV blocks T-cell proliferation.

Studying the effect of RSV on T-cells in the laboratory, however, has been very difficult. That's because when RSV is put into the same culture as T-cells, it blocks them from multiplying as they would naturally do when they are stimulated. To get past this problem, most researchers kill RSV with ultraviolet light before adding the virus to T-cell cultures. However we did not have the option of killing the RSV because that would have prevented us from determining the virus's role in triggering asthma.

Our first major discovery was that RSV causes the release from certain immune system cells of signaling molecules called Type I and Type III interferons that can suppress T-cell proliferation (*Journal of Virology* 80:5032–5040; 2006).

Conclusion

The hygiene hypothesis suggests that a newborn baby's immune system must be educated so it will function properly during infancy and the rest of life. One of the key elements of this education is a switch on T cells called TLR4. The bacterial protein LPS normally plays a key role by flipping that switch into the "on" position.

Prior research suggested that since RSV flips the TLR4 switch, RSV should educate the child's immune system to defend against infections just like LPS does.

But it turns out that RSV does not flip the TLR switch in the same way as LPS. This difference in switching on TLR, combined with other characteristics of RSV, can prevent proper education of the immune system.

One difference in the way that RSV flips the TLR4 switch may be through the release of interferons, which suppresses the proliferation of T-cells. We still do not know whether these interferons are part of the reason the immune system is not properly educated or simply an indicator of the problem. Therefore, we plan to continue our studies about how RSV can contribute to the development of asthma according to the hygiene hypothesis.

Chapter 3

Allergies Impact Daily Life

Chapter Contents

Section 3.1

Allergies and Cognitive Impairment

Sneezing, wheezing, watery eyes, and runny nose aren't the only symptoms of allergic diseases. Many people with allergic rhinitis also report feeling "slower" and drowsy. When their allergies are acting up, they have trouble concentrating and remembering.

For instance, allergic rhinitis can be associated with:

- decreased ability to concentrate and function;
- activity limitation;
- decreased decision-making capacity;
- impaired hand-eye coordination;
- problems remembering things;
- irritability;
- sleep disorders;
- fatigue;
- missed days at work or school;
- more motor vehicle accidents;
- more school or work injuries.

Many parents of children with allergic rhinitis observe increased bad moods and irritability in their child's behavior during the allergy season. Since children cannot always express their uncomfortable or painful symptoms verbally, they may express their discomfort by acting up at school and at home. In addition, some kids feel that having an allergic disease is a stigma that separates them from other kids.

It is important that the irritability or other symptoms caused by ear, nose, or throat trouble are not mistaken for attention deficit disorder. With proper treatment, symptoms can be kept under control and disruptions in learning and behavior can be avoided.

Causes

Experts believe the top two culprits contributing to cognitive impairment of people with allergic rhinitis are sleep interruptions and sedating antihistamine (OTC) medications.

Secondary factors, such as blockage of the Eustachian tube (ear canal), also can cause hearing problems that have a negative impact on learning and comprehension. Constant nose blowing and coughing can interrupt concentration and the learning process, and allergy-related absences can cause people to miss school or work and subsequently fall behind.

Sleep Disruption

Chronic nasal congestion can cause difficulty in breathing, especially at night. Waking is a hard-wired reflex to make you start breathing again. If you have bad allergic rhinitis, you may waken a dozen times a night. Falling back asleep can be difficult, cutting your total number of sleep hours short.

The average person needs about 8 hours of sleep per night to function normally the next day. Losing just a few hours of sleep can lead to a significant decrease in your ability to function. Prolonged loss of sleep can cause difficulty in concentration, inability to remember things, and can contribute to automotive accidents. Night after night of interrupted sleep can cause serious decreases in learning ability and performance in school or on the job.

Over-the-Counter Medications

Most allergy therapies don't take into account the effects of allergic rhinitis on mental functioning—they treat the more obvious physical symptoms. Some allergy therapies may even cause some cognitive or mental impairment.

In a recent poll in which allergy sufferers were asked how they treat their symptoms, about 50 percent responded that they use over-the-counter (OTC) medications. The most commonly used OTC medications for allergy symptoms are decongestants and first generation antihistamines, such as diphenhydramine (Benadryl)—both of which can cause sleep disturbances.

Decongestants

Decongestants constrict small blood vessels in the nose. This opens the nasal passageways and lets you breathe easier. Some decongestants are available over-the-counter, while higher strength formulas are available with a prescription. In some people, oral decongestants can cause problems with getting to sleep, appetite loss, and irritability, which can contribute to allergy problems. If you have any of these symptoms, discuss them with your doctor.

Antihistamines

Antihistamines block the effects of histamine, a chemical produced by the body in response to allergens. Histamine is responsible for the symptoms of allergic rhinitis, including an itchy runny nose, sneezing, and itchy eyes. First generation OTC antihistamines available in the United States also can cause drowsiness. Regularly taking OTC antihistamines can lead to a feeling of constant sluggishness, affecting learning, memory, and performance.

Newer second generation antihistamines such as Claritin (loratadine) and Zyrtec (cetirizine) which are OTC and Clarinex (desloratadine), Allegra (fexofenadine), and Xyzal (levocetirizine) by prescription are non or low sedating and are designed to minimize drowsiness while still blocking the effects of histamine.

Solutions

With all the allergic diseases, the best way to control your symptoms is to avoid coming into contact with your triggers—the substances that cause you to have an allergic reaction. This is often easier said than done. Sometimes it is impossible to avoid the substances that cause symptoms, especially when you are not in control of your environment.

If your allergens can't be avoided, your doctor can help you to create an allergy treatment plan. People who are allergic to indoor things like dust mites or animal dander may need medication on a daily basis, while people who have seasonal symptoms may only need treatment at certain times during the year. An allergist-immunologist can help you determine to which substances you are allergic.

Several types of non-sedating medications are available to help control allergies. One nonsedating nasal spray, NasalCrom (cromolyn), is available without a prescription. Your doctor may also prescribe nasal steroid sprays to treat nasal inflammation. Nasal steroid sprays are highly effective in treating allergy symptoms. The most common side effect associated with nasal sprays is headache.

If medications are not effective or cause unwanted side effects, your doctor may suggest immunotherapy, or allergy shots. Immunotherapy is used to treat allergy to pollen, ragweed, dust mites, animal dander, and other allergens. This process gradually desensitizes you to these substances by changing the way that your body's immune system responds to them. For example, if you are allergic to ragweed, immunotherapy treatments would involve injecting a tiny amount of ragweed pollen extract under your skin every week.

Immunotherapy treatments usually last 3 to 5 years or longer. Once your body is able to tolerate the substance without producing the symptoms of an allergy, immunotherapy can be stopped, and the need for oral medications should be gone or greatly reduced.

Remember

If allergies are affecting your ability to concentrate or function, several treatment options may be beneficial. Getting allergy symptoms under control can help you sleep at night and function during the day.

If you suspect that you or a family member may have an allergic disorder, make an appointment with your doctor for proper diagnosis. Treating allergies sooner rather than later can help prevent disruptions in learning and behavior.

Section 3.2

Allergen Exposure Interrupts Sleep

Nocturnal asthma. Many parents know all too well the coughing, choking, wheezing, and congestion that can keep their children—and the rest of the family—awake at night.

"When my 3-year-old's asthma acts up, it definitely disrupts his sleep and mine," says AANMA (Allergy and Asthma Network Mothers of Asthmatics) member Rachel Gerke. "I know it is bothering him when he is really restless at night, crying or moaning and hitting the sides of the bed when rolling. And when I go in to listen to him he is either breathing faster, usually from his belly, his chest not rising, or I hear a whistle at the end of his breaths."

Rachel's family is not alone. More than 20 million Americans are affected by nocturnal asthma—also called nighttime or sleep-related asthma. The condition has been reported in medical literature for centuries.

AANMA consulted sleep experts—including parents!—for advice to help you and your family get a good night's sleep.

Why We're Losing Sleep

When you breathe in, the lungs transport oxygen into the bloodstream, where it's carried to the rest of the body. When you breathe out, they transport the waste product—carbon dioxide—out of the bloodstream. How well this process works varies throughout the day as part of the body's natural circadian rhythm—an internal clock that regulates body mechanics over a 24-hour period. Lungs work best during the day, with peak lung function at about 4 p.m. Several studies show that 12 hours later—around 4 a.m.—lung function is at its lowest. The fluctuation is usually less than 10 percent. However, people with asthma can have up to a 50 percent difference between daytime and nighttime lung function.

In addition to rhythmic fluctuations, other factors contribute to worsening asthma symptoms during sleep. According to Eli Meltzer, MD, of the Allergy and Asthma Medical Group and Research Center in San Diego, California, "These factors include changes in the degree of inflammation, the amount of allergen exposure, and the responsiveness patients have to their medications. Not only do short-acting bronchodilators wear off while patients are asleep, their effect over the 4–6 hours of their activity is less at night than in the day. These conditions result in patients waking up short of breath because they need to take another dose."

Gastroesophageal reflux (often called acid reflux or reflux), a backwash of stomach acid into the esophagus, is also a contributing factor to sleep disturbance. AANMA member Carol O'Leary found reflux to be the cause of her son's sleep problems. "After two and a half years of sleepless nights, my son's acid reflux was finally diagnosed and treated. An effective treatment plan helped our whole family start sleeping better."

Researchers aren't sure exactly how reflux and asthma interact, but they do see a connection—adult studies suggest as many as 75 percent of adults with asthma also have reflux. Reflux can set off asthma symptoms. Because reflux is more common when a person is lying down, people with asthma may have more difficulty during sleep.

Another sleep-related condition that can worsen nighttime asthma is sleep apnea. This sleep disorder causes repeated pauses in breathing throughout the night—a serious problem in itself, but also one that can set off or worsen asthma symptoms. A recent study by the Cincinnati Children's Hospital Medical Center showed that women with asthma are twice as likely to have symptoms of sleep apnea as women without asthma.

"Please don't rule out sleep apnea as a cause of poor sleep—even in children!" says AANMA member Laurie Soares. "My 10-year-old son has asthma and allergies. He snored, was a mouth breather at night, was tired a lot, and had poor height and weight growth. His father has sleep apnea, so with all those factors present we had my son's tonsils and adenoids removed. Since then, he sleeps quietly, is gaining weight, and reports that he now has dreams!"

Allergens—like pollen or mold that cause allergic reactions—can also play a role in sleep problems. Exposure to allergens during the day may set off a chain reaction in the immune system that produces symptoms hours later, as can allergens in the bedroom like dust mites or animal dander.

Studies show that postnasal drip and congestion from allergies can cause multiple nighttime "micro-arousals." These awakenings are so brief that the sleeper doesn't even remember them, but they affect alertness the following day.

The Next Day

The effects of nighttime asthma and allergy symptoms reach beyond the bedroom. Children with nighttime asthma miss more time from school—and their parents more time from work—than healthy children. School and work performance can suffer when the family can't sleep. Children whose rest is disturbed by asthma symptoms have a higher incidence of psychological problems and poor school performance. Studies show that these children score lower on memory and time-limited tests. The most obvious signs that asthma is disturbing someone's sleep are fatigue, irritability, and reduced alertness the following day. According to Dr. Meltzer, other signs to look for include morning headaches, depression, and impaired concentration.

Doctors use the term "allergic fatigue" to describe the tiredness and general lack of energy experienced by people with nasal allergies. This condition is often blamed on antihistamine medications, many of which cause sedation. But recent studies show that, in addition to other factors, poor sleep quality contributes to the exhaustion people with allergies may feel all day long.

Clean Sleep

Eliminating allergens and potential asthma triggers in the bedroom can make a big difference in your child's quality of sleep. Allergy testing, combined with your child's symptom history, will help your doctor determine which specific allergens are triggering your child's asthma or allergy symptoms. Then you can focus your efforts on eliminating exposure to those specific allergens. AANMA member Rachel Clarke reports, "We were amazed at the huge difference in our children's quality of sleep once we removed our carpeting and installed wooden floors. It was expensive—but well worth it."

Jan Frey concurs. After finding out her son was allergic to dust mites and mold, she says, "We ripped out carpeting, removed drapes, and stuffed animals and got rid of the clutter that collects dust. We allergy-proofed not only his bed but also his brother's bed in the same room and our bed. We were amazed at the immediate improvement. His nightly wheezing and asthma flare-ups cleared and he now sleeps more deeply and soundly."

Christine Noriega took a multi-step approach to helping her son get a good night's sleep. "My son's eczema would flare up and keep him scratching all night and his asthma would get worse. First, we found out he had food allergies and eliminated those foods. This helped calm his eczema. We also found he was allergic to dust mites. We put dust mite covers on his mattress and pillows, wash his bedding frequently in hot water and put a HEPA [high efficiency particulate air] filter in his room. When he comes in after playing outdoors, we get him into the bath right away to get rid of the pollen and other allergens. Then we rub Vaseline all over his body and put on cotton pajamas. This helps his eczema. All of these steps are helping calm his asthma and he's finally getting a good night's sleep."

If cleaning up the bedroom isn't enough to curb allergy symptoms, work with an allergist on treatment options, including immunotherapy (allergy shots), oral and nasal antihistamines, and nasal corticosteroids. Children 12 and older can also be tested to see if they qualify for a medication that reduces the number of antibodies responsible for allergic reactions.

Ensuring Sleep

If you think your child is having trouble sleeping due to asthma or allergies, monitor his symptoms, encourage him to report any problems to you, and keep a sleep journal (this can be part of his daily symptom diary). Talk to your child's doctor about nighttime problems. "We need to control asthma both during the day and at night to maximize a patient's health-related quality of life," emphasizes Dr. Meltzer. If you notice excessive napping or drowsiness, school problems, hyperactivity, or distractibility, ask your doctor to assess your child's nighttime symptoms. Talk about your child's sleep schedule, sleep environment, sleep-related symptoms, and behavioral issues. You should also carefully monitor your child's use of medication: Is he taking all doses on time? Adept at using a metered-dose inhaler or nebulizer? Check his inhaler technique at the next medical appointment and talk to the doctor about other medical conditions—like reflux and sleep apnea—that could be contributing to sleep problems.

Rachel Gerke says, "It has taken us all 3 years of his life, but we've finally started to get my son's asthma symptoms under control." Rachel makes regular appointments for her son with his allergist and asthma program coordinator. "He's had fewer asthma symptoms now that we fine-tuned his medication plan, put wood flooring in his room, removed all stuffed animals, started washing his bedding frequently, and put dust mite-proof covers on his mattress and pillow cases. I also think that it made a difference to take the diaper wipes warmer out of his room—it gave off a scent from the wipes that I believe irritated his airways. It is all those little things that a lot of people don't think about doing in their sleeping environment that make a world of difference."

Asthma and allergies don't have to keep your family from getting the sleep you need. Work with your child's medical care team to determine what's causing sleep problems and how you can solve them.

Dealing with Dust Mites

Most children and even teenagers have well-loved stuffed animals that are full of dust mites. How do you get rid of those dust mites? You could turn the hot water heater up to 130 degrees Fahrenheit on laundry day. Or you can make your child's stuffed animals "allergy friendly" by sticking them in the freezer overnight. This tip was first reported by AANMA president and founder Nancy Sander in "A Parent's Guide to Asthma" in 1989. After the deep freeze, wash and dry the stuffed animals to get rid of dust mite body parts and fecal pellets.

What's on Your Bed?

With all the mattress and pillow options available today, are some better than others for people with asthma and allergies? It depends on what's causing your sneezing and wheezing.

If you have dust mite allergy, the keys to a good night's sleep are using mattress and pillow encasements and monitoring humidity levels. Dust mites need two things to thrive: water (which they absorb from the air) and food (which they get from you in the form of dead skin cells). Keeping your bedroom's humidity below 50 percent will deprive dust mites of their water source, and a special cover over your mattress and pillow will deprive them of food. The mattress and pillow encasements will also protect you from allergens in mite body parts and poop.

A word about mattress and pillow encasements: Old-style pillow and mattress encasements were made of plastic; they didn't allow air to flow through, so you'd end up sweaty, and they made a lot of noise when you rolled over. New encasements are made of tightly woven fabric that's soft and silent. Small pores allow air to pass through but are too small for dust mites and allergens to get through. When shopping for encasements, look for bound seams and a pore size (the amount of space between fabric threads) of 10 microns or less. Avoid coatings or lamination that can wear off in the wash.

New allergy-free and hypoallergenic pillows may not solve your slumber problems. According to the American Academy of Allergy, Asthma and Immunology, both synthetic pillows and feather pillows promote dust mite growth. And allergy to feathers is actually very rare. So select the pillow that's most comfortable for you and use a tightly woven pillow encasement.

Chapter 4

Allergies in Children

Chapter Contents

Section 4.1

How Allergies Affect Your Child

Dust, cats, peanuts, cockroaches. An odd grouping, but one with
a common thread: allergies—a major cause of illness in the United
States. Up to 50 million Americans, including millions of kids, have
some type of allergy. In fact, allergies account for the loss of an estimated 2 million schooldays per year.

About Allergies

An allergy is an overreaction of the immune system to a substance
that's harmless to most people. But in someone with an allergy, the
body's immune system treats the substance (called an allergen) as an
invader and reacts inappropriately, resulting in symptoms that can
be anywhere from annoying to possibly harmful to the person.

In an attempt to protect the body, the immune system of the allergic person produces antibodies called immunoglobulin E (IgE). Those
antibodies then cause mast cells and basophils (allergy cells in the
body) to release chemicals, including histamine, into the bloodstream
to defend against the allergen "invader."

It's the release of these chemicals that causes allergic reactions,
affecting a person's eyes, nose, throat, lungs, skin, or gastrointestinal tract as the body attempts to rid itself of the invading allergen.
Future exposure to that same allergen (things like nuts or pollen
that you can be allergic to) will trigger this allergic response again.
This means every time the person eats that particular food or is
exposed to that particular allergen, he or she will have an allergic
reaction.

Who Gets Allergies?

The tendency to develop allergies is often hereditary, which means it can be passed down through your genes. However, just because you, your partner, or one of your children might have allergies doesn't mean that all of your kids will definitely get them, too. And someone usually doesn't inherit a particular allergy, just the likelihood of having allergies.

But a few kids have allergies even if no family member is allergic. A child who is allergic to one substance is likely to be allergic to others as well.

Common Airborne Allergens

Some of the most common things people are allergic to are airborne (carried through the air):

- **Dust mites** are one of the most common causes of allergies. These microscopic insects live all around us and feed on the millions of dead skin cells that fall off our bodies every day. Dust mites are the main allergic component of house dust, which is made up of many particles and can contain things such as fabric fibers and bacteria, as well as microscopic animal allergens. Dust mites are present year-round in most parts of the United States (although they don't live at high altitudes), and live in bedding, upholstery, and carpets.

- **Pollen** is another major cause of allergies (most people know pollen allergy as hay fever or rose fever). Trees, weeds, and grasses release these tiny particles into the air to fertilize other plants. Pollen allergies are seasonal, and the type of pollen a child is allergic to determines when symptoms will occur. For example, in the mid-Atlantic states, tree pollination begins in February and lasts through May, grass from May through June, and ragweed from August through October; so people with these allergies are likely to experience increased symptoms during those times. Pollen counts measure how much pollen is in the air and can help people with allergies determine how bad their symptoms might be on any given day. Pollen counts are usually higher in the morning and on warm, dry, breezy days, whereas they're lowest when it's chilly and wet. Although not always exact, the local weather report's pollen count can be helpful when planning outside activities.

- **Molds,** another common allergen, are fungi that thrive both indoors and out in warm, moist environments. Outdoors, molds may be found in poor drainage areas, such as in piles of rotting leaves or compost piles. Indoors, molds thrive in dark, poorly ventilated places such as bathrooms and damp basements, and in clothes hampers or under kitchen sinks. A musty odor suggests mold growth. Although molds tend to be seasonal, many can grow year-round, especially those indoors.

- **Pet allergens** from warm-blooded animals can cause problems for kids and parents alike. When the animal—often a household pet—licks itself, the saliva gets on its fur or feathers. As the saliva dries, protein particles become airborne and work their way into fabrics in the home. Cats are the worst offenders because the protein from their saliva is extremely tiny and they tend to lick themselves more than other animals as part of grooming. Pet allergens are also present in dander, hair, and urine. Cockroaches are also a major household allergen, especially in inner cities. Exposure to cockroach-infested buildings may be a major cause of the high rates of asthma in inner-city kids.

Common Food Allergens

The American Academy of Allergy, Asthma, and Immunology estimates that up to 2 million, or 8%, of kids in the United States are affected by food allergies, and that eight foods account for most of those food allergy reactions in kids: eggs, fish, milk, peanuts, shellfish, soy, tree nuts, and wheat.

- **Cow's milk (or cow's milk protein):** Between 1% and 7.5% of infants are allergic to the proteins found in cow's milk and cow's milk-based formulas. About 80% of formulas on the market are cow's milk-based. Cow's milk protein allergy (also called formula protein allergy) means that the infant (or child or adult) has an abnormal immune system reaction to proteins found in the cow's milk used to make standard baby formulas, cheeses, and other milk products. Milk proteins can also be a hidden ingredient in many prepared foods.

- **Eggs:** One of the most common food allergies in infants and young children, egg allergy can pose many challenges for parents. Because eggs are used in many of the foods kids eat—and in many cases they're "hidden" ingredients—an egg allergy is hard to diagnose. An egg allergy usually begins when kids are very young, but most outgrow the allergy by age 5. Most kids with an egg allergy are allergic to the proteins in egg whites, but some can't tolerate proteins in the yolk.

- **Seafood and shellfish:** The proteins in seafood can cause a number of different types of allergic reactions. Seafood allergy is one of the more common adult food allergies and one that you don't always grow out of.

- **Peanuts and tree nuts:** Peanuts are one of the most severe food allergens, often causing life-threatening reactions. About 1.5 million people in the United States are allergic to peanuts. (Peanuts are not a true nut, but a legume—in the same family as peas and lentils, although people with peanut allergy don't usually have cross-reactions to other legumes). Half of those allergic to peanuts are also allergic to tree nuts, such as almonds, walnuts, pecans, cashews, and often sunflower and sesame seeds. Like seafood allergy, peanut allergy is one you don't always grow out of.

- **Soy:** Like peanuts, soybeans are legumes. Soy allergy is more prevalent among babies than older children; about 30% to 40% of infants who are allergic to cow's milk are also allergic to the protein in soy formulas. Soy proteins, such as soya, are often a hidden ingredient in prepared foods.

- **Wheat:** Wheat proteins are found in many of the foods we eat— some are more obvious than others. As with any allergy, an allergy to wheat can happen in different ways and to different degrees. Although wheat allergy is often confused with celiac disease, there is a difference. Celiac disease is caused by a sensitivity to gluten, which is found in wheat, oat, rye, and barley. It typically develops between 6 months and 2 years of age and the sensitivity causes damage to the small intestine in a different way to the usual allergic reaction.

Other Common Allergens

- **Insect stings:** For most kids, being stung by an insect means swelling, redness, and itching at the site of the bite. But for those with insect venom allergy, an insect bite can cause more severe symptoms. Although some doctors and parents have believed that most kids eventually outgrow insect venom allergy, a recent study found that insect venom allergies often persist into adulthood. An allergy evaluation is needed if wheezing and other signs of anaphylaxis are present after an insect sting or bite.

- **Medicines:** Antibiotics—medications used to treat infections—
  are the most common types of medicines that cause allergic
  reactions. Many other medicines, including over-the-counter
  medications, can also cause allergic reactions. If you suspect a
  medicine allergy, talk to your doctor first before assuming a reaction is a sign of allergy.

- **Chemicals:** Some cosmetics or laundry detergents can cause
  people to break out in an itchy rash. Usually, this is because
  someone has a reaction to the chemicals in these products. Dyes,
  household cleaners, and pesticides used on lawns or plants can
  also cause allergic reactions in some people.

Some kids also have what are called cross-reactions. For example,
kids who are allergic to birch pollen might have reactions when they
eat an apple because that apple is made up of a protein similar to one
in the pollen. Another example is that kids who are allergic to latex
(as in gloves or certain types of hospital equipment) are more likely to
be allergic to kiwifruit, water chestnuts, or bananas.

Signs and Symptoms

The type and severity of allergy symptoms vary from allergy to allergy and child to child. Allergies may show up as itchy eyes or an itchy
nose, sneezing, nasal congestion, throat tightness, trouble breathing,
and even shock (faintness or passing out).

Symptoms can range from minor or major seasonal annoyances (for
example, from pollen or certain molds) to year-round problems (from
allergens like dust mites or food). Allergies to dust mites are common to
the eastern parts of the United States, but not in areas of high-altitude
and low humidity (for example, like Colorado).

Because different allergens are more prevalent in different parts of
the country and the world, allergy symptoms can also vary, depending
on where you live. For example, peanut allergy is unknown in Scandinavia, where they don't eat peanuts, but is common in the United
States, where peanuts are not only a popular food, but are also found
in many of the things we eat.

Airborne Allergy Symptoms

Airborne allergens can cause something known as allergic rhinitis,
which occurs in about 15% to 20% of Americans. It develops by 10 years
of age and reaches its peak in the early twenties, with symptoms often
disappearing between the ages of 40 and 60.

Symptoms can include:

- sneezing;

- itchy nose and/or throat;

- nasal congestion;

- coughing.

These symptoms are often accompanied by itchy, watery, and/or red eyes, which is called allergic conjunctivitis. (When dark circles are present around the eyes, they're called allergic "shiners.") Those who react to airborne allergens usually have allergic rhinitis and/or allergic conjunctivitis. If a person has wheezing and shortness of breath, the allergy may have progressed to become asthma.

Food Allergy Symptoms

The severity of food allergy symptoms and when they develop depends on:

- how much of the food is eaten;

- the person's sensitivity to the food.

Symptoms of food allergies can include:

- itchy mouth and throat when food is swallowed (some kids have only this symptom—called "oral allergy syndrome");

- hives (raised, red, itchy bumps);

- eczematous rash;

- runny, itchy nose;

- abdominal cramps accompanied by nausea and vomiting or diarrhea (as the body attempts to flush out the food allergen);

- difficulty breathing;

- shock.

Insect Venom Allergy Symptoms

Being stung by an insect that a child is allergic to may cause some of these symptoms:

- Throat swelling

- Hives over the entire body

- Difficulty breathing
- Nausea
- Diarrhea
- Shock

About Anaphylaxis

In rare instances, if the sensitivity to an allergen is extreme, a child may experience anaphylaxis (or anaphylactic shock)—a sudden, severe allergic reaction involving various systems in the body (such as the skin, respiratory tract, gastrointestinal tract, and cardiovascular system).

Severe symptoms or reactions to any allergen, from certain foods to insect bites, require immediate medical attention and can include:

- difficulty breathing;
- swelling (particularly of the face, throat, lips, and tongue in cases of food allergies);
- rapid drop in blood pressure;
- dizziness;
- unconsciousness;
- hives;
- tightness of the throat;
- hoarse voice;
- lightheadedness.

Anaphylaxis can happen just seconds after being exposed to a triggering substance or can be delayed for up to 2 hours if the reaction is from a food. It can involve various areas of the body.

Fortunately, though, severe or life-threatening allergies occur in only a small group of kids. In fact, the annual incidence of anaphylactic reactions is small—about 30 per 100,000 people—although those with asthma, eczema, or hay fever are at greater risk of experiencing them.

Most anaphylactic reactions—up to 80%—are caused by peanuts or tree nuts.

Diagnosing Allergies

Some allergies are fairly easy to identify because the pattern of symptoms following exposure to certain allergens can be hard to miss. But other allergies are less obvious because they can masquerade as other conditions.

If your child has cold-like symptoms lasting longer than a week or two or develops a "cold" at the same time every year, consult your doctor, who will likely ask questions about the symptoms and when they appear. Based on the answers to these questions and a physical exam, the doctor may be able to make a diagnosis and prescribe medications or may refer you to an allergist for allergy skin tests and more extensive therapy.

To determine the cause of an allergy, allergists usually perform skin tests for the most common environmental and food allergens. These tests can be done in infants, but they're more reliable in kids over 2 years old.

A skin test can work in one of two ways:

1. A drop of a purified liquid form of the allergen is dropped onto the skin and the area is pricked with a small pricking device.

2. A small amount of allergen is injected just under the skin. This test stings a little but isn't extremely painful. After about 15 minutes, if a lump surrounded by a reddish area appears (like a mosquito bite) at the injection site, the test is positive.

If reactions to a food or other allergen are severe, a blood test may be used to diagnose the allergy so as to avoid exposure to the offending allergen. Skin tests are less expensive and more sensitive than blood tests for allergies. But blood tests may be required in children with skin conditions or those who are extremely sensitive to a particular allergen.

Even if a skin test and/or a blood test shows an allergy, a child must also have symptoms to be definitively diagnosed with an allergy. For example, a toddler who has a positive test for dust mites and sneezes frequently while playing on the floor would be considered allergic to dust mites.

Treating Allergies

There is no real cure for allergies, but it is possible to relieve symptoms. The only real way to cope with them is to reduce or eliminate exposure to allergens. That means that parents must educate their kids early and often, not only about the allergy itself, but also about what reaction they will have if they consume or come into contact with the allergen.

Informing any and all caregivers (childcare personnel, teachers, extended family members, parents of your child's friends, etc.) about your child's allergy is equally important.

If reducing exposure isn't possible or is ineffective, medications may be prescribed, including antihistamines (which you can also buy over the counter) and inhaled or nasal spray steroids.

In some cases, an allergist may recommend immunotherapy (allergy shots) to help desensitize your child. However, allergy shots are only helpful for allergens such as dust, mold, pollens, animals, and insect stings. They're not used for food allergies, and someone with food allergies must avoid that food.

Here are some things that can help kids avoid airborne allergens:

- Keep family pets out of certain rooms, like your child's bedroom, and bathe them if necessary.

- Remove carpets or rugs from your child's room (hard floor surfaces don't collect dust as much as carpets do).

- Don't hang heavy drapes and get rid of other items that allow dust to accumulate.

- Clean frequently.

- Use special covers to seal pillows and mattresses if your child is allergic to dust mites.

- For kids allergic to pollen, keep the windows closed when the pollen season is at its peak, change their clothing after they've been outdoors, and don't let them mow the lawn.

- Keep kids who are allergic to mold away from damp areas, such as basements, and keep bathrooms and other mold-prone areas clean and dry.

Injectable Epinephrine

Food allergies usually aren't lifelong (although those to peanuts, tree nuts, and seafood can be). Avoiding the food is the only way to avoid symptoms while the sensitivity persists.

Doctors often recommend that caregivers of kids who are extremely sensitive to a particular food, have asthma in addition to the food allergy, or are allergic to insect venom carry injectable epinephrine (adrenaline) to counteract any allergic reactions.

Available in an easy-to-carry container that looks like a pen, injectable epinephrine is carried by millions of parents (and older kids) everywhere they go. With one injection into the thigh, the device administers epinephrine to ease the allergic reaction.

An injectable epinephrine prescription usually includes two auto-injectors and a "trainer" that contains no needle or epinephrine, but allows you and your child (if he or she is old enough) to practice using the device. It's vital that you familiarize yourself with the procedure by practicing with the trainer. Your doctor also can provide instructions on how to use and store injectable epinephrine.

Make sure kids 12 years or older keep injectable epinephrine readily available at all times. If your child is younger than 12, talk to the school nurse, teachers, and your childcare provider about keeping injectable epinephrine on hand in case of an emergency.

It's also important to ensure that injectable epinephrine devices are available in your home and in the homes of friends and family members if your child spends time there. Your doctor may also encourage your child to wear a medical alert bracelet. It's also wise to carry an over-the-counter antihistamine, which can help alleviate allergy symptoms in some people. But antihistamines should not be used as a replacement for the epinephrine pen.

Kids who have had to take injectable epinephrine should go immediately to a medical facility or hospital emergency department, where additional treatment can be given if needed. Up to one third of anaphylactic reactions can have a second wave of symptoms several hours following the initial attack, so these kids might need to be observed in a clinic or hospital for 4 to 8 hours following the reaction even though they seem well.

The good news is that only a very small group of kids will experience severe or life-threatening allergies. With proper diagnosis, preventive measures, and treatment, most kids can keep their allergies in check and live happy, healthy lives.

Section 4.2

Will Your Child Outgrow His or Her Allergies?

One of the first things parents ask when their child is diagnosed
with food allergy is, "When will he outgrow it?" That's because it's been
conventional wisdom that most children outgrow food allergies—particularly milk and egg—within a few years. Today, however, research
shows that food allergies persist into childhood longer.

Two studies highlighted in the *Journal of Allergy and Clinical Immunology* (November and December 2007) followed the progress of
more than 800 children with milk allergy and almost 900 children
with egg allergy over 13 years. The results showed a major shift in
how these allergies progressed in children.

Early research suggested that three out of four children would
outgrow milk allergy by age 3. In the new studies, only one out of five
children outgrew milk allergy by age 4, and less than half the children
had outgrown it by age 8. By age 16, almost 80 percent of the children
were free of milk allergy. Egg allergy followed similar trends.

What's causing this shift in allergy rates? "The 'why' is still an unanswered question," says Robert Wood, MD, lead investigator of the
studies and one of the foremost U.S. experts on food allergies. "I am
definitely seeing this in my practice, which is why we did the studies.
I suspect that the same factors that have led to the increase in food
allergies are also related to the greater persistence. I believe that food
allergy is a different disease than it was 20 or 30 years ago."

The important question for parents is what they should do about
it. The answer: Monitor your child's diet carefully and work with an
allergist for accurate diagnosis and a management plan.

Dr. Wood says he tracks his patients' allergies with blood tests at
least once a year. Blood tests measure the amount of allergy-specific
IgE antibodies (a sign of allergy) in a patient's blood—the higher the
milk IgE count, for instance, the more likely the patient is to be allergic
to milk. If the IgE count begins to decrease, it may mean the patient

will eventually be able to drink milk without an allergic reaction. It's important to work with a board-certified allergist specializing in food allergies, who is trained to interpret these numbers accurately and should be up-to-date on the most recent research in the field.

If blood tests indicate your child's allergy may be going away, your allergist is likely to recommend a food challenge (a.k.a., taste test done at the doctor's office) to see whether your child is able to consume the food without an allergic reaction.

If all goes well during the food challenge, Dr. Wood recommends parents gradually add more and more of the food to the child's diet. "It's important to follow the doctor's instructions carefully and proceed slowly," he writes in his book, *Food Allergies for Dummies®*. "Once you can tolerate a full serving of the food over a period of several days, your doctor is likely to lift all restrictions, so you can consume all forms of the food."

Dr. Wood advises parents to be watchful for signs of allergy, even after it seems to have gone away. Recurrences of milk and egg allergy are rare, he says, but peanut allergy is known to return.

There's so much we don't know about food allergies. Research is adding to our understanding every day, but we have a long way to go. That's why it's important to work closely with a specialist, follow instructions carefully, and listen to what your body tells you.

Section 4.3

Colic May Be Linked to Allergies

Researchers at The University of Texas Health Science Center at Houston say one organism discovered during their study may unlock the key to what causes colic, inconsolable crying in an otherwise healthy baby.

"Right now, pediatric gastroenterologists can treat just about anything that comes through the door," said J. Marc Rhoads, MD, professor of pediatrics at The University of Texas Medical School at Houston, which is part of the UT Health Science Center at Houston. "With colic, there is no evidence-based treatment we can offer. Colic can be a dangerous situation for a baby. The parent's frustration over the crying can lead to maternal frustration, postpartum depression, and even thoughts of harming the baby."

Published in the [July 23, 2009] online edition of the *Journal of Pediatrics,* the study pointed to an organism called Klebsiella, a normally occurring bacterium that can be found in the mouth, skin, and intestines. In the study of 36 babies, half of which had colic, researchers found the bacterium and gut inflammation in the intestines of the babies with colic.

"We believe that the bacterium may be sparking an inflammatory reaction, causing the gut inflammation," said Rhoads, the lead investigator for the study. "Inflammation in the gut of colicky infants closely compared to levels in patients with inflammatory bowel disease. Colic could prove to be a precursor to other gastrointestinal conditions such as irritable bowel syndrome, celiac disease, and allergic gastroenteropathies."

Babies in the study were fed breast milk and/or formula. Previous research articles have not shown significant data supporting the theory that breastfeeding protects infants against colic. The babies in the study were recruited from UT Physicians' pediatric clinics and Kelsey-Seybold clinics.

Colic is defined as unexplained and severe crying in an otherwise healthy newborn. It usually occurs in infants 3 months old or younger and lasts for more than 3 hours daily for at least 3 days a week. "Colic is a very common condition. It affects about 15 percent of normal, healthy infants. More than half of infanticides fall into the age category of colic. We may be able to prevent deaths if we can find a treatment," Rhoads said.

Right now, pediatricians prescribe special hypoallergenic infant formula to try and treat colic, but none of it has been proven in studies to be effective in treating the condition.

"During our study, we also found that the babies that didn't have colic had more types of bacteria in their intestines. The presence of more bacteria may indicate that specific bacterial species (phylotypes) are beneficial to humans," Rhoads said.

The study was funded by the Gerber Foundation.

A larger study is needed to examine Klebsiella and the use of a probiotic, which is a dietary supplement made up of good bacteria, to control the gut inflammation. Before that can begin, Rhoads said an adult trial will take place to examine the safety of the probiotics in healthy adults. For that study, UT researchers are recruiting 40 adult patients.

Other research personnel at the UT Medical School included Nicole Fatheree, research coordinator; Yuying Liu, PhD, researcher; Joseph Lucke, PhD, and Jon E. Tyson, MD, professor of pediatrics and obstetrics and Michelle Bain Distinguished Professor in Medicine and Public Health.

Section 4.4

Urban Environment and Childhood Allergen Exposure

Excerpted from "Urban Environment and Childhood Asthma,"
a report by the National Institute of Allergy and Infectious Diseases
(NIAID, www.niaid.nih.gov), September 12, 2007.

Asthma is more prevalent, and may be more severe, in the inner city, even after controlling for differences in ethnicity and socioeconomic status, thus strongly suggesting that environmental factors that are unique to the inner city may promote the development of more severe asthma in early childhood. Although there are comprehensive studies of allergen exposure in the inner city environment, information relating early life exposures to viral infections and stress in the inner city to the development of asthma are lacking. Furthermore, despite studies which link asthma to abnormal development of the immune system and patterns of cytokine secretion, there has been no prospective evaluation of the effects of the unique environmental exposures unique to the inner city on immune development and the incidence of asthma. As a result, a number of important questions remain unanswered:

- Does dysregulation of innate immune responses, which may already be present at birth, increase the risk of allergen sensitization (adaptive immune responses) and asthma, and if so, which cytokines are key in this process?

- How do lower respiratory infections in infancy affect the subsequent risk of recurrent wheezing and asthma in inner city children?

- Is the immune system of inner city children already abnormal at birth, due to a unique prenatal environment?

- Of the many unique features associated with the inner city environment, which are the principal factors that adversely affect immune development, and thereby increase the risk of asthma?

- Does the inner city environment (e.g., increased stress and pollution) increase the frequency or severity of lower respiratory infections (LRI), and if so, what are the relevant mechanisms (immune modulation versus lung-specific effects)?

- Do environmental factors interact at a critical time point to establish a particular wheezing phenotype with future infections and/or exposures?

There is increasing evidence that allergy and asthma are associated with abnormal patterns of cellular immunity, as evidenced by a distinct and abnormal pattern of cytokine secretion. Since the pattern of cytokine secretion changes rapidly during the first few years of life, it is likely that the environment influences the development of the immune system in infancy, and this in turn modifies the risk for developing allergies and asthma. Differences in the inner city environment are numerous, and include prenatal factors (e.g., maternal stress, placental insufficiency), and numerous postnatal exposures. Some of the differences in postnatal exposures are well-documented, such as increased exposure to cockroach and tobacco smoke, while there is less specific information related to patterns of stress, exposure of young children to other pollutants and endotoxin, and the development of viral infections in the first years of life. If primary prevention of asthma is to be achieved, establishing the relationship of these factors to the onset of infantile wheezing, as well as their impact on the evolution to recurrent childhood wheezing (or asthma) will be critical.

Do respiratory viruses increase the risk of developing asthma?

There are experimental data to suggest that lower respiratory infections at a critical period during the development of the immune system or lungs could have long-lasting effects. For example, young mice infected with RSV [respiratory syncytial virus] have a propensity to develop Th2 rather than Th1 recall responses to virus, which could enhance inflammation and impair antiviral responses upon reexposure to the virus. In addition, CMV [cytomegalovirus] infections specifically inhibit expression of the epithelial growth factor receptor. This finding implies that infection during early infancy, a time period of continued lung and epithelial differentiation, could have detrimental and long-term effects on lung structure and function. Other infections (e.g., mycoplasma, chlamydia, adenovirus) have also been implicated in the promotion of chronic airway inflammation and/or recurrent wheezing, or conversely (e.g., hepatitis A), have been associated with reduced prevalence of allergies and asthma. However, based on the experimental design, these observations could not determine if these changes had been present or "programmed" (i.e., cytokine dysregulation) prior to the onset of the infection.

There is a close association between RSV infections and wheezing syndromes in infants. Although nearly all infants are infected with RSV during the first 3 years of life, only a subset of infants develop wheezing illnesses, and consequently other risk factors including small lung size and genetic factors, such as polymorphisms in the IL-8 [interleukin-8] gene, are also involved. In animal models, enhanced lower airway responses to Sendai virus infection have been related to reduced interferon (IFN) production, and preliminary data from a cohort of suburban infants (the Childhood Origins of Asthma [COAST] study) suggest that reduced cytokine responses (e.g., IL-13) by cord blood mononuclear cells may also increase the risk for wheezing with RSV infection.

Children who develop wheezing with RSV infection are at an increased risk of recurrent wheezing and asthma in childhood. Most of the risk factors for developing asthma after bronchiolitis in infancy relate to other signs or indicators of allergy, such as atopic dermatitis, food allergy, or allergic rhinitis. In addition, immunologic responses at the time of infection which have been associated with recurrent wheezing after bronchiolitis include eosinophilic inflammation in airway secretions, reduced IFN production from peripheral blood mononuclear cells (PBMC) ex vivo, and increased ex vivo PBMC IL-10 secretion during convalescence. It has yet to be established whether this pattern of immune responses is a preexisting condition or whether abnormalities in immune responses develop in response to environmental influences. One of the keys to understanding the relationship between viral infections in infancy and asthma will be to determine the temporal sequence of these events, and the interplay with the unique pattern of environmental factors (stress, allergens, microbial products) in the inner city that could modify the clinical response to, and consequences of, viral respiratory infections. One final consideration is that the pattern of infectious diseases, and the age at which they are contracted, may be distinct in the inner city. This raises the possibility that a unique pattern of infections could modify lung and/or immunologic development in children, and that this could affect the risk of allergy and asthma.

How does the hygiene hypothesis relate to asthma in inner city children?

There are indications that some viral infections might actually protect against the subsequent development of allergies and asthma. This controversial theory, termed the "hygiene hypothesis," was first suggested by David Strachan, who noted that the risk of developing allergies and asthma is inversely related to the number of children in the family, leading to speculation that infectious diseases, which are more likely to be transmitted in large families, modulate the development of the immune system to reduce the chances of developing allergies. This hypothesis implies that the immune system is skewed towards a Th2-like response pattern at birth. This may in part be due to suppression of Th1-like responses by immunologically active factors in the intrauterine environment. According to the theory, each viral infection would provide a stimulus for the development of Th1-like immune responses, and with this repetitive stimulation, the polarization would shift away from Th2 over-expression and thus reduce the risk for developing allergies.

Although early reports suggesting that contracting a single infectious disease, such as measles, can protect against allergies and asthma have not been confirmed, the hygiene hypothesis is supported by studies that demonstrate an inverse relationship between attendance at day care centers, where exposure to viral infections is quite high, and a reduction in subsequent rates of allergy and asthma. There is also evidence that it is not only the type of infection that is important, but also the route of exposure, as food-borne or enteric infections may have greater effects on allergy than respiratory infections.

It is possible that distinct patterns of exposure to infectious diseases in inner city children could modify the incidence of allergy and asthma, and there are, in fact, several examples of differences in the epidemiology or clinical expression of infectious diseases that are related to ethnicity or culture. For instance, African-American and Native American populations acquire cytomegalovirus infections at an earlier age compared to middle-income Caucasian groups. Furthermore, the seropositivity rates for other herpes viruses such as HHV-6 [human herpesvirus 6] and EBV [Epstein-Barr virus] can vary between ethnic groups. There may also be differences in the clinical severity of disease after infection: Although RSV infections are nearly ubiquitous in the first 3 years of life, the rate of hospitalization is greater for African-American children, and those with low socioeconomic status. Whether distinct patterns of infectious diseases in inner city infants affect the risk for developing allergy and asthma has not yet been determined.

In addition to infectious diseases, exposure to microbes or microbial products in the environment has been related to wheezing, allergy, and asthma, although this relationship is complex. For example, elevated endotoxin levels in house dust has been associated with an increased risk of wheezing in the first year of life, and increased severity of asthma in children. On the other hand, growing up on a farm, and/or having exposure to higher levels of lipopolysaccharide (LPS), are associated with reduced rates of allergy and asthma. Collectively, these findings suggest that exposure to microbial products in infancy may enhance respiratory illnesses to some degree in the short term, but may promote immune development and respiratory health in the long term. Unfortunately, there is very little information about the quantity and quality of innate stimuli in inner city homes.

The innate immune response is initiated by recognition of pathogen associated molecular patterns (PAMPs) through the toll-like receptors (TLRs). Much attention has focused on endotoxin, which binds primarily to TLR4. TLR2 in combination with TLR6 or TLR1 responds to a wide range of PAMPs including peptidoglycans and microbial lipoproteins. The fungal wall polysaccharides are probably also transduced by toll-like receptors. Because the signaling from TLR4 and from the other toll-like receptors is not identical—there is a MyD88 independent pathway for TLR4 not activated by other TLRs—it may be important to have a broad panel of markers to adequately characterize the environmental stimuli to innate immunity early in life.

How does allergen exposure affect asthma?

More than 80% of asthmatic children in the United States are allergic to one or more allergens. Despite this well-established relation between asthma and allergy, far less is known about whether allergens contribute to the development of asthma. Specific patterns of allergy are particular to asthmatic children in the inner city with higher rates of exposure to cockroach and rodents, as well as sensitization to these allergens compared to asthmatic children from other communities.

Several recent prospective epidemiologic studies have demonstrated that increased home allergen exposure increases asthma morbidity in asthmatic children specifically sensitized to the allergen. Exposure to indoor allergens may not only be a risk factor for aggravating existing disease, but for the development of childhood asthma as well. For example, birth studies have demonstrated that exposure to dust mite allergen in early life was associated with an increased risk of asthma at age 11 years, and that exposure to cockroach allergen is associated with an increased incidence of wheeze in the first year of life and incident asthma among the sibling of the index children.

However, there is limited information regarding the role of allergens in the development of asthma in the inner city.

What is the relationship between stressful life events and asthma?

Stress has been associated with a number of effects on the developing immune system and respiratory health, and could be an important cofactor in the development or disease activity of asthma. In fact, there are indications that the effects of stress on developmental immunology could begin in utero. Both the prenatal and postnatal environments exert long-term influences through pathways connecting the autonomic nervous system, endocrine regulation, and the immune system by triggering the release of immunoreactive hormones and neuropeptides. By modifying the production of cytokines, psychological stress influences cell trafficking, T-cell function, and lymphocyte production. It has been speculated that stress-induced alterations in the maternal or infant hormonal response may affect T cell differentiation towards a Th2 cell predominance.

Epidemiological data also links early life stress to childhood asthma phenotypes. Wright and colleagues have demonstrated that caregiver stress prospectively predicts early onset of wheezing in infancy and persistent wheezing at age 5 years among 505 children. In this same birth cohort, these authors have shown that children living in households reporting high-level chronic stress have increased IgE expression and a more pronounced allergen-induced lymphocyte proliferative response compared with their counterparts living in low stress households.

This proposed study will consider pervasive sources of stress unique to inner-city populations. Differential experiencing of stress including unique stressors in high-risk inner city environments may in part explain socioeconomic disparities in the asthma burden. It may be that stress experienced as early as the prenatal period 'primes' the maturing immune system towards a Th2 phenotype which is further potentiated by subsequent environmental exposures (e.g., allergens, viruses). A potential consequence of stress-induced changes in immune response is suppression of host resistance to infectious agents, particularly viral agents. Psychological stress has been associated with the incidence of viral respiratory infection, with increasing stress related in a dose-response manner to increasing risk of infection. In this context, stress may be hypothesized to not only increase susceptibility to viral respiratory illnesses but also may potentiate the inflammatory response in a multiplicative manner.

How does pollution relate to asthma in the inner city?

Several different pollutants have been linked to acute exacerbations of asthma, and studies of selected pollutants, suggest an effect on initiation of asthma as well. For example, exposure to ETS [environmental tobacco smoke] in early childhood has been linked to an increased frequency of respiratory infection, increased respiratory symptoms, and slightly reduced rates of lung function growth in childhood. In addition, a growing body of data suggests that tobacco smoke exposure in utero and in infancy may influence the risk of asthma. Smoking remains an even larger public health problem in inner-city communities than in other segments of the U.S. population, and ETS is therefore likely to be a particularly important exposure variable to consider in a study of asthma pathogenesis in this community.

Nitrogen dioxide (NO_2) is a combustion product of both gas stoves and automobiles. In very high concentrations, NO_2 and other reactive nitrogen species formed during combustion can damage respiratory epithelium and induce airway inflammation. Investigators have demonstrated relatively high levels of indoor NO_2 in the homes of inner-city asthmatic children and have shown a significant association between high indoor NO_2 levels and asthma morbidity in this population. Indoor NO_2 exposure has been linked to an increased risk of asthma exacerbation following upper respiratory infection in asthmatic children, and among subjects with allergic asthma, exposure to NO_2 may enhance the response to inhaled allergen. Collectively, these data indicate that there are significant adverse effects of NO_2 on persons with existing asthma, and suggest that NO_2 can involve other environmental factors to exacerbate airway symptoms. NO_2 exposure in inner city homes is particularly high, due to the frequent use of gas stoves and heaters. Collectively, these data suggest that NO_2 could be an important contributor to respiratory symptoms and asthma disease in children raised in an inner city environment.

Other pollutants of potential importance to asthma in the inner city include fine particulate matter suspended in the air, and diesel exhaust particles (DEP). For example, recent studies have revealed an association between the proximity of the home to roadways and the occurrence of childhood asthma. Considerable attention has recently been focused on DEP as a potential risk factor for allergic sensitization and asthma. The concentration of DEP in outdoor air varies greatly in relation to proximity to motor vehicle sources, and inner-city communities often have particularly high exposures because of their proximities to highways, industrial sites, and public transportation stations and routes.

What about asthma and cytokine dysregulation?

Recent observations have stimulated research efforts to further define the relative importance and pathophysiologic contributions of cytokine dysregulation (so-called Th1/Th2 imbalance) to the development of various atopic phenotypes, including asthma. Although questions remain as to the full impact of a Th1/Th2 dysregulation in established asthma, the contribution of cytokine polarization to the inception and evolution of various atopic diseases including asthma has received more uniform support. At birth, cytokine profiling of cord blood suggests that the newborn infant's mononuclear cell responses are not fully developed, and this includes both Th1 and Th2 cytokine responses. Although these changes are apparent in all newborns, those who later go on to develop clinical or serological evidence of atopy appear to have a distinct pattern of immune responses at birth or in early infancy. The observed abnormalities have included diminished IFN production, and surprisingly, reduced Th2-like responses (e.g., IL-13) as well. This has led to the concept that immune development, including both Th1 and Th1-like responses, in atopic children may be delayed. Following the neonatal period, there appears to be a progressive skewing of immune responses to allergen (and perhaps other stimuli) towards a Th2 phenotype. Although genetic factors, and especially genes that contribute to the regulation of the innate immune system, contribute to the differentiation of adapted immune responses to allergens, observations in clinical studies (e.g., the hygiene hypothesis) and animal models suggest that environmental factors during early infancy may shape the development of cytokine responses, and thereby modify the risk of developing allergy and asthma. Although studies of immune development as it relates to childhood allergies and asthma have been conducted in several countries around the world, and have stimulated insights into the nature of these disorders, there is a striking lack of data from American inner cities.

Specific cytokines may play key roles in the pathogenesis of asthma in early childhood. Innate immune responses may play important roles in establishing tolerance to proteins in the environment, and the roles of CD14 [cluster of differentiation 14], IL-12, and IL-10 have been studied in this regard. Production of IL-10 by T regulatory cells may be particularly important in preventing hyperresponsiveness and promoting tolerance to allergens in the airway. In addition, IL-4 and IL-13 play critical roles in IgE [immunoglobulin E] antibody isotype switching, and IL-13 is of particular interest as it has been implicated in murine models with enhanced inflammation, mucus secretion, subepithelial fibrosis, and airway hyperresponsiveness. IL-12 and IFN are antagonistic to many Th2 cytokine responses, and IFN is an important component of the antiviral response. Taken together, these observations strongly support continued study of the ontogeny of innate and allergen-specific cytokine responses, especially as they relate to the roles of viral infections and allergen sensitization in the inception of asthma.

What about the genetics of asthma?

Asthma has long been known to be a familial condition. Genome screen linkage studies of asthma and related phenotypes have been performed in families from various populations, and a growing number of linkages to various chromosomal regions have been reported. Linkage of asthma, serum total IgE, and/or nonspecific bronchial responsiveness to the chromosomal region 5q has been observed in most but not all populations studied. This region includes genes for IL-4, -5, -9, and -13, cytokines that appear to play important roles in asthma pathophysiology. Other putative genes in this region include the adrenergic receptor and 5-lipoxygenase. Linkage of regulators of innate immune responses to atopy and asthma have recently been reported, and may have particular relevance to the onset of allergies and asthma in infancy and early childhood.

The frequency of many genetic polymorphisms varies among racial and ethnic groups, but there is no clear evidence at present that excess asthma prevalence or severity in inner-city populations is explained by genetic variation. In all populations it is undoubtedly the case that gene-by-environment and gene-by-gene interactions are crucial determinants of asthma occurrence and severity. The specific combinations of genetic factors and environmental exposures that predispose to asthma and severe asthma are as yet unknown and are the focus of investigations now underway. Such investigations hold the promise of targeting specific immune-based therapies to the asthma patients most likely to benefit on the basis of their genetic profile.

One of the barriers to investigating the genetics of asthma is that asthma seems to be a collection of different disorders that have several features in common, including airway inflammation, hyperresponsiveness, and eventual remodeling. Perhaps the clearest demonstration that asthma is a syndrome instead of a uniform disease process is in early childhood. This has greatly influenced the design of the URECA study, as one of the major goals of this study is to provide a clear phenotypic and immunologic characterization of recurrent wheezing in infancy and early childhood. Once these, and perhaps new, asthma phenotypes have been defined in inner city children, this will provide the basis for investigating genetic linkages with specific asthma phenotypes. As part of the URECA protocol, genetic studies will be conducted to evaluate polymorphisms in genes that regulate both innate (i.e., IL-8, TLR-3, -4, and -9) and adaptive (i.e., IL-4, IL-13, IL-10, IFN-?) immune responses that may be involved in the pathogenesis of virus-induced wheezing illnesses, asthma, and other allergic diseases.

Chapter 5

Economic Costs and Trends in Allergic Disease

Allergic Rhinitis: Trends in Use and Expenditures

Allergic rhinitis is a collection of symptoms such as coughing, sneezing, watery eyes, itching in eyes and nose, headache, and wheezing in people allergic to airborne particles of dust, dander, or plant pollens. When these symptoms are caused by pollen, the allergic rhinitis is commonly called hay fever.

Number of reported cases for allergic rhinitis, by sex

In 2005, 7.3 percent of the U.S. population or 22 million persons reported experiencing related symptoms, visiting a physician, or obtaining a prescription drug to treat allergic rhinitis. In 2000, the same was reported by 6.3 percent of the population. In both 2000 and 2005, more females reported experiencing allergic rhinitis than males (7.6 percent versus 4.9 percent in 2000 and 8.2 percent versus 6.4 percent in 2005).

This chapter includes text from "Allergic Rhinitis: Trends in Use and Expenditures, 2000 and 2005," by the Agency for Healthcare Research and Quality (AHRQ, www.ahrq.gov), May 2008, and text excerpted from "Food Allergy Among U.S. Children: Trends in Prevalence and Hospitalizations," by the National Center for Health Statistics (NCHS, www.cdc.gov/nchs), Centers for Disease Control and Prevention, October 2008.

Total and average reported mean health care expenditures on allergic rhinitis, by age

A total of $6.1 billion (in 2005 dollars) was spent on health care and treatment of allergic rhinitis in 2000 (excluding over-the-counter medications). By 2005, total expenditures to treat allergic rhinitis almost doubled to $11.2 billion. Average expenditures per person for those with an allergic rhinitis related expense increased from $253 to $434 for those under age 18, from 2000 to 2005, and for those ages 18–64 from $381 to $566.

Total and average mean health care expenditures on allergic rhinitis, by type of service

There was a 73 percent increase in the ambulatory expenditures on allergic rhinitis from 2000 to 2005. In 2000, a total of $2.3 billion (in 2005 dollars) was spent on ambulatory visits related to allergic rhinitis compared to $4.0 billion in 2005.

Among those who received treatment for allergic rhinitis, $350 (in 2005 dollars), on average, was spent for treatment in 2000. In 2005, per person expenditures increased to $520. An average of $207 was spent per person on prescription medicines for allergic rhinitis in 2000, as compared to an average of $305 in 2005.

Distribution of average annual health care expenditures for allergic rhinitis, by type of service

For the treatment of allergic rhinitis in both 2000 and 2005, more than half (59.1 percent and 58.7 percent, respectively) of the total was spent on prescription medications and more than one third was spent on ambulatory visits (38.1 percent and 35.9 percent, respectively).

Note: These expenditures do not include over-the-counter medications used for treatment of allergic rhinitis. (Many popular prescription medications such as Zyrtec and Claritin used for treatment of allergic rhinitis are currently sold as over the counter were sold as prescription drugs only in years 2000 and 2005, thus are included in the expenditures).

Food Allergy Among U.S. Children: Trends in Prevalence and Hospitalizations

Food allergy is a potentially serious immune response to eating specific foods or food additives. Eight types of food account for over 90% of allergic reactions in affected individuals: milk, eggs, peanuts, tree nuts, fish, shellfish, soy, and wheat. Reactions to these foods by an allergic person can range from a tingling sensation around the mouth and lips and hives to death, depending on the severity of the allergy. The mechanisms by which a person develops an allergy to specific foods are largely unknown. Food allergy is more prevalent in children than adults, and a majority of affected children will "outgrow" food allergies with age. However, food allergy can sometimes become a lifelong concern. Food allergies can greatly affect children and their families' well-being. There are some indications that the prevalence of food allergy may be increasing in the United States and in other countries.

Four out of every 100 children have a food allergy.

In 2007, an estimated 3 million children under age 18 years (3.9%) had a reported food allergy.

Children under age 5 years had higher rates of reported food allergy compared with children 5 to 17 years of age. Boys and girls had similar rates of food allergy.

Hispanic children had lower rates of reported food allergy than non-Hispanic white or non-Hispanic black children.

Food allergy among children in the United States is becoming more common over time.

In 2007, the reported food allergy rate among all children younger than 18 years was 18% higher than in 1997. During the 10-year period 1997 to 2006, food allergy rates increased significantly among both preschool-aged and older children.

Children with food allergy are more likely to have asthma or other allergic conditions.

In 2007, 29% of children with food allergy also had reported asthma compared with 12% of children without food allergy.

Approximately 27% of children with food allergy had reported eczema or skin allergy, compared with 8% of children without food allergy.

Over 30% of children with food allergy also had reported respiratory allergy, compared with 9% of children with no food allergy.

Recent data show hospitalizations with diagnoses related to food allergies have increased among children.

From 2004 to 2006, there were an average of 9,537 hospital discharges per year with a diagnosis related to food allergy among children 0 to 17 years.

Hospital discharges with a diagnosis related to food allergy increased significantly over time from 1998–2000 through 2004–2006.

Part Two

Types of Allergic Reactions

Chapter 6

Allergic Rhinitis (Hay Fever)

Chapter Contents

Section 6.1

What Is Rhinitis?

Allergic rhinitis is a collection of symptoms, mostly in the nose and eyes, which occur when you breathe in something you are allergic to, such as dust, dander, or pollen.

This text focuses on allergic rhinitis due to outdoor triggers, such as plant pollen. This type of allergic rhinitis is commonly called hay fever.

Causes

An allergen is something that triggers an allergy. When a person with allergic rhinitis breathes in an allergen such as pollen or dust, the body releases chemicals, including histamine. This causes allergy symptoms such as itching, swelling, and mucus production.

Hay fever involves an allergic reaction to pollen. (A similar reaction occurs with allergy to mold, animal dander, dust, and similar inhaled allergens.)

The pollens that cause hay fever vary from person to person and from region to region. Large, visible pollens are seldom responsible for hay fever. Tiny, hard to see pollens more often cause hay fever. Examples of plants commonly responsible for hay fever include:

- trees (deciduous and evergreen);

- grasses;

- ragweed.

The amount of pollen in the air can play a role in whether hay fever symptoms develop. Hot, dry, windy days are more likely to have increased amounts of pollen in the air than cool, damp, rainy days when most pollen is washed to the ground.

Some disorders may be associated with allergies. These include eczema and asthma.

Allergies are common. Your genes and environment may make you more prone to allergies.

Whether or not you are likely to develop allergies is often passed down through families. If both your parents have allergies, you are likely to have allergies. The chance is greater if your mother has allergies.

Symptoms

Symptoms that occur shortly after you come into contact with the substance you are allergic to may include:

- itchy nose, mouth, eyes, throat, skin, or any area;
- problems with smell;
- runny nose;
- sneezing;
- tearing eyes.

Symptoms that may develop later include:

- stuffy nose (nasal congestion);
- coughing;
- clogged ears and decreased sense of smell;
- sore throat;
- dark circles under the eyes;
- puffiness under the eyes;
- fatigue and irritability;
- headache;
- memory problems and slowed thinking.

Exams and Tests

The health care provider will perform a physical exam and ask you questions about your symptoms. Your history of symptoms is important in diagnosing allergic rhinitis, including whether the symptoms vary according to time of day or the season, exposure to pets or other allergens, and diet changes.

Allergy testing may reveal the specific substances that trigger your symptoms. Skin testing is the most common method of allergy testing.

If your doctor determines you cannot undergo skin testing, special blood tests may help with the diagnosis. These tests can measure the levels of specific allergy-related substances, especially one called immunoglobulin E (IgE).

A complete blood count (CBC), specifically the eosinophil white blood cell count, may also help reveal allergies.

Treatment

The best treatment is to avoid what causes your allergic symptoms in the first place. It may be impossible to completely avoid all your triggers, but you can often take steps to reduce exposure.

There are many different medications available to treat allergic rhinitis. Which one your doctor prescribes depends on the type and severity of your symptoms, your age, and whether you have other medical conditions (such as asthma).

For mild allergic rhinitis, a nasal wash can be helpful for removing mucus from the nose. You can purchase a saline solution at a drug store or make one at home using 1 cup of warm water, 1/2 tsp of salt, and a pinch of baking soda.

Treatments for allergic rhinitis include:

Antihistamines: Antihistamines work well for treating allergy symptoms, especially when symptoms do not happen very often or do not last very long.

Antihistamines taken by mouth can relieve mild to moderate symptoms, but can cause sleepiness. Many may be bought without a prescription. Talk to your doctor before giving these medicines to a child, as they may affect learning.

Newer antihistamines cause little or no sleepiness. Some are available over the counter. They usually do not interfere with learning. These medications include fexofenadine (Allegra), and cetirizine (Zyrtec).

Azelastine (Astelin) is an antihistamine nasal spray that is used to treat allergic rhinitis.

Corticosteroids: Nasal corticosteroid sprays are the most effective treatment for allergic rhinitis.

They work best when used nonstop, but they can also be helpful when used for shorter periods of time.

Many brands are available. They are safe for children and adults.

Decongestants: Decongestants may also be helpful in reducing symptoms such as nasal congestion.

Nasal spray decongestants should not be used for more than 3 days.

Be careful when using over-the-counter saline nasal sprays that contain benzalkonium chloride. These may actually worsen symptoms and cause infection.

Other treatments: The leukotriene inhibitor Singulair is a prescription medicine approved to help control asthma and to help relieve the symptoms of seasonal allergies.

Specific illnesses that are caused by allergies (such as asthma and eczema) may require other treatments.

Allergy shots: Allergy shots (immunotherapy) are occasionally recommended if the allergen cannot be avoided and if symptoms are hard to control. This includes regular injections of the allergen, given in increasing doses (each dose is slightly larger than the previous dose) that may help the body adjust to the antigen.

Outlook (Prognosis)

Most symptoms of allergic rhinitis can be treated. More severe cases require allergy shots.

Some people (particularly children) may outgrow an allergy as the immune system becomes less sensitive to the allergen. However, as a general rule, once a substance causes allergies for an individual, it can continue to affect the person over the long term.

Possible Complications

- Sinusitis

When to Contact a Medical Professional

Call for an appointment with your health care provider if severe symptoms of allergies or hay fever occur, if previously successful treatment has become ineffective, or if your symptoms do not respond to treatment.

Prevention

Symptoms can sometimes be prevented by avoiding known allergens. During the pollen season, people with hay fever should remain indoors in an air-conditioned atmosphere whenever possible:

- Most trees produce pollen in the spring.

- Grasses usually produce pollen during the late spring and summer.

- Ragweed and other late-blooming plants produce pollen during late summer and early autumn.

Section 6.2

Postnasal Drip Often Caused by Rhinitis

"Allergies, Sinus Infections, and Postnasal Drip," © 2010 Duke University Health System (www.dukehealth.org). Reprinted with permission.

Allergies can be seasonal or year-round. People who suffer from allergies may experience irritation to the lining of the nose and sinus cavities. This may lead to a runny nose, mucus drainage into the throat (postnasal drip), and infection of the lining in the sinus cavities (sinusitis).

These symptoms can lead to changes in the voice quality. Postnasal drip can impact the quality of your voice by irritating the vocal folds, increasing the stiffness of the vocal folds, and altering the resonance of your voice.

It can also increase the thickness of your mucus, which may lead to throat clearing (another behavior which can cause vocal fold swelling and irritation).

The health of your voice is dependent on the control of your allergy and sinus symptoms. If you have any of the following symptoms, talk to your doctor, as these may be signs of allergies or sinusitis. These may also be symptoms of other conditions, so proper diagnosis by your doctor is important.

- Postnasal drip
- Thick mucus in the throat (despite drinking plenty of water)
- Runny or stuffy nose
- Headache (in the front of your face)
- Nighttime cough
- Pain in the upper jaw or teeth
- Chronic sore throat

Treatment may include a sinus rinse and medications to reduce irritation and/or infection. Keep in mind that over-the-counter nasal sprays are not usually recommended as some of these are addictive.

Also, some allergy medications taken by mouth have a drying effect (particularly ones with a decongestant ingredient), which can contribute to your voice problem. Your doctor will help you understand the causes of your symptoms and help to find the best care for you and your voice.

Section 6.3

Cough Caused by Rhinitis

Cough, cough, cough. That maddening cough that never goes away. The cough that makes people in the grocery store cover their carts as they speed past you. The cough that hammers a classroom of students trying to take a test or learn a new concept. Why do we cough? What can we do about it? Minnesota allergist Pramod Kelkar, MD, chair of the American Academy of Allergy, Asthma & Immunology Cough Committee, answers our cough questions.

What are the different causes of coughs?

Dr. Kelkar: Coughing is a reflex and usually happens involuntarily; it's your body's natural reaction to an irritated airway. Often, it is a symptom of an underlying disease. For instance, chronic "it-won't-go-away" coughing can indicate that asthma, allergies, or GERD (gastroesophageal reflux disease) is out of control.

Coughing is also the body's way of clearing mucus in the airways or getting rid of foreign materials such as allergens, irritating pollutants, or secondhand smoke that enter the respiratory tract (the nose, throat, larynx, sinuses, or lungs).

Physicians divide coughs into three categories:

1. Acute cough is a cough that lasts less than 2–3 weeks. Most often it is caused by the common cold or other upper respiratory tract viral infections, bronchitis, pneumonia, allergies, asthma, or sinusitis.

2. Subacute cough is a cough that lasts from 3 to 8 weeks. It is often caused by the same diseases that cause acute cough but becomes more serious if not treated.

3. Chronic cough is a cough that lasts longer than 8 weeks (or 4 weeks in children). The three most common causes of chronic cough are postnasal drip/drainage, asthma, and GERD.

73

Can you tell what's causing a cough by how it sounds or feels?

Dr. Kelkar: Not really. Figuring out the exact cause of cough can be challenging. Whooping cough will obviously have whooping sound in most cases (but not always). Barking or honking cough in children can sometimes be from habit (again, not always). In adults, the types of cough do not give a specific indication about a specific diagnosis.

That's why it's important to consider all symptoms. For example, allergies are associated with nose and sinus problems; asthma can produce chest tightness, wheezing, and shortness of breath; and GERD often causes heartburn and a sour taste in the mouth. Having said that, it is important to keep in mind that all these diseases can occur with cough as the only symptom and multiple conditions can occur in the same patient (such as asthma and GERD).

When should patients see a doctor about a cough?

Dr. Kelkar: Cough in children less than 6 months old must always be evaluated. In other children, any wet cough or coughing while feeding should be checked by a physician.

Many cold- and virus-related coughs go away within a couple of weeks. If a cough lasts more than 2 weeks, however, you should see your healthcare provider.

For patients of all ages, seek medical help as soon as possible if you experience any of the following:

- Coughing up blood or yellow-green sputum/phlegm
- A temperature higher than 101 degrees Fahrenheit
- Losing weight
- Night sweats
- Feeling short of breath and tight in the chest
- No relief from over-the-counter medications or other medicines
- Coughing all night long
- Coughing that changes in character or becomes worse/deeper
- Coughing accompanied by a high-pitched sound or stridor while inhaling

What type of physician should patients see for a cough?

Dr. Kelkar: Common types of acute and subacute cough can be treated initially by any healthcare professional. If the cough lasts more than four weeks, however, your physician may suggest you consult a specialist, such as an allergist. Trained to treat upper and lower respiratory disorders, allergists can be an important part of your healthcare team, guiding patients to specific testing, referrals, and a comprehensive treatment plan.

What should you expect at your visit with a healthcare provider?

Dr. Kelkar: First of all, your provider will gather information from you, like how long you've had the cough, how it started, what triggers it, accompanying symptoms, when the cough occurs, whether there is fever, and whether there is any phlegm/sputum and what color it is. This will be followed by a detailed physical examination to detect signs of any underlying disease such as swelling in your nose, drainage on the back of your throat from allergies, or wheezing from asthma.

Some patients may require an x-ray or specialized tests based on the suspected cause of the cough: skin prick tests for allergies, breathing tests and spirometry for asthma, or imaging study (CAT scans) for sinuses. Your healthcare provider may refer you to an appropriate specialist like an allergist or pulmonologist for some of these tests.

What medications might a physician prescribe for coughing?

Dr. Kelkar: Your physician will diagnose and treat the cause of your cough, not just the cough itself. Sometimes, your physician will recommend trying a particular medication to see if it's effective before doing expensive and invasive testing.

For instance, allergies can be treated by oral antihistamines, corticosteroid nose sprays, and allergy shots. Asthma can be treated with bronchodilator inhalers and inhaled corticosteroids and by avoiding allergens and irritants that cause symptoms. (Asthma patients who need daily medications for their breathing symptoms should see an allergist to identify specific allergies.) GERD requires medications as well as a change in diet and lifestyle such as avoiding caffeinated beverages, alcohol, acidic fruit juices, chocolate, and smoking and not lying down immediately after a meal.

Are there issues with chronic cough that are specific to children?

Dr. Kelkar: Coughing in children may occur from a variety of causes, some of which are specific to children, including croup, bronchiolitis,

RSV [respiratory syncytial virus] infection, a tic disorder manifesting as a dry cough, and exposure to cigarette smoke from parents/caregivers. Sometimes a foreign body such as a toy or a food item will get stuck in a child's airway and cause a cough that goes on for days or weeks before it is detected.

Because young children cannot communicate in detail, it is challenging to treat coughs at home without a physician's guidance. Parents and caregivers should talk with their healthcare team before using over-the-counter medications in children and not give more than the label recommends. Parents should also watch their children for signs of respiratory distress between coughing spells, especially if the child has asthma.

To repeat, any child with a cough should see a physician if:

- the child is less than 6 months old;
- the cough sounds wet and mucousy;
- the child is coughing at night.

Will any over-the-counter (OTC) medicines help with cough?

Dr. Kelkar: Two types of cough medications are available without prescription: antitussives and expectorants. Antitussives (such as dextromethorphan) help suppress cough by blocking the cough reflex. Expectorants or mucolytics (such as guaifenesin) help thin mucus so the cough can get rid of thick accumulations. Some medications combine these two products. However, recent guidelines from the American College of Chest Physicians say that OTC cough medicines don't work very well and can be dangerous for children.

The Food and Drug Administration (FDA) now says cough and cold medicines should not be used in children under the age of 4.

Cough and cold medicines can be dangerous for people of all ages if used incorrectly. While pharmacies now restrict the sale of cold medicines that contain pseudoephedrine or ephedrine, which can be used to make methamphetamine, experts also warn that dextromethorphan is a problem. Numerous studies by The Partnership for a Drug-Free America and others show increasing numbers of young people are using this easily available cough suppressant to get high.

Are there any "home remedies" patients can use to relieve cough symptoms until they can see a doctor?

Dr. Kelkar: Home treatments can be tried but should never take the place of consulting your healthcare provider. Some things that might help you feel better include:

- drinking adequate hot/warm liquids, which can soothe the throat, and help keep the body hydrated and thin mucus;

- using a cool mist humidifier in the patient's room;

- avoiding carbonated or citrus drinks, which can sometimes irritate the throat and lead to more coughing;

- following asthma medication regimens and action plans, as well as monitoring progress;

- using cough drops to soothe sore throats (for older children and adults only; they are a choking hazard for young children).

Talk with your physician before using any herbal remedies. Although some herbs are harmless, it is better to consult your doctor before trying them out. Pramod Kelkar, MD, chairs the American Academy of Allergy, Asthma and Immunology Cough Committee. He is a graduate of the Mayo Clinic and is in private practice at Allergy and Asthma Care, PA, in Maple Grove, Minnesota.

Chapter 7

Sinusitis

Chapter Contents

Section 7.1

What Is Sinusitis?

From "Sinus Infection (Sinusitis)," by the National Institute of
Allergy and Infectious Diseases (NIAID, www.niaid.nih.gov), part
of the National Institutes of Health, March 2010.

Your nose is stuffy, you're coughing, and you feel tired and achy. You
think you might be getting a cold. Later, when the medicines you've been
taking to relieve symptoms of the common cold are not working and you
now have a terrible headache, you finally drag yourself to the doctor. After
listening to your history of symptoms, examining your face and forehead,
and perhaps doing a sinus x-ray, the doctor says you have sinusitis.

Sinusitis simply means your sinuses are infected or inflamed. But
this gives little indication of the misery and pain this condition can
cause. Health experts usually divide sinusitis cases into the following:

- Acute, which last up to 4 weeks
- Subacute, which last 4 to 12 weeks
- Chronic, which last more than 12 weeks and can continue for
  months or even years
- Recurrent, with several acute attacks within a year

The Centers for Disease Control and Prevention estimates that
close to 31 million adults suffer from chronic sinusitis, resulting in 15
billion doctor visits and more than 200,000 sinus surgical procedures
every year. Acute sinusitis is more common, though there are no good
estimates for the number of people who experience an episode of acute
sinusitis every year.

Where Are Your Sinuses?

When people say, "my sinuses are killing me," they usually are
referring to symptoms of congestion and achiness in one or more of
four pairs of cavities, or sinuses, known as paranasal sinuses. These
cavities, located within the skull or bones of the head surrounding the
nose, include the following (see Figures 7.1 and 7.2):

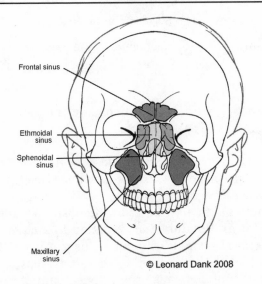

Figure 7.1. *Front view of the nose and sinuses.*

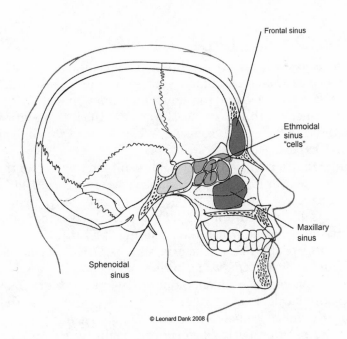

Figure 7.2. *Side view of the structure of the nose and sinuses.*

81

- Frontal sinuses over the eyes in the brow area

- Maxillary sinuses inside each cheekbone

- Ethmoid sinuses just behind the bridge of the nose, between the eyes

- Sphenoid sinuses behind the ethmoids in the upper region of the nose and behind the eyes

Each sinus has an opening into the nose for the free exchange of air and mucus, and each is joined with the nasal passages by a continuous mucous membrane lining.

Anything that causes a swelling in the nose—an infection, an allergic reaction, or an inflammatory reaction to a chemical to which you may get exposed—can affect your sinuses. Air trapped within a blocked sinus, along with pus or other secretions may cause pressure on the sinus wall that can cause the intense pain of a sinus attack. Similarly, when air is prevented from entering a paranasal sinus by a swollen membrane at the opening, a vacuum can be created that also causes pain.

Cause

Acute Sinusitis

Most cases of acute sinusitis start with a common cold, which is caused by a virus. Colds can inflame your sinuses and cause symptoms of sinusitis. Both the cold and the sinus inflammation usually go away without treatment within 2 weeks. However, if the inflammation produced by the cold leads to a bacterial infection, then this infection is what health experts call acute sinusitis.

The inflammation caused by the cold results in swelling of the mucous membranes (linings) of your sinuses, trapping air and mucus behind the narrowed sinus openings. When mucus stays inside your sinuses and is unable to drain into your nose, it can become the source of nutrients for bacteria, which then can multiply.

Most healthy people harbor bacteria, such as *Streptococcus pneumoniae* and *Haemophilus influenzae*, in their noses and throats. Usually, these bacteria cause no problems. But when sniff or blow your nose when you have a cold, these actions create pressure changes that can send typically harmless bacteria inside the sinuses. If your sinuses then stop draining properly, bacteria can begin to multiply in your sinuses, causing acute sinusitis.

People who have allergies or other chronic problems that affect the nose are also prone to episodes of acute sinusitis. Chronic nasal problems cause the nasal membranes to swell and the sinus passages to become blocked. The normally harmless bacteria in your nose and throat again lead to acute sinusitis.

Fungal infections very rarely cause acute sinusitis because the human body has a natural resistance to fungi. However, in people whose immune systems are not functioning properly, fungi can cause acute sinusitis.

In general, people who have reduced immune function, such as those with primary immune deficiencies or HIV [human immunodeficiency virus] infection, or abnormalities in mucus secretion or mucus movement, such as those with cystic fibrosis, are more likely to suffer from sinusitis.

Chronic Sinusitis

In chronic sinusitis, the membranes of both the paranasal sinuses and the nose are thickened because they are constantly inflamed. Most experts now use the term chronic rhinosinusitis to describe this condition. They also recommend that the condition be divided into rhinosinusitis with or without nasal polyps. (Polyps are grape-size growths of the sinus membranes that protrude into the sinuses or into the nasal passages.) Polyps make it even more difficult for the sinuses to drain and for air to pass through the nose.

The causes of chronic rhinosinusitis are largely unknown. The condition often occurs in people with asthma, many of whom also have allergies. It is possible that constant exposure to airborne allergens (substances that cause allergic reactions) from house dust mites, pets, mold (a kind of fungus), and cockroaches cause chronic inflammation of the lining of the nose and the sinuses.

An allergic reaction to certain fungi may be responsible for some cases of chronic rhinosinusitis; this condition is called allergic fungal sinusitis. However, at least half of all people with chronic rhinosinusitis do not have allergies.

Although most health experts believe that chronic rhinosinusitis is not an infectious disease, like acute sinusitis, if you suffer from frequent episodes of acute sinusitis, you may be prone to develop chronic rhinosinusitis. Other health care experts believe that chronic rhinosinusitis is caused by an exaggerated immune response to fungi that normally are found in most people's sinuses.

As with acute sinusitis, other causes of chronic rhinosinusitis may be an immune deficiency disorder or cystic fibrosis.

Another group of people who may develop chronic rhinosinusitis are those with significant variations in the anatomical structure inside the nose that lead to blockage of mucus.

Symptoms

One of the most common symptoms of acute or chronic sinusitis is pain, and the location depends on which sinus is affected:

- If you have pain in your forehead over the frontal sinuses, your frontal sinuses may be inflamed.

- If you have pain in your upper jaw and teeth and your cheeks are tender to the touch, your maxillary sinuses may be infected.

- If you have pain between your eyes, sometimes with swelling of the eyelids and tissues around your eyes, stuffy nose, loss of smell, and tenderness when you touch the sides of your nose, your ethmoid sinuses may be inflamed.

- If you have pain in your neck, with earaches and deep achiness at the top of your head, your sphenoid sinuses may be infected, though these sinuses are less frequently affected.

However, most people with sinusitis have pain or tenderness in several locations, and their symptoms usually do not clearly point out which sinuses are inflamed. Pain is not as common in chronic rhinosinusitis as it is in acute sinusitis.

In addition to the pain, people with sinusitis (acute or chronic) frequently have thick nasal secretions that are yellow, green, or blood-tinged. Sometimes these secretions, referred to as postnasal drip, drain in the back of the throat and are difficult to clear. Also, acute and chronic rhinosinusitis are strongly associated with a stuffy nose, as well as with a general feeling of fullness over the entire face.

Less common symptoms of sinusitis (acute or chronic) can include the following:

- Tiredness
- Decreased sense of smell
- Cough that may be more severe at night

- Sore throat
- Bad breath
- Fever

On very rare occasions, acute sinusitis can result in brain infection and other serious complications.

Diagnosis

Your healthcare provider can usually diagnose acute sinusitis by noting your symptoms and doing a physical examination of your nose and face. If your symptoms are vague or persistent, your healthcare provider may order a CT (computed tomography) scan, a form of x-ray, to confirm that you have sinusitis.

Laboratory tests your healthcare provider may use to assess possible causes of chronic sinusitis include the following:

- Blood tests to rule out conditions associated with sinusitis, like an immune deficiency disorder

- A sweat test or a blood test to rule out cystic fibrosis

- Tests on the material that is inside your sinuses to look for bacterial or fungal infection

- Biopsy (taking a small sample) of the membranes (linings) of the nose or sinuses to find out the health of the cells lining these cavities

Because your nose can get stuffy when you have a condition like the common cold, you may confuse simple nasal congestion with sinusitis. A cold, however, usually lasts about 7 to 14 days and goes away without treatment. Acute sinusitis often lasts longer and typically causes more symptoms than a cold.

Treatment

After diagnosing sinusitis and identifying a possible cause, your healthcare provider can suggest various treatments.

Acute Sinusitis

If you have acute sinusitis, your healthcare provider may recommend the following:

- Antibiotics to control a bacterial infection, if present
- Pain relievers to reduce any pain
- Decongestants to reduce congestion

Even if you have acute sinusitis, your healthcare provider may choose not to use an antibiotic because many cases of acute sinusitis will end on their own. But if you do not feel better after a few days, you should contact your healthcare provider again.

Follow your healthcare provider's instructions on how to use over-the-counter or prescription decongestant nose drops and sprays. You should use these medicines for only for few days because longer-term use can lead to even more congestion and swelling of your nasal passages.

If you have an allergic disease, such as hay fever, along with sinusitis, your healthcare provider may recommend medicine to control allergies. This may include a nasal steroid spray that reduces the swelling around the sinus passages and allows the sinuses to drain. If you already have asthma and then get sinusitis, your asthma may worsen. You should contact your healthcare provider, who may recommend a change in your asthma treatment.

Chronic Rhinosinusitis

Healthcare providers often find it difficult to treat chronic rhinosinusitis successfully. They have two options to offer: medicine and surgery.

Medicine: Medicines prescribed for chronic rhinosinusitis include the following:

- Nasal steroid sprays are helpful for many people, but most people still do not get full relief of symptoms with these medicines.

- A long course of antibiotics may be recommended, but clinical trial results do not support their use.

- Saline (saltwater) washes or sprays in the nose help remove thick secretions and allow the sinuses to drain. However, current evidence for the long-term benefit of saline washes is not strong.

- Oral steroids, such as prednisone, may be prescribed for severe chronic rhinosinusitis. However, oral steroids are powerful medicines with significant side effects, and they are typically prescribed only when other medicines have failed.

- Research is needed to develop new, more effective treatments.

Surgery: When medicine fails, surgery may be the only alternative for treating chronic rhinosinusitis. The goal of surgery is to improve sinus drainage and reduce blockage of the nasal passages. Surgery is usually done through the nose to:

- enlarge the natural opening of the sinuses;

- remove polyps (Polyps are grape-size growths of the sinus membranes that protrude into the sinuses or into the nasal passages);

- correct significant structural problems inside the nose and the sinuses that contribute to the obstruction.

Although most people have fewer symptoms and a better quality of life after surgery, problems can return, sometimes even after a short period of time.

In children, problems can sometimes be eliminated by removing the adenoids. These gland-like tissues, located in the throat behind and above the roof of the mouth, can obstruct nasal-sinus passages.

Prevention

There are no methods that have been tested scientifically and proven to prevent acute or chronic sinusitis. However, your healthcare provider may recommend a variety of measures that may offer you some benefit, such as the following:

- Keep your nose as moist as possible with frequent use of saline (saltwater) sprays.

- Avoid very dry indoor environments and use a humidifier, if necessary. You should be aware that a humid environment may also increase the amount of mold, house dust mite, or cockroach allergens in your home.

- Avoid exposure to irritants such as cigarette and cigar smoke or strong odors from chemicals.

- Avoid exposure to substances to which you have allergies.

- If you have not been tested for allergies and you are getting frequent sinus infections, ask your healthcare provider to give you an allergy evaluation or to refer you to an allergy specialist.

- Avoid long periods of swimming in pools treated with chlorine, which can irritate the lining of the nose and sinuses.

- Avoid water diving, which forces water into the sinuses from the nasal passages.

Air travel may pose a problem if you are suffering from acute or chronic sinusitis. As air pressure in a plane is reduced, pressure can build up in your head, blocking your sinuses or the eustachian tubes in your ears. As a result, you might feel discomfort in your sinuses or middle ear during the plane's ascent or descent. Some health experts recommend using decongestant nose drops or sprays before a flight to avoid this problem.

Research

The National Institute of Allergy and Infectious Diseases (NIAID) supports research to better understand the immune system in health and disease, and to develop new treatments.

The vast majority of people with moderate to severe asthma also have chronic sinusitis, suggesting that these two diseases may be the same disease occurring in the two different parts of the respiratory system—upper and lower. NIAID supports research to understand the causes of chronic airway inflammation in asthma that will aid in our understanding of chronic rhinosinusitis and lead to the development of more effective treatments and ways to prevent the disease.

At least two thirds of acute sinusitis cases are caused by two bacteria, *Streptococcus pneumoniae* and *Haemophilus influenzae*. NIAID supports studies to better understand the basis of how these bacteria infect people as well as identify potential targets for future vaccination strategies that could eliminate the diseases they cause.

NIAID funds projects that examine the causes of thickening and inflammation of the lining of the sinuses and the nasal passages. These projects also focus on the cells that produce mucus and that line the sinuses and nasal passages.

In many people with chronic rhinosinusitis, especially those with nasal polyps, eosinophils (white blood cells that have strong inflammatory properties) can be found in abundance in the tissues that line the sinuses and nasal passages. NIAID funds several projects that examine the role of eosinophils and the chemical messengers they produce in causing chronic sinus inflammation and chronic rhinosinusitis with polyps.

NIAID supports research to test the theory that chronic rhinosinusitis is caused by an exaggerated immune response to fungi. One study already has shown that when blood cells from people with chronic rhinosinusitis are exposed to fungal material, these cells make chemicals that produce inflammation.

NIAID supports a project to identify the human genes and proteins found in patients with chronic rhinosinusitis. The results will help us understand the causes of chronic rhinosinusitis and develop new treatments. For example, research has found that some people with chronic rhinosinusitis have certain alterations in the gene that causes cystic fibrosis.

Section 7.2

Allergies Cause Sinus Headaches

"Headache and Sinus Disease," by Howard Levine, MD, Mt. Sinai Nasal-Sinus Center, Cleveland, OH. © 2010 American Rhinologic Society (www.american-rhinologic.org). Reprinted with permission.

Headache is a common complaint that is often associated with sinusitis. However, the true cause for a headache may be difficult to determine because headaches have many causes. The United States Center for Disease Control reports that sinusitis affects over 30 million people and is the most common chronic disease in this country. Thus, many sinus sufferers will also suffer headaches. While headaches and sinusitis are common problems sometimes headaches occur with sinusitis and sometimes they do not.

The Nasal Sinus Problem

Typically, a nasal and/or sinus problem will have congestion and stuffiness, often with nasal drainage. If an infection is present there will be discolored, thick drainage in the front of the nose and down the back of the throat. If a headache is present, it is usually a pressure sensation varying in intensity from almost non-existent to somewhat severe.

Generally, a sinus headache will be located over the sinuses (forehead, corners of the eye, and cheek areas). On occasion, the pain will be felt behind the eyes, in the back of the neck, or may extend into the upper teeth. Head movement usually worsens this headache.

The true cause for headache may be difficult to determine; sometimes headaches occur with sinusitis and sometimes not.

Non-Sinus Headaches

Non-sinus headaches may give these same symptoms thus making it difficult to determine if the headache is truly from a sinus problem. For example, tension headaches will occur in the forehead and neck; migraine headaches often occur in and around the eyes.

It is unusual for a person with a sinus or nasal problem to only have a headache. A sinus headache is nearly always accompanied by nasal stuffiness, congestion, obstruction, or drainage. When headache is the only symptom, it is rarely sinus related.

Sinus Headaches

The main cause of nasal and sinus headaches is the nasal turbinates—nasal structures that swell and contract throughout the day giving the feeling of nasal congestion and occasionally pressure. Worsened by irritants such as perfume, cigarette smoke, or allergens, the internal swelling causes facial pressure. When the turbinates swell, not only is the breathing passage blocked, but also normal sinus draining passages are blocked creating a "back-up" situation.

Drainage remains "trapped" in the sinus cavity causing the pain and pressure you feel over the sinuses. It may also cause an infection.

Oral decongestants (i.e., pseudoephedrine) or a nasal spray (i.e. Neo-Synephrine, oxymetazoline) will often give relief. However, these sprays should not be used for more than a few days since they can cause even more congestion when their effect wears off.

Caution is needed when using decongestant pills, especially if a person has a history of heart disease or high blood pressure. These adrenaline-like medications can cause a rapid heart rate or increased blood pressure.

If over-the-counter medical management for nasal congestion is not effective, a physician may choose to prescribe a steroid nasal spray.

If medical management fails or cannot be tolerated, surgery to reduce the turbinates is extremely successful.

Another cause for a sinus headache is the common cold, which may seem to be a sinus infection. If over-the-counter cold remedies fail and the symptoms continue beyond several days or if there are other debilitating medical problems, a physician should be called.

Section 7.3

Allergic Fungal Sinusitis

"Fungal Sinusitis," by Daniel Carothers, MD,
Northwestern Nasal and Sinus, Chicago, IL. © 2010.
Reprinted with permission.

Is there a fungus among us? In short, yes. Fungi as a group are found nearly everywhere on the planet, including the human body. Of the approximately 50,000 kinds of fungi, only a few dozen have been implicated in human illness. In most cases, these various fungi coexist in a natural balance with other microorganisms that colonize our bodies. However, in certain circumstances, fungi can cause infection ranging from minor to life-threatening in severity. Inflammation or infection of the sinuses by fungi is termed fungal sinusitis. Fungal sinusitis can be classified into four types:

- Fungal ball
- Allergic fungal sinusitis
- Chronic invasive sinusitis
- Acute invasive sinusitis

Fungal Ball

A fungal ball is an overgrowth of fungal elements which typically occur in the maxillary (or cheek) sinus. The organism involved is most often from the common bread mold family, Aspergillus. Patients with this condition may have a history of recurrent sinus infections, and the symptoms may be similar to bacterial sinusitis. A radiologic study (x-ray, CT [computed tomography], MRI [magnetic resonance imaging]) ordered to investigate this will show blockage of the involved sinus(es), without any damage to the surrounding bone. Treatment consists of removal of the fungal ball. In most cases, this is possible with a minimally invasive procedure termed endoscopic sinus surgery, with excellent cure rates.

Allergic Fungal Sinusitis

The most common type of fungal infection is termed allergic fungal sinusitis. The fungi involved are mainly from the Dematiaceous family, including Bipolaris, Curvularia, and Alternaria, which are common in the environment. As in fungal ball, the symptoms can be similar to bacterial sinusitis. Nasal polyps and thick drainage are usually found on examination of the nose. Radiologic studies will show blockage of the affected sinuses and can show impressive bony thinning and occasionally bony destruction. Treatment consists of removal of the fungal elements, with re-establishment of sinus drainage. As in fungal ball, endoscopic sinus surgery is possible in most cases. Recurrence rates are higher than in fungal ball, due to the allergic component, inflammation, and nasal polyps associated with this condition. In many cases, lifelong medical and intermittent surgical management is necessary. Although the treatment of this condition is controversial, typical adjuncts to surgical removal may include systemic and/or topical steroids, antihistamines, antibiotics, antifungal medications, allergy immunotherapy, and irrigations.

Invasive Fungal Sinusitis

Acute and chronic invasive sinusitis are the most serious types of fungal sinusitis, and fortunately the least common. Acute invasive fungal sinusitis is a quickly advancing process that grows deeply into the sinus tissues and bones. Chronic invasive fungal sinusitis is a similar, but much slower infection. Patients who are affected with acute invasive sinusitis typically have a compromised immune system, such as after chemotherapy, or patients with uncontrolled diabetes. In contrast, most patients with chronic invasive sinusitis have a normal immune system. Common environmental fungi from the families Rhizopus, Mucor, and Aspergillus are frequently found in this type of infection. Symptoms of this condition, like all types of fungal sinusitis, can be similar to bacterial sinusitis. On examination of the nose, mold spores and areas of dying tissue can be seen. The area involved in the infection can extend far beyond the confines of the nasal cavity and sinuses. Radiologic studies will show blockage of the involved sinuses, destruction of bone, and swelling in the affected areas of the facial tissues. A combination of surgery and antifungal medications are required in this often-fatal infection.

Few Final Comments

Indeed, as in humans' interaction with other microorganisms, our interaction with fungi varies from benign coexistence to deadly infection. Fungal sinusitis has been felt to be uncommon, however, recently published data contradicts previous reports. A topic of much debate, the diagnosis and treatment of fungal sinusitis continues to frustrate physicians and their patients. For more information regarding sinus infections, fungal or otherwise, contact your local otorhinolaryngology specialist.

Section 7.4

Nasal Polyps

"Nasal Polyps," by Howard Levine, MD, Mt. Sinai Nasal-Sinus Center, Cleveland, OH. © 2010 American Rhinologic Society (www.american-rhinologic.org). Reprinted with permission.

Blocked nose? Food seem less tasty? Thick, discolored nasal drainage? You might be suffering from nasal polyps—a treatable nasal problem.

Nasal polyps are noncancerous growths occurring in the nose or sinuses. Other types of polyps occur in the bowel or urinary bladder, but have no relationship to those in the nose and sinuses. Polyps in the bowel or bladder have a chance of being cancerous; polyps in the nose and sinuses are rarely malignant.

Polyps can cause nasal blockage making it hard to breathe, but most nasal polyp problems can be helped.

While some polyps are a result of swelling from an infection, most of the time, the cause for the nasal polyps is never known. A few individuals may have a combination of asthma, aspirin sensitivity, and nasal polyps. If aspirin is taken, the asthma and nasal polyps may worsen.

Because polyps block the nose, patients often notice a decrease in the sense of smell. Since much of our sense of taste is related to our sense of smell, patients with nasal polyps may describe a loss of both taste and smell.

Nasal polyps also cause nasal obstruction and may also block the pathways where the sinuses drain into the nose. This blockage by the polyps causes the mucus (which normally forms and drains through the nose) to remain in the sinuses. When this mucus stays in the sinuses too long, it can become infected. It is this infected mucus that the patient experiences as a thick, discolored drainage in the nose and down the throat. This type of nasal obstruction and infection may also cause pressure over the forehead and face.

Many people with nasal polyps have no symptoms and therefore require no treatment. For those patients whose polyps are causing symptoms, medical or surgical management is available.

Medical management to reduce the size of the polyps often requires a series of steroid pills and nasal steroid sprays. Since the nasal steroid sprays have very little absorption into the blood stream, there are few, if any, side effects. For those patients whose polyps cannot be managed medically or choose not to manage them medically, surgery is usually effective.

Surgery for nasal polyps is usually done as an outpatient in an ambulatory surgery center where patients go home the same day as surgery. The polyps are removed from the nose and sinuses using small nasal telescopes, which not only removes the diseased tissue but also preserves the normal structures and reconstructs the normal inflow, outflow, and function of the sinuses.

While most patients with nasal polyps and asthma or nasal polyps, asthma, and aspirin sensitivity have the same 90% improvement, 18 months after surgery 40% of patients with asthma and nasal polyps report continued improvement, and 35% of patients with the combination of aspirin sensitivity, asthma, and nasal polyps report still feeling well.

The asthmatic patient with nasal polyps is the most difficult to cure, but by using the endoscopic technique, as well as ongoing management with medication after surgery, we are able to help many patients breathe easier, regain their sense of smell, eliminate facial pressure, and have their asthma better controlled.

Chapter 8

Allergic Conjunctivitis (Eye Allergies)

Eye allergies often are hereditary, and occur due to processes associated with other types of allergic responses.

When an allergic reaction takes place, your eyes may be overreacting to a substance perceived as harmful, even though it may not be. For example, dust that is harmless to most people can cause excessive production of tears and mucus in eyes of overly sensitive, allergic individuals.

Allergies can trigger other problems, such as conjunctivitis (pink eye) and asthma. Combined nasal and eye allergies create a condition known as rhinoconjunctivitis.

About 30 percent to 50 percent of U.S. residents have allergy symptoms. And about 75 percent of those symptoms affect the eyes.

Allergy Symptoms and Signs

Common signs of allergies include:

- red, swollen, or itchy eyes;

- runny nose;

- sneezing and coughing;

- itchy nose, mouth, or throat;

- headache from sinus congestion.

"Eye Allergies," reprinted with permission from www.allaboutvision.com. © 2009 Access Media Group LLC. All rights reserved.

Beyond more obvious symptoms, you also may feel fatigued and could suffer from lack of sleep.

What Causes Eye Allergies?

Many allergens are in the air, where they come in contact with your eyes and nose. Airborne allergens include pollen, mold, dust, and pet dander.

Other causes of allergies, such as certain foods or bee stings, do not typically affect the eyes the way airborne allergens do. Adverse reactions to certain cosmetics or drugs such as antibiotic eye drops also may cause eye allergies.

Some people actually are allergic to the preservatives in eye drops such as those used to lubricate dry eyes. In this case, you may need to use a preservative-free brand.

General Eye Allergy Treatment

Avoidance: The most common "treatment" is to avoid what's causing your eye allergy. Itchy eyes? Keep your home free of pet dander and dust and keep pets off the furniture. Stay inside with the air conditioner on when a lot of pollen is in the air. Air conditioners filter out allergens, though you must clean the filters from time to time.

Make sure you wear wraparound sunglasses to help shield your eyes from allergens, and drive with the windows closed.

Medications: If you're not sure what's causing your eye allergies, or you're not having any luck avoiding them, your next step probably will be medication to alleviate the symptoms.

Over-the-counter and prescription medications each have their advantages; for example, over-the-counter products are often less expensive, while prescription ones are often stronger.

Eye drops are available as simple eye washes, or they may have one or more active ingredients such as antihistamines, decongestants, or mast cell stabilizers that inhibit inflammation. Antihistamines relieve many symptoms caused by airborne allergens, such as itchy, watery eyes, runny nose, and sneezing. Decongestants help shrink swollen nasal passages for easier breathing.

Relief for Watery, Itchy Eyes

Common causes of excessively watery eyes are allergies and dry eye syndrome—two very different problems.

With allergies, your body's release of histamine causes your eyes to water, just as it may cause your nose to run. It may seem illogical that watery eyes would result from dry eye syndrome. But this is sometimes true, because the excessive dryness works to overstimulate production of the watery component of your eye's tears.

Decongestants clear up redness. They contain vasoconstrictors, which simply make the blood vessels in your eyes smaller, lessening the apparent redness. They treat the symptom, not the cause.

In fact, with extended use, the blood vessels can become dependent on the vasoconstrictor to stay small. When you discontinue the eye drops, the vessels actually get bigger than they were in the beginning. This process is called rebound hyperemia, and the result is that your red eyes worsen over time.

Some products have ingredients that act as mast cell stabilizers, which alleviate redness and swelling. Mast cell stabilizers are similar to antihistamines. But while antihistamines are known for their immediate relief, mast cell stabilizers are known for their long-lasting relief.

Antihistamines, decongestants, and mast cell stabilizers are available in pill form, but pills don't work as quickly as eye drops or gels to bring eye relief.

Nonsteroidal anti-inflammatory drug (NSAID) eye drops may be prescribed to decrease swelling, inflammation, and other symptoms associated with seasonal allergic conjunctivitis, also called hay fever.

Prescription corticosteroid eye drops also may provide similar, quick relief. However, steroids have been associated with side effects such as increased inner eye pressure (intraocular pressure) leading to glaucoma and damage to optic nerves. Steroids also have been known to cause the eye's natural lens to become cloudy, producing cataracts.

Check the product label or insert for a list of side effects of over-the-counter medications. For prescription medication, ask your doctor. In some cases, combinations of medications may be used.

You may benefit from immunotherapy, in which an allergy specialist injects you with small amounts of the allergen to help you gradually build up immunity.

Eye Allergies and Contact Lenses

Even if you are generally a successful contact lens wearer, allergy season can make your contacts uncomfortable. Airborne allergens can get on your lenses, causing discomfort. Allergens also can stimulate the excessive production of natural substances in your tears, which bind to your contacts and also become uncomfortable. Pollen maps can help you determine when allergens are present.

Ask your eye doctor about eye drops that can help relieve your symptoms and keep your contact lenses clean. Certain drops can discolor or damage certain lenses, so it makes sense to ask first before trying out a new brand.

Another alternative is daily disposable contact lenses, which are discarded nightly. Because you replace them so frequently, these types of lenses are unlikely to develop irritating deposits that can build up over time and cause or heighten allergy-related discomfort.

Resources

Allergic diseases of the eye. *Medical Clinics of North America.* January 2006.

Ocular allergy overview. *Immunology and Allergy Clinics of North America.* February 2008.

Chapter 9

Allergic Asthma

Chapter Contents

Section 9.1

What Is Asthma?

From "Asthma," by the National Heart, Lung, and Blood
Institute (NHLBI, www.nhlbi.nih.gov), part of the National
Institutes of Health, September 2008.

Asthma is a chronic (long-term) lung disease that inflames and narrows the airways. Asthma causes recurring periods of wheezing (a whistling sound when you breathe), chest tightness, shortness of breath, and coughing. The coughing often occurs at night or early in the morning.

Asthma affects people of all ages, but it most often starts in childhood. In the United States, more than 22 million people are known to have asthma. Nearly 6 million of these people are children.

Overview

The airways are tubes that carry air into and out of your lungs. People who have asthma have inflamed airways. This makes the airways swollen and very sensitive. They tend to react strongly to certain substances that are breathed in.

When the airways react, the muscles around them tighten. This causes the airways to narrow, and less air flows to your lungs. The swelling also can worsen, making the airways even narrower. Cells in the airways may make more mucus than normal. Mucus is a sticky, thick liquid that can further narrow your airways.

This chain reaction can result in asthma symptoms. Symptoms can happen each time the airways are irritated.

Sometimes symptoms are mild and go away on their own or after minimal treatment with an asthma medicine. At other times, symptoms continue to get worse. When symptoms get more intense and/or additional symptoms appear, this is an asthma attack. Asthma attacks also are called flare-ups or exacerbations.

It's important to treat symptoms when you first notice them. This will help prevent the symptoms from worsening and causing a severe asthma attack. Severe asthma attacks may require emergency care, and they can cause death.

Outlook

Asthma can't be cured. Even when you feel fine, you still have the disease and it can flare up at any time.

But with today's knowledge and treatments, most people who have asthma are able to manage the disease. They have few, if any, symptoms. They can live normal, active lives and sleep through the night without interruption from asthma.

For successful, comprehensive, and ongoing treatment, take an active role in managing your disease. Build strong partnerships with your doctor and other clinicians on your health care team.

What Causes Asthma?

The exact cause of asthma isn't known. Researchers think a combination of factors (family genes and certain environmental exposures) interact to cause asthma to develop, most often early in life. These factors include the following:

- An inherited tendency to develop allergies, called atopy

- Parents who have asthma

- Certain respiratory infections during childhood

- Contact with some airborne allergens or exposure to some viral infections in infancy or in early childhood when the immune system is developing

If asthma or atopy runs in your family, exposure to airborne allergens (for example, house dust mites, cockroaches, and possibly cat or dog dander) and irritants (for example, tobacco smoke) may make your airways more reactive to substances in the air you breathe.

Different factors may be more likely to cause asthma in some people than in others. Researchers continue to explore what causes asthma.

The "Hygiene Hypothesis"

One theory researchers have for what causes asthma is the "hygiene hypothesis." They believe that our Western lifestyle—with its emphasis on hygiene and sanitation—has resulted in changes in our living conditions and an overall decline in infections in early childhood.

Many young children no longer experience the same types of environmental exposures and infections as children did in the past. This affects the way that the immune systems in today's young children develop during very early childhood, and it may increase their risk for atopy and asthma. This is especially true for children who have close family members with one or both of these conditions.

Who Is at Risk for Asthma?

Asthma affects people of all ages, but it most often starts in childhood. In the United States, more than 22 million people are known to have asthma. Nearly 6 million of these people are children.

Young children who have frequent episodes of wheezing with respiratory infections, as well as certain other risk factors, are at the highest risk of developing asthma that continues beyond 6 years of age. These risk factors include having allergies, eczema (an allergic skin condition), or parents who have asthma.

Among children, more boys have asthma than girls. But among adults, more women have the disease than men. It's not clear whether or how sex and sex hormones play a role in causing asthma.

Most, but not all, people who have asthma have allergies.

Some people develop asthma because of exposure to certain chemical irritants or industrial dusts in the workplace. This is called occupational asthma.

What Are the Signs and Symptoms of Asthma?

Common asthma symptoms include the following:

- Coughing—Coughing from asthma is often worse at night or early in the morning, making it hard to sleep.

- Wheezing—Wheezing is a whistling or squeaky sound that occurs when you breathe.

- Chest tightness—This may feel like something is squeezing or sitting on your chest.

- Shortness of breath—Some people who have asthma say they can't catch their breath or they feel out of breath. You may feel like you can't get air out of your lungs.

Not all people who have asthma have these symptoms. Likewise, having these symptoms doesn't always mean that you have asthma. A lung function test, done along with a medical history (including type and frequency of your symptoms) and physical exam, is the best way to diagnose asthma for certain.

The types of asthma symptoms you have, how often they occur, and how severe they are may vary over time. Sometimes your symptoms may just annoy you. Other times they may be troublesome enough to limit your daily routine.

Severe symptoms can threaten your life. It's vital to treat symptoms when you first notice them so they don't become severe.

With proper treatment, most people who have asthma can expect to have few, if any, symptoms either during the day or at night.

What Causes Asthma Symptoms to Occur?

A number of things can bring about or worsen asthma symptoms. Your doctor will help you find out which things (sometimes called triggers) may cause your asthma to flare up if you come in contact with them. Triggers may include:

- Allergens found in dust, animal fur, cockroaches, mold, and pollens from trees, grasses, and flowers

- Irritants such as cigarette smoke, air pollution, chemicals or dust in the workplace, compounds in home décor products, and sprays (such as hairspray)

- Certain medicines such as aspirin or other nonsteroidal anti-inflammatory drugs and nonselective beta-blockers

- Sulfites in foods and drinks

- Viral upper respiratory infections such as colds

- Exercise (physical activity)

Other health conditions—such as runny nose, sinus infections, reflux disease, psychological stress, and sleep apnea—can make asthma more difficult to manage. These conditions need treatment as part of an overall asthma care plan.

Asthma is different for each person. Some of the factors listed may not affect you. Other factors that do affect you may not be on the list. Talk to your doctor about the things that seem to make your asthma worse.

How Is Asthma Diagnosed?

Your primary care doctor will diagnose asthma based on your medical history, a physical exam, and results from tests. He or she also will figure out what your level of asthma severity is—that is, whether it's intermittent, mild, moderate, or severe. Your severity level will determine what treatment you will start on.

You may need to see an asthma specialist if the following are true:

- You need special tests to be sure you have asthma.
- You've had a life-threatening asthma attack.
- You need more than one kind of medicine or higher doses of medicine to control your asthma, or if you have overall difficulty getting your asthma well controlled.
- You're thinking about getting allergy treatments.

Medical History

Your doctor may ask about your family history of asthma and allergies. He or she also may ask whether you have asthma symptoms, and when and how often they occur. Let your doctor know if your symptoms seem to happen only during certain times of the year or in certain places, or if they get worse at night.

Your doctor also may want to know what factors seem to set off your symptoms or worsen them.

Your doctor may ask you about related health conditions that can interfere with asthma management. These conditions include a runny nose, sinus infections, reflux disease, psychological stress, and sleep apnea.

Physical Exam

Your doctor will listen to your breathing and look for signs of asthma or allergies. These signs include wheezing, a runny nose or swollen nasal passages, and allergic skin conditions such as eczema.

Keep in mind that you can still have asthma even if you don't have these signs on the day that your doctor examines you.

Diagnostic Tests

Lung function test: Your doctor will use a test called spirometry to check how your lungs are working. This test measures how much air you can breathe in and out. It also measures how fast you can blow air out. Your doctor also may give you medicines and then test you again to see whether the results have improved.

If the starting results are lower than normal and improve with the medicine, and if your medical history shows a pattern of asthma symptoms, your diagnosis will likely be asthma.

Other tests: Your doctor may order other tests if he or she needs more information to make a diagnosis. Other tests may include the following:

- You may need allergy testing to find out which allergens affect you, if any.

- You may need a test to measure how sensitive your airways are. This is called a bronchoprovocation test. Using spirometry, this test repeatedly measures your lung function during physical activity or after you receive increasing doses of cold air or a special chemical to breathe in.

- You may need a test to show whether you have another disease with the same symptoms as asthma, such as reflux disease, vocal cord dysfunction, or sleep apnea.

- You may need a chest x-ray or an EKG (electrocardiogram). These tests will help find out whether a foreign object or other disease may be causing your symptoms.

Diagnosing Asthma in Young Children

Most children who have asthma develop their first symptoms before 5 years of age. However, asthma in young children (aged 0 to 5 years) can be hard to diagnose. Sometimes it can be difficult to tell whether a child has asthma or another childhood condition because the symptoms of both conditions can be similar.

Also, many young children who have wheezing episodes when they get colds or respiratory infections don't go on to have asthma after they're 6 years old. These symptoms may be due to the fact that infants have smaller airways that can narrow even further when they get a cold or respiratory infection. The airways grow as a child grows older, so wheezing no longer occurs when the child gets a cold.

A young child who has frequent wheezing with colds or respiratory infections is more likely to have asthma if:

- one or both parents have asthma;

- the child has signs of allergies, including the allergic skin condition eczema;

- the child has allergic reactions to pollens or other airborne allergens; or

- the child wheezes even when he or she doesn't have a cold or other infection.

A lung function test along with a medical history and physical exam is the most certain way to diagnose asthma. However, this test is hard to do in children younger than 5 years. Thus, doctors must rely on children's medical histories, signs and symptoms, and physical exams to make a diagnosis. Doctors also may use a 4- to 6-week trial of asthma medicines to see how well a child responds.

How Is Asthma Treated and Controlled?

Asthma is a long-term disease that can't be cured. The goal of asthma treatment is to control the disease. Good asthma control will do the following:

- Prevent chronic and troublesome symptoms such as coughing and shortness of breath

- Reduce your need of quick-relief medicines

- Help you maintain good lung function

- Let you maintain your normal activity levels and sleep through the night

- Prevent asthma attacks that could result in your going to the emergency room or being admitted to the hospital for treatment

To reach this goal, you should actively partner with your doctor to manage your asthma or your child's asthma. Children aged 10 or older—and younger children who are able—also should take an active role in their asthma care.

Taking an active role to control your asthma involves working with your doctor and other clinicians on your health care team to create and follow an asthma action plan. It also means avoiding factors that can make your asthma flare up and treating other conditions that can interfere with asthma management.

An asthma action plan gives guidance on taking your medicines properly, avoiding factors that worsen your asthma, tracking your level of asthma control, responding to worsening asthma, and seeking emergency care when needed.

Asthma is treated with two types of medicines: long-term control and quick-relief medicines. Long-term control medicines help reduce airway inflammation and prevent asthma symptoms. Quick-relief, or "rescue," medicines relieve asthma symptoms that may flare up.

Your initial asthma treatment will depend on how severe your disease is. Followup asthma treatment will depend on how well your asthma action plan is working to control your symptoms and prevent you from having asthma attacks.

Your level of asthma control can vary over time and with changes in your home, school, or work environments that alter how often you are exposed to the factors that can make your asthma worse. Your doctor may need to increase your medicine if your asthma doesn't stay under control.

On the other hand, if your asthma is well controlled for several months, your doctor may be able to decrease your medicine. These adjustments either up or down to your medicine will help you maintain the best control possible with the least amount of medicine necessary.

Asthma treatment for certain groups of people, such as children, pregnant women, or those for whom exercise brings on asthma symptoms, will need to be adjusted to meet their special needs.

Follow an Asthma Action Plan

You can work with your doctor to create a personal written asthma action plan. The asthma action plan shows your daily treatment, such as what kind of medicines to take and when to take them. The plan explains when to call the doctor or go to the emergency room.

If your child has asthma, all of the people who care for him or her should know about the child's asthma action plan. This includes babysitters and workers at daycare centers, schools, and camps. These caretakers can help your child follow his or her action plan.

Avoid Things That Can Worsen Your Asthma

A number of common things (sometimes called asthma triggers) can set off or worsen your asthma symptoms. Once you know what these factors are, you can take steps to control many of them.

For example, if exposure to pollens or air pollution makes your asthma worse, try to limit time outdoors when the levels of these substances are high in the outdoor air. If animal fur sets off your asthma symptoms, keep pets with fur out of your home or bedroom.

If your asthma symptoms are clearly linked to allergies, and you can't avoid exposure to those allergens, then your doctor may advise you to get allergy shots for the specific allergens that bother your asthma. You may need to see a specialist if you're thinking about getting allergy shots. These shots may lessen or prevent your asthma symptoms, but they can't cure your asthma.

Several health conditions can make asthma more difficult to manage. These conditions include runny nose, sinus infections, reflux disease, psychological stress, and sleep apnea. Your doctor will treat these conditions as well.

Medicines

Your doctor will consider many things when deciding which asthma medicines are best for you. Doctors usually use a stepwise approach to prescribing medicines. Your doctor will check to see how well a medicine works for you; he or she will make changes in the dose or medicine, as needed.

Asthma medicines can be taken in pill form, but most are taken using a device called an inhaler. An inhaler allows the medicine to go right to your lungs.

Not all inhalers are used the same way. Ask your doctor and other clinicians on your health care team to show you the right way to use your inhaler. Ask them to review the way you use your inhaler at every visit.

Long-Term Control Medicines

Most people who have asthma need to take long-term control medicines daily to help prevent symptoms. The most effective long-term medicines reduce airway inflammation.

These medicines are taken over the long term to prevent symptoms from starting. They don't give you quick relief from symptoms.

Inhaled corticosteroids: Inhaled corticosteroids are the preferred medicines for long-term control of asthma. These medicines are the most effective long-term control medicine to relieve airway inflammation and swelling that makes the airways sensitive to certain substances that are breathed in.

Reducing inflammation helps prevent the chain reaction that causes asthma symptoms. Most people who take these medicines daily find they greatly reduce how severe symptoms are and how often they occur.

Inhaled corticosteroids are generally safe when taken as prescribed. They're very different from the illegal anabolic steroids taken by some athletes. Inhaled corticosteroids aren't habit-forming, even if you take them every day for many years.

But, like many other medicines, inhaled corticosteroids can have side effects. Most doctors agree that the benefits of taking inhaled corticosteroids and preventing asthma attacks far outweigh the risks of side effects.

One common side effect from inhaled corticosteroids is a mouth infection called thrush. You can use a spacer or holding chamber to avoid thrush. A spacer or holding chamber is attached to your inhaler when taking medicine to keep the medicine from landing in your mouth or on the back of your throat.

Work with your health care team if you have any questions about how to use a spacer or holding chamber. Rinsing your mouth out with water after taking inhaled corticosteroids also can lower your risk of thrush.

If you have severe asthma, you may have to take corticosteroid pills or liquid for short periods to get your asthma under control. If taken for long periods, these medicines raise your risk for cataracts and osteoporosis. A cataract is the clouding of the lens in your eye. Osteoporosis is a disorder that makes your bones weak and more likely to break.

Your doctor may have you add another long-term control asthma medicine to lower your dose of corticosteroids. Or, your doctor may suggest you take calcium and vitamin D pills to protect your bones.

Other long-term control medicines: Other long-term control medicines include the following:

- Inhaled long-acting beta$_2$-agonists—These medicines open the airways and may be added to low-dose inhaled corticosteroids to improve asthma control. An inhaled long-acting beta$_2$-agonist shouldn't be used alone.

- Leukotriene modifiers—These medicines are taken by mouth. They help block the chain reaction that increases inflammation in your airways.

- Cromolyn and nedocromil—These inhaled medicines also help prevent inflammation and can be used to treat asthma of mild severity.

- Theophylline—This medicine is taken by mouth and helps open the airways.

If your doctor prescribes a long-term control medicine, take it every day to control your asthma. Your asthma symptoms will likely return or get worse if you stop taking your medicine.

Long-term control medicines can have side effects. Talk to your doctor about these side effects and ways to monitor or avoid them.

Quick-relief medicines: All people who have asthma need a quick-relief medicine to help relieve asthma symptoms that may flare up. Inhaled short-acting beta$_2$-agonists are the first choice for quick relief.

These medicines act quickly to relax tight muscles around your airways when you're having a flare-up. This allows the airways to open up so air can flow through them.

You should take your quick-relief medicine when you first notice your asthma symptoms. If you use this medicine more than two days a week, talk with your doctor about how well controlled your asthma is. You may need to make changes in your asthma action plan.

Carry your quick-relief inhaler with you at all times in case you need it. If your child has asthma, make sure that anyone caring for him or her and the child's school has the child's quick-relief medicines. They should understand when and how to use them and when to seek medical care for your child.

You shouldn't use quick-relief medicines in place of prescribed long-term control medicines. Quick-relief medicines don't reduce inflammation.

Track Your Asthma

To track your asthma, keep records of your symptoms, check your peak flow number using a peak flow meter, and get regular asthma checkups.

Record your symptoms: You can record your asthma symptoms in a diary to see how well your treatments are controlling your asthma. Asthma is "well controlled" if:

- You have symptoms no more than 2 days a week and they don't wake you from sleep more than 1 or 2 nights a month.

- You can carry out all your normal activities.

- You take quick-relief medicines no more than 2 days a week.

- You have no more than one asthma attack a year that requires you to take corticosteroids by mouth.

- Your peak flow doesn't drop below 80 percent of your personal best number.

If your asthma isn't well controlled, contact your doctor. He or she may need to change your asthma action plan.

Use a peak flow meter: This small, handheld device shows how well air moves out of your lungs. You blow into the device and it gives you a score, or peak flow number. Your score shows how well your lungs are working at the time of the test.

Your doctor will tell you how and when to use your peak flow meter. He or she also will teach you how to take your medicines based on your score.

Your doctor and other clinicians on your health care team may ask you to use your peak flow meter each morning and keep a record of your results. It may be particularly useful to record peak flow scores for a couple of weeks before each medical visit and take the results with you.

When first diagnosed with asthma, it's important to find out your "personal best" peak flow number. To do this, you record your score each day for a 2- to 3-week period when your asthma is under good control. The highest number you get during that time is your personal best. You can compare this number to future numbers to make sure your asthma is under control.

Your peak flow meter can help warn you of an asthma attack, even before you notice symptoms. If your score falls to a number that shows that your breathing is getting worse, you should take your quick-relief medicines the way your asthma action plan directs. Then you can use the peak flow meter to check how well the medicine worked.

Get asthma checkups: When you first begin treatment, you will see your doctor about every 2 to 6 weeks. Once your asthma is under control, your doctor may want to see you anywhere from once a month to twice a year.

During these checkups, your doctor or nurse will ask whether you've had an asthma attack since the last visit or any changes in symptoms or peak flow measurements. You will also be asked about your daily activities. This will help them assess your level of asthma control.

Your doctor or nurse also will ask whether you have any problems or concerns with taking your medicines or following your asthma action plan. Based on your answers to these questions, your doctor may change the dose of your medicine or give you a new medicine.

If your control is very good, you may be able to take less medicine. The goal is to use the least amount of medicine needed to control your asthma.

Emergency Care

Most people who have asthma, including many children, can safely manage their symptoms by following the steps for worsening asthma provided in the asthma action plan. However, you may need medical attention. Call your doctor for advice if the following occur:

- Your medicines don't relieve an asthma attack.
- Your peak flow is less than half of your personal best peak flow number.

Call 911 for an ambulance to take you to the emergency room of your local hospital if the following are true:

- You have trouble walking and talking because you're out of breath.

- You have blue lips or fingernails.

At the hospital, you will be closely watched and given oxygen and more medicines, as well as medicines at higher doses than you take at home. Such treatment can save your life.

Asthma Treatment for Special Groups

The treatments described in this section generally apply to all people who have asthma. However, some aspects of treatment differ for people in certain age groups and those who have special needs.

Children: It's hard to diagnose asthma in children younger than 5 years old. Thus, it's hard to know whether young children who wheeze or have other asthma symptoms will benefit from long-term control medicines. (Quick-relief medicines tend to relieve wheezing in young children whether they have asthma or not.)

Doctors will treat infants and young children who have asthma symptoms with long-term control medicines if the child's asthma health assessment indicates that the symptoms are persistent and likely to continue after 6 years of age.

Inhaled corticosteroids are the preferred treatment for young children. Montelukast or cromolyn are alternative options. Treatment may be given for a trial period of 1 month to 6 weeks. The treatment usually is stopped if benefits aren't seen during that time and the doctor and parents are confident the medicine was used properly.

Inhaled corticosteroids can possibly slow the growth of children of all ages. If this slowed growth occurs, it usually is apparent in the first several months of treatment, is generally small, and doesn't get worse over time. Poorly controlled asthma also may reduce a child's growth rate.

Most experts think the benefits of inhaled corticosteroids for children who need them to control their asthma far outweigh the risk of slowed growth.

Older adults: Doctors may need to adjust asthma treatment for older adults who take certain other medicines, such as beta-blockers, aspirin and other pain relievers, and anti-inflammatory medicines. These medicines can prevent asthma medicines from working properly and may worsen asthma symptoms.

Be sure to tell your doctor about all of the medicines you take, including over-the-counter medicines.

Older adults may develop weak bones from using inhaled corticosteroids, especially at high doses. Talk to your doctor about taking calcium and vitamin D pills and other ways to help keep your bones strong.

Pregnant women: Pregnant women who have asthma need to control the disease to ensure a good supply of oxygen to their babies. Poor asthma control raises the chance that a baby will be born early and have a low birth weight. Poor asthma control can even risk the baby's life.

Studies show that it's safer to take asthma medicines while pregnant than to risk having an asthma attack.

Talk to your doctor if you have asthma and are pregnant or planning to get pregnant. Your level of asthma control may get better or it may get worse while you're pregnant. Your health care team will check your asthma control often and adjust your treatment as needed.

People whose asthma symptoms occur with physical activity: Physical activity is an important part of a healthy lifestyle. Adults need physical activity to maintain good health. Children need it for growth and development.

In many people, however, physical activity may set off asthma symptoms. If this happens to you or your child, talk to your doctor about the best ways to control asthma so you can stay active.

The following medicines may help to prevent asthma symptoms due to physical activity:

- **Short-acting beta$_2$-agonists** (quick-relief medicine) taken shortly before physical activity can last 2 to 3 hours and prevent exercise-related symptoms in most people who take them.

- **Long-acting beta$_2$-agonists** can be protective up to 12 hours. However, with daily use, they will no longer give up to 12 hours of protection. Also, frequent use for physical activity may be a sign that asthma is poorly controlled.

- **Leukotriene modifiers** are pills taken several hours before physical activity. They help relieve asthma symptoms brought on by physical activity in up to half of the people who take them.

- **Cromolyn or nedocromil** are medicines taken shortly before physical activity to help control asthma symptoms.

- **Long-term control medicines** reduce inflammation. Frequent or severe symptoms due to physical activity may indicate poorly controlled asthma and the need to either start or increase long-term control medicines that reduce inflammation. This will help prevent exercise-related symptoms.

Easing into physical activity with a warmup period also may be helpful. You also may want to wear a mask or scarf over your mouth when exercising in cold weather.

If you use your asthma medicines as your doctor directs, you should be able to take part in any physical activity or sport you choose.

People having surgery: Asthma may add to the risk of having problems during and after surgery. For instance, having a tube put into your throat may cause an asthma attack.

Tell your surgeon about your asthma when you first consult him or her. The surgeon can take steps to lower your risks, such as giving you asthma medicines before or during surgery.

Can Asthma Be Prevented?

Currently, there isn't a way to prevent asthma from starting in the first place. However, you can take steps to control the disease and prevent its symptoms.

- Learn about your asthma and how to control it.
- Follow your written asthma action plan.
- Use medicines as your doctor directs.
- Identify and avoid things that make your asthma worse (as much as you can).
- Keep track of your asthma symptoms and level of control.
- Get regular checkups for your asthma.

Living with Asthma

Asthma is a long-term disease that requires long-term care. Successful asthma treatment requires you to take an active role in your care and follow your asthma action plan.

Learn How to Manage Your Asthma

Most people who have asthma can successfully manage their symptoms at home by following their asthma action plans and having regular checkups. However, it's important to know when to seek emergency medical care.

Learn how to use your medicines correctly. If you take inhaled medicines, you should practice using your inhaler at your doctor's office. If you take long-term control medicines, take them daily as your doctor prescribes.

Record your asthma symptoms as a way to track how well your asthma is controlled. Also, you may use a peak flow meter to measure and record how well your lungs are working.

Your doctor may ask you to keep records of your symptoms or peak flow results daily for a couple of weeks before an office visit and bring these records with you to the visit.

These steps will help you keep track over time of how well you're controlling your asthma. This will help you spot problems early and prevent or relieve asthma attacks. Recording your symptoms and peak flow results to share with your doctor also will help him or her decide whether to adjust your treatment.

Ongoing Care

Have regular asthma checkups with your doctor so he or she can assess your level of asthma control and adjust your treatment if needed. Remember, the main goal of asthma treatment is to achieve the best control of your asthma using the least amount of medicine. This may require frequent adjustments to your treatments.

If it's hard to follow your plan or the plan isn't working well, let your health care team know right away. They will work with you to adjust your plan to better suit your needs.

Get treatment for any other conditions that can interfere with your asthma management.

Watch for Signs That Your Asthma Is Getting Worse

Your asthma may be getting worse if the following occur:

- Your symptoms start to occur more often, are more severe, and/ or bother you at night and cause you to lose sleep.

- You're limiting your normal activities and missing school or work because of your asthma.

- Your peak flow number is low compared to your personal best or varies a lot from day to day.

- Your asthma medicines don't seem to work well anymore.

- You have to use your quick-relief inhaler more often. If you're using quick-relief medicine more than 2 days a week, your asthma isn't well controlled.

- You have to go to the emergency room or doctor because of an asthma attack.

If you have any of these signs, see your doctor. He or she may need to change your medicines or take other steps to control your asthma.

Partner with your health care team and take an active role in your care. This can help control asthma so it doesn't interfere with your activities and disrupt your life.

Section 9.2

Do Allergies Cause Asthma?

"Do Allergies Cause Asthma?," June 2007, reprinted with permission from www.kidshealth.org. Copyright © 2007 The Nemours Foundation. This information was provided by KidsHealth, one of the largest resources online for medically reviewed health information written for parents, kids, and teens. For more articles like this one, visit www.KidsHealth.org, or www .TeensHealth.org.

Although allergies and asthma are separate conditions, they are related. People who have allergies—particularly those that affect the nose and eyes—are more likely to have asthma. If you have allergies or asthma, your child is more likely to have it, too, because the tendency to develop these conditions is often inherited.

But not everyone who has allergies has asthma, and not all cases of asthma are related to allergies. About 75% of kids who have asthma also have an allergy to something. And many people who have asthma find their symptoms get worse when they're exposed to specific allergens (things that can cause allergic reactions in some people).

With any kind of allergy, the immune system overreacts to normally harmless substances such as pollen or dust mites. As part of this overreaction, the body produces an antibody of the immunoglobulin E (IgE) type, which specifically recognizes and attaches to the allergen when the body is exposed to it.

When that happens, it sets a process in motion that results in the release of certain substances in the body. One of them is histamine, which causes allergic symptoms that can affect the eyes, nose, throat, skin, gastrointestinal tract, or lungs. When the airways in the lungs are affected, symptoms of asthma can occur.

Future exposure to the same allergens can cause the reaction to happen again. So if your child has asthma, it's wise to explore whether allergies may be triggering some of the symptoms. Talk with your doctor about how to identify possible triggers, which can be things other than allergens, such as cold air, pets, or tobacco smoke. Your doctor might also recommend visiting an allergist for allergy tests. If your child is allergic to something, that substance may be causing or contributing to asthma symptoms (coughing, wheezing, and trouble breathing).

If it does look like allergens are an important trigger for the asthma symptoms, do what you can to help your child avoid exposure to the allergens involved. If this doesn't control the asthma symptoms adequately, the doctor may also prescribe medications or allergy shots.

Section 9.3

Immunoglobulin E's Role in Allergic Asthma

Immunoglobulin E (IgE) is a type of antibody that is present in minute amounts in the body but plays a major role in allergic diseases. IgE binds to allergens and triggers the release of substances from mast cells that can cause inflammation. When IgE binds to mast cells, a cascade of allergic reaction can begin.

- **Allergen exposure:** Repeated exposure to a particular allergen can be the first step in developing a reaction to it. Some allergens trigger strong allergic reactions, while others trigger milder reactions.

- **T cell action:** Allergens induce T cells to activate B cells, which develop into plasma cells that produce and release more antibodies.

Binding of IgE to Mast Cells

The surfaces of mast cells contain special receptors for binding IgE. The IgE antibody fits to this receptor like a module docking with the mother ship. This arrangement is such that when two adjacent mast-cell-linked IgE antibodies are in place, the allergen is drawn to both and attaches itself to both, cross-linking the two IgEs. When a critical mass of IgEs become cross-linked, the mast cell releases histamine and other inflammatory substances, and the allergic cascade begins.

The Allergic Cascade

Following exposure to an allergen, a series of initial reactions in the immune system occurs. This early-phase response is followed by a second, more severe reaction known as a late-phase response.

Typically, the allergic cascade follows this pattern:

1. Sensitization to an allergen

2. Early-phase response upon re-exposure to an allergen

3. Late-phase response to an allergen

1. Sensitization to an Allergen: Being Exposed for the First Time

You might be initially exposed to an allergen by:

- inhalation (of pollen, mold, dust mites, etc.);

- ingestion (swallowing a type of food or medication);

- touch (coming into contact with poison ivy, latex, or certain metals, such as nickel);

- injection (receiving a medication or being stung by an insect).

Your body produces IgE designed specifically for that particular allergen, but you won't experience a reaction yet.

- If you are atopic (meaning, you've inherited a predisposition toward allergic disease), your T cells are quick to stimulate B cells.

- When stimulated, B cells develop into plasma cells.

- Plasma cells produce IgE antibodies, which are targeted to that specific allergen.

- The IgE binds to special receptors on mast cells.

- Your system is now sensitized. Your mast cells are like little bombs that are armed and ready for detonation.

2. Early-Phase Response upon Re-exposure to an Allergen

When you are re-exposed to an allergen:

- The IgE of mast cells binds to the allergen, cross-linking the IgE.

- When enough cross-linking occurs, the mast cells explode with histamine and other inflammatory substances, called mediators. The mediators speed through your system.

- It happens. You wheeze, sneeze, cough, get itchy eyes, have a runny nose, become short of breath—in other words, you experience the whole unpleasant range of symptoms known as the allergic response.

And all of this occurs within an hour after initial exposure.

3. Late-Phase Response to an Allergen

The late-phase response actually begins at the same time as the early-phase response, but it takes longer to see. In some individuals, the body rallies its immune system for this second phase, which can happen relatively soon after the initial reaction—anywhere from about 3 to 10 hours later. Often, this late-phase response involves immune cells known as eosinophils and it can last for 24 hours or so before subsiding. During the late-phase response, congestion and certain other symptoms can be more severe than those seen during the initial response.

Consequences of Chronic Allergic Reaction in Asthma

With repeated allergen exposure and allergic response, some damage can be done to the tissues involved. To remedy this damage, researchers are exploring the issue of airway remodeling, or scarring of the airways in the lungs of asthma patients. Long-term controller medications that aggressively attack inflammation and maintain maximum lung function are also believed to reduce the risk of permanent damage.

Although allergic disease is not curable, it is treatable enough to live with. Healthcare providers can be significant allies in this effort—particularly allergists, pulmonologists, and certain other specialists. In addition, many research organizations make studying allergic disease their top priority, and can be excellent sources of information on the immune system. The more you know about how an allergic response occurs, the better armed you'll be to meet its challenges.

Section 9.4

Asthma and Its Environmental Triggers

From text by the National Institute of Environmental Health Sciences (NIEHS, www.niehs.nih.gov), part of the National Institutes of Health, May 2006.

Once considered a minor ailment affecting only a few, asthma is now the most common chronic disorder in childhood, affecting an estimated 6.2 million children under the age of 18. Despite improvements in diagnosis and management, and a better understanding of the causes of the disease, the prevalence of asthma has progressively increased over the past 15 years. In the United States alone, 30.8 million people—10.6 percent of adults and 12.2 percent of children—have been diagnosed with asthma.

Asthma is an inflammatory disease of the lung. This inflammatory process can occur along the entire airway from the nose to the lung. Once the airway becomes swollen and inflamed, it becomes narrower, and less air gets through to the lung tissue. This causes symptoms like wheezing, coughing, chest tightness, and trouble breathing. During an asthma attack, the muscles around the airways tighten up, and the asthma symptoms become even worse than usual.

Environmental Triggers: The National Allergen Survey

The fact that asthma runs in families suggests that genetic factors play an important role in the development of the disease. If one or both parents have asthma, the child is much more likely to develop the condition—this is known as genetic susceptibility. However, environmental

120

factors also contribute to the disease process. Asthma can be triggered by a wide range of substances called allergens.

Recent studies also show that exposure to indoor allergens from house dust mites, cockroaches, dogs, cats, rodents, molds, and fungi are among the most important environmental triggers for asthma. From 1998 to 2002, NIEHS scientists, along with researchers from the Department of Housing and Urban Development, conducted an extensive survey to assess the prevalence of these indoor allergens in American homes.

The results of this survey, known as the National Survey of Lead and Allergens in Housing, showed that more than 46 percent of the homes surveyed had levels of dust mite allergens high enough to produce allergic reactions, while nearly a quarter of the homes had allergen levels high enough to trigger asthma symptoms in genetically susceptible individuals. The survey results also showed that nearly two thirds of American homes have detectable levels of cockroach allergens, with higher allergen concentrations in high-rise apartments, urban settings, older homes, and homes of low-income households. Approximately 10 percent of homes had cockroach levels above the threshold for triggering asthma symptoms. One of the most surprising findings from the national survey was that 100 percent of U.S. homes had detectable levels of dog and cat allergens, even though dogs were present in only 32 percent of the surveyed homes, and cat ownership was reported in only 24 percent. Most homes had levels of dog and cat allergen that exceeded the threshold for allergic sensitization, while about one third of homes had allergen levels high enough to produce asthma symptoms.

Asthma Intervention: Reducing Indoor Exposures

In addition to their research on indoor allergens, NIEHS scientists are collaborating with researchers from other asthma research centers to develop intervention strategies aimed at reducing asthma symptoms. These strategies are based on simple methods that are designed to reduce exposure to the allergens that trigger asthma. Recent evidence suggests that exposure to cockroach allergen might be the most important risk factor for asthma in inner-city households.

In 2001, NIEHS researchers conducted a 6-month trial to test a new intervention method for reducing cockroach allergen levels in low-cockroach allergen levels in low-income, urban homes. The intervention included cockroach extermination, thorough professional cleaning, and in-home visits to educate the occupants about asthma management.

At the end of 6 months, cockroach allergen levels were reduced by 84 percent on bedroom floors and in the beds, well below the threshold for producing asthma symptoms. The researchers also observed a 96 percent reduction in allergen levels on kitchen floors, although allergen levels remained above the asthma threshold. A follow-up study conducted in 2005 showed that these reductions in allergen levels could be maintained with continued cockroach control, and that effective cockroach extermination alone could reduce allergen concentrations to a comparable level.

Other intervention studies have targeted allergens produced by house dust mites, microscopic creatures that reside in bedding, carpets, and upholstery. In 1999, Institute researchers collaborated with scientists from Harvard University and the University of Washington to evaluate some practical methods for lowering these allergens in the bedrooms of low-income Seattle homes. The research showed that some simple steps—washing the bedding in hot water, putting allergen-impermeable covers on the pillows, box springs and mattresses, and vacuuming and steam cleaning the carpets and upholstered furniture—can significantly reduce dust mite allergen levels.

The results of the indoor allergen surveys also showed that the construction and operation of the homes may have a significant impact on allergen levels. For example, indoor humidity and age of the house were the best predictors of dust mite allergen levels.

Helping Minority Populations: The Inner-City Asthma Study

In order to address the rising incidence of asthma among inner-city children, NIEHS has partnered with the National Institute of Allergy and Infectious Diseases to conduct the National Cooperative Inner-City Asthma Study, a long-term project that includes seven asthma study centers across the country. The study has enrolled more than 900 children, ages 5 to 11, with moderate to severe asthma. The goal of the study is to develop and implement a comprehensive, cost-effective intervention program aimed at reducing asthma incidence among children living in low socioeconomic areas.

Begun in the early 1990s, the study has already provided researchers with some positive results. Scientists developed an intervention program that targets six major classes of allergens that trigger asthma symptoms—dust mites, cockroaches, pet dander, rodents, passive smoking, and mold. The environmental interventions are tailored to each child's sensitivity to the selected allergens as determined by allergy testing. They include allergen-impermeable covers on the child's mattress, box spring and pillows, air purifiers, vacuum cleaners with HEPA [high-efficiency particulate air] filters, and professional pest control. Children who received the intervention had 19 percent fewer unscheduled clinic visits, a 13 percent reduction in the use of albuterol inhalers, and 38 more symptom-free days over the course of the study than those in the control group.

The Role of Outdoor Air Pollution

While much of the asthma research has focused on indoor allergens, scientists are realizing that outdoor pollutants also play a major role. NIEHS-funded researchers at the University of Southern California's Keck School of Medicine studied air pollution levels in 10 Southern California cities, and found that the closer children live to a freeway, the greater their chances of being diagnosed with asthma. The researchers also found that children who had higher levels of nitrogen dioxide in the air around their homes were more likely to develop asthma symptoms.

Nitrogen dioxide is one of many pollutants emitted from the tailpipes of motor vehicles.

Armed with a better understanding of asthma's environmental triggers, researchers want to learn more about how genes interact with these exposures to influence disease risk. To address this need, NIEHS has launched a new research program to identify the genetic risk factors that predispose people to asthma. Using a technique called gene expression profiling, the researchers will screen thousands of genes to identify which genes are activated when a patient's airways become obstructed or inflamed. The ultimate goal of this program is to determine which genes make people susceptible to different types of asthma, which may help explain why some people develop asthma while others remain unaffected.

Section 9.5

Occupational Asthma Due to Allergen Exposure at Work

"OSH Answers: Asthma," http://www.ccohs.ca/oshanswers/disease/asthma .html, Canadian Centre for Occupational Health and Safety (CCOHS), © 2005. Reproduced with permission of CCOHS. Reviewed by David A. Cooke, MD, FACP, August 3, 2010.

What is occupational asthma?

Asthma is a respiratory disease. It creates narrowing of the air passages that results in difficult breathing, tightness of the chest, coughing, and breath sounds such as wheezing.

Occupational asthma refers to asthma that is caused by breathing in specific agents in the workplace. An abnormal response of the body to the presence of an agent in the workplace causes occupational asthma.

The abnormal response, called sensitization, develops after variable periods of workplace exposure to certain dusts, fumes, or vapors.

This sensitization may not show any symptoms of disease or it may be associated with skin rashes (urticaria), hay fever-like symptoms, or a combination of these symptoms.

Not all workers react with an asthmatic response when exposed to industrial agents. Asthma strikes only a fraction of workers. Asthmatic attacks can be controlled either by ending exposure to the agent responsible or by medical treatment.

How does asthma develop?

Asthma is triggered in several ways and most of them are not completely understood. For simplicity, we categorize them into two groups: allergic and non-allergic.

Allergic asthma: Allergic asthma involves the body's immune system. This is a complex defense system that protects the body from harm caused by foreign substances or microbes. Among the most important elements of the defense mechanism are special proteins called antibodies. These are produced when the human body contacts an alien substance or microbe. Antibodies react with substances or microbes to destroy them. Antibodies are often very selective, acting only on one particular substance or type of microbe.

But antibodies can also respond in a wrong way and cause allergic disorders such as asthma. After a period of exposure to an industrial substance, either natural or synthetic, a worker may start producing too many of the antibodies called immunoglobulin E (IgE). These antibodies attach to specific cells in the lung in a process known as sensitization.

When re-exposure occurs, the lung cells with attached IgE antibodies react with the substance. This reaction results in the release of chemicals such as leukotrienes that are made in the body. Leukotrienes provoke the contraction of some muscles in the airways. This causes the narrowing of air passages which is characteristic of asthma.

Non-allergic asthma: Following repeated exposure to an industrial chemical, substances such as leukotrienes are released in the lungs. Again, the leukotriene causes narrowing of air passages typical of asthma. The reasons for such release are still not clear because no antibody reaction seems to be involved.

Other types of asthma: In certain circumstances, symptoms of asthma may develop suddenly (within 24 hours) following exposure to high airborne concentrations of respiratory irritants such as chlorine. This condition is known as reactive airways dysfunction syndrome (RADS). The symptoms may persist for months or years when the sensitized person is re-exposed to irritants. RADS is controversial because of its rarity and the lack of good information on how the lungs are affected and the range of substances which cause it.

How long does asthma take to develop?

There is no fixed period of time in which asthma can develop. Asthma as a disease may develop from a few weeks to many years after the initial exposure. Studies carried out on some platinum refinery workers show that in most cases asthma develops in 6 to 12 months. But it may occur within 10 days or be delayed for as long as 25 years.

Analysis of the respiratory responses of sensitized workers has established three basic patterns of asthmatic attacks, as follows:

- **Immediate** typically develops within minutes of exposure and is at its worst after approximately 20 minutes; recovery takes about 2 hours.

- **Late** can occur in different forms. It usually starts several hours after exposure and is at its worst after about 4 to 8 hours with recovery within 24 hours. However, it can start 1 hour after exposure with recovery in 3 to 4 hours. In some cases, it may start at night, with a tendency to recur at the same time for a few nights following a single exposure.

- **Dual or combined** is the occurrence of both immediate and late types of asthma.

How common is asthma?

The frequency of occupational asthma is unknown, although various estimates are available. In Japan, 15 percent of asthma in males is believed to be occupational. In the United States, two percent of all cases of asthma are thought to be of occupational origin. The number of cases of occupational asthma varies from country to country and from industry to industry. About six percent of animal handlers develop asthma due to animal hair or dust. Between 10 and 45 percent of workers who process subtilisins, the proteolytic enzymes like *Bacillus subtilis* in the detergent industry develop asthma. However, preparations of the enzymes in granulated form, which is less readily inhaled, have reduced the likelihood of asthma. Approximately five percent of workers exposed to such chemicals as isocyanates and certain wood dusts develop asthma.

What factors increase the chances of developing asthma?

Some workplace conditions seem to increase the likelihood that workers will develop asthma, but their importance is not fully known. Factors such as the properties of the chemicals, and the amount and duration of exposure are obviously important. However, because only a fraction of exposed workers are affected, factors unique to individual workers can also be important. Such factors include the ability of some people to produce abnormal amounts of IgE antibodies. The contribution of cigarette smoking to asthma is not known. But smokers are more likely than nonsmokers to develop respiratory problems in general.

For more information about the causes of occupational asthma, see Tables 9.1–9.6.

How does the doctor know if a worker has asthma?

Sufferers from occupational asthma experience attacks of difficult breathing, tightness of the chest, coughing, and breath sounds such as wheezing, which is associated with air-flow obstruction. Such symptoms should raise the suspicion of asthma. Typically these symptoms are worse on working days, often awakening the patient at night, and improving when the person is away from work. While off work, sufferers from occupational asthma may still have chest symptoms when exposed to airway irritants such as dusts, or fumes, or upon exercise. Itchy and watery eyes, sneezing, stuffy and runny nose, and skin rashes are other symptoms often associated with asthma.

Lung function tests and skin tests can help to confirm the disease. But some patients with occupational asthma may have normal lung function as well as negative skin tests.

The diagnosis of work-related asthma needs to be confirmed objectively. This can be done by carrying out pulmonary function tests at work and off work. Specific inhalation challenges can demonstrate the occupational origin of asthma and may identify the agents responsible when the cause is uncertain. Specific inhalation challenge tests require breathing in small quantities of industrial agents that may induce an attack of asthma. But they are safe when performed by experienced physicians in specialized centers.

How can we control occupational asthma?

Although there are drugs that may control the symptoms of asthma, it is important to stop exposure. If the exposure to the causal agent is not stopped, treatment will be needed continuously and the breathing problems may become permanent. People may continue to suffer from occupational asthma even after removal from exposure.

For example, a follow-up study of 75 patients with asthma caused by red cedar dust showed that only half the patients recovered. The remaining half continued to have asthmatic attacks for a period of 1 to 9 years after the termination of exposure.

Dust masks and respirators can help to control workplace exposure. However, these protective devices, in order to be effective, must be carefully selected, properly fitted, and well maintained. Preventing further exposure might involve a change of job. If a job change is not feasible, relocation to another area of the plant with no exposure may be essential.

Table 9.1. Causes of Occupational Asthma: Grains, Flours, Plants, and Gums

Occupation	Agent
Bakers, millers	Wheat
Chemists, coffee bean baggers and handlers, gardeners, millers, oil industry workers, farmers	Castor beans
Cigarette factory workers	Tobacco dust
Drug manufacturers, mold makers in sweet factories, printers	Gum acacia
Farmers, grain handlers	Grain dust
Gum manufacturers, sweet makers	Gum tragacanth
Strawberry growers	Strawberry pollen
Tea sifters and packers	Tea dust
Tobacco farmers	Tobacco leaf
Woollen industry workers	Wool

Table 9.2. Causes of Occupational Asthma: Animals, Insects, and Fungi

Occupation	Agent
Bird fanciers	Avian proteins
Cosmetic manufacturers	Carmine
Entomologists	Moths, butterflies
Feather pluckers	Feathers
Field contact workers	Crickets
Fish bait breeders	Bee moths
Flour mill workers, bakers, farm workers, grain handlers	Grain storage mites, Alternaria, aspergillus
Laboratory workers	Locusts, cockroaches, grain weevils, rats, mice, guinea pigs, rabbits
Mushroom cultivators	Mushroom spores
Oyster farmers	Hoya
Pea sorters	Mexican bean weevils
Pigeon breeders	Pigeons
Poultry workers	Chickens
Prawn processors	Prawns
Silkworm sericulturers	Silkworms
Zoological museum curators	Beetles

Table 9.3. Causes of Occupational Asthma: Chemicals/Materials

Occupation	Agent
Aircraft fitters	Triethyl tetramine
Aluminum cable solderers	Aminoethylethanolamine
Aluminum pot room workers	Fluorine
Auto body workers	Acrylates (resins, glues, sealants, adhesives)
Brewery workers	Chloramine-T
Chemical plant workers, pulp mill workers	Chlorine
Dye weighers	Leva fix brilliant yellow, dramarin brilliant yellow and blue, Ciba chrome brilliant scarlet
Electronics workers	Colophony
Epoxy resin manufacturers	Tetrachlorophthalic anhydride
Foundry mold makers	Furan-based resin binder systems
Fur dyers	Para-phenylenediamine
Hairdressers	Per sulphate salts
Health care workers	Glutaraldehyde, latex
Laboratory workers, nurses, phenolic resin molders	Formalin/formaldehyde
Meat wrappers	Polyvinyl chloride vapor
Paint manufacturers, plastic molders, tool setters	Phthalic anhydride
Paint sprayers	Dimethyl ethanolamine
Photographic workers, shellac manufacturers	Ethylenediamine
Refrigeration industry workers	CFCs [chlorofluorocarbons]
Solderers	Polyether alcohol, polypropylene glycol

How can we prevent occupational asthma?

The best way to prevent occupational asthma is to replace dangerous substances with less harmful ones. Where this is not possible, exposure should be minimized through engineering controls such as ventilation and enclosures of processes.

Education of workers is also very important. Proper handling procedures, avoidance of spills, and good housekeeping reduce the occurrence of occupational asthma.

Table 9.4. Causes of Occupational Asthma: Isocyanates and Metals

Occupation	Agent
Boat builders, foam manufacturers, office workers, plastics factory workers, refrigerator manufacturers, TDI [toluene diisocyanate] manufacturers/users, printers, laminators, tinners, toy makers	Toluene diisocyanate
Boiler cleaners, gas turbine cleaners	Vanadium
Car sprayers	Hexamethylene diisocyanate
Cement workers	Potassium dichromate
Chrome platers, chrome polishers	Sodium bichromate, chromic acid, potassium chromate
Nickel platers	Nickel sulphate
Platinum chemists	Chlor platinic acid
Platinum refiners	Platinum salts
Polyurethane foam manufacturers, printers, laminators	Diphenylmethane diisocyanate
Rubber workers	Naphthalene diisocyanate
Tungsten carbide grinders	Cobalt
Welders	Stainless steel fumes

Table 9.5. Causes of Occupational Asthma: Drugs and Enzymes

Occupation	Agent
Ampicillin manufacturers	Phenylglycine acid chloride
Detergent manufacturers	*Bacillus subtilis*
Enzyme manufacturers	Fungal alpha-amylase
Food technologists, laboratory workers	Papain
Pharmacists	Gentian powder, flaviastase
Pharmaceutical workers	Methyldopa, salbutamol, dichloramine, piperazine dihydrochloride, spiramycin, penicillins, sulphathiazole, sulphonechloramides, chloramine-T, phosdrin, pancreatic extracts
Poultry workers	Amprolium hydrochloride
Process workers, plastic polymer production workers	Trypsin, bromelin

What occupations are at risk for asthma?

Some of the occupations where asthma has been seen are listed in Tables 9.1–9.6. It should be noted that the lists of occupational substances and microbes which can cause asthma are not complete. New causes continue to be added. New materials and new processes introduce new exposures and create new risks.

Table 9.6. Causes of Occupational Asthma: Woods

Occupation	Agent
Carpenters, timber millers, woodworkers	Western red cedar, cedar of Lebanon, iroko, California redwood, ramin, African zebra wood
Sawmill workers, pattern makers	Mansonia, oak, mahogany, abiurana
Wood finishers	Cocabolla
Wood machinists	Kejaat

Section 9.6

Aspergillosis:
People with Asthma at Highest Risk

"Aspergillosis," © 2010 A.D.A.M., Inc. Reprinted with permission.

Aspergillosis is an infection, growth, or allergic response due to the *Aspergillus fungus*.

Causes

Aspergillosis is caused by a fungus (*Aspergillus*), which is commonly found growing on dead leaves, stored grain, compost piles, or in other decaying vegetation. It can also be found on marijuana.

Although most people are frequently exposed to aspergillus, infections caused by the fungus rarely occur in people with a normal immune system. The rare infections caused by aspergillus include pneumonia and fungus ball (aspergilloma).

There are several forms of aspergillosis:

- Pulmonary aspergillosis—allergic bronchopulmonary type—is an allergic reaction to the fungus that usually develops in people who already have lung problems (such as asthma or cystic fibrosis).

- Aspergilloma is a growth (fungus ball) that develops in an area of previous lung disease or lung scarring (such as tuberculosis or lung abscess).

- Pulmonary aspergillosis–invasive type is a serious infection with pneumonia that can spread to other parts of the body. This infection occurs almost exclusively in people with weakened immune systems due to cancer, AIDS [acquired immunodeficiency syndrome], leukemia, organ transplantation, chemotherapy, or other conditions or medications that lower the number of normal white blood cells or weaken the immune system.

Symptoms

Symptoms depend on the type of infection.
Symptoms of allergic bronchopulmonary aspergillosis may include:

- cough;
- coughing up blood or brownish mucous plugs;
- fever;
- generalized ill feeling (malaise);
- wheezing;
- weight loss;
- recurrent episodes of lung airway obstruction.

Additional symptoms seen in invasive aspergillosis depend on the part of the body affected, and may include:

- bone pain;
- blood in the urine;
- chest pain;
- chills;
- decreased urine output;
- endocarditis;
- headaches;
- increased sputum production, which may be bloody;
- meningitis;
- shortness of breath;
- sinusitis;
- skin sores (lesions);
- vision problems.

It is difficult to identify exactly how many people are affected by atopic dermatitis. Many people report that they have symptoms, but never have received a diagnosis from a doctor. An estimated 10 to 20 percent of infants and young children experience symptoms of the disease. Roughly 60 percent of these infants continue to have one or more symptoms of atopic dermatitis in adulthood. In adults, the prevalence is thought to be 1 to 3 percent, with an overall lifetime prevalence of about 7 percent.

Types of Eczema (Dermatitis)

- **Allergic contact eczema (dermatitis):** A red, itchy, weepy reaction where the skin has come into contact with a substance that the immune system recognizes as foreign, such as poison ivy or certain preservatives in creams and lotions.

- **Atopic dermatitis:** A chronic skin disease characterized by itchy, inflamed skin.

- **Contact eczema:** A localized reaction that includes redness, itching, and burning where the skin has come into contact with an allergen (an allergy-causing substance) or with an irritant such as an acid, a cleaning agent, or other chemical.

- **Dyshidrotic eczema:** Irritation of the skin on the palms of hands and soles of the feet characterized by clear, deep blisters that itch and burn.

- **Neurodermatitis**: Scaly patches of the skin on the head, lower legs, wrists, or forearms caused by a localized itch (such as an insect bite) that become intensely irritated when scratched.

- **Nummular eczema:** Coin-shaped patches of irritated skin— most common on the arms, back, buttocks, and lower legs—that may be crusted, scaling, and extremely itchy.

- **Seborrheic eczema:** Yellowish, oily, scaly patches of skin on the scalp, face, and occasionally other parts of the body.

- **Stasis dermatitis:** A skin irritation on the lower legs, generally related to circulatory problems.

Cost of Atopic Dermatitis

In a recent analysis of the costs associated with atopic dermatitis in the United States, researchers reviewed studies evaluating both direct costs (doctor visits, hospitalizations, and medicine) and indirect costs (over-the-counter remedies, lubricants, and days lost from work). They found that direct costs totaled about 25 percent, and indirect costs totaled about 75 percent of costs. Per patient, the costs averaged about $600 per year. On the whole, direct costs alone may exceed $3 billion per year.

Causes of Atopic Dermatitis

The cause of atopic dermatitis is not known, but the disease seems to result from a combination of genetic (hereditary) and environmental factors.

Children are more likely to develop this disorder if a parent has had it or another atopic disease like asthma or hay fever. If both parents have an atopic disease, the likelihood increases. Although some people outgrow skin symptoms, approximately half of children with atopic dermatitis go on to develop hay fever or asthma. Environmental factors can bring on symptoms of atopic dermatitis at any time in individuals who have inherited the atopic disease trait.

Atopic dermatitis is also associated with malfunction of the body's immune system, the system that recognizes and helps fight bacteria and viruses that invade the body. Scientists have found that people with atopic dermatitis have a low level of a cytokine (a protein) that is essential to the healthy function of the body's immune system and a high level of other cytokines that lead to allergic reactions. The immune system can become misguided and create inflammation in the skin even in the absence of a major infection. This can be viewed as a form of autoimmunity, where a body reacts against its own tissues.

In the past, doctors thought that atopic dermatitis was caused by an emotional disorder. We now know that emotional factors, such as stress, can make the condition worse, but they do not cause the disease.

Symptoms of Atopic Dermatitis

Symptoms (signs) vary from person to person. The most common symptoms are dry, itchy skin and rashes on the face, inside the elbows and behind the knees, and on the hands and feet. Itching is the most important symptom of atopic dermatitis. Scratching and rubbing in response to itching irritates the skin, increases inflammation, and actually increases itchiness. Itching is a particular problem during sleep when conscious control of scratching is lost.

The appearance of the skin that is affected by atopic dermatitis depends on the amount of scratching and the presence of secondary skin infections. The skin may be red and scaly, be thick and leathery, contain small raised bumps, or leak fluid and become crusty and infected.

Atopic dermatitis may also affect the skin around the eyes, the eyelids, and the eyebrows and lashes. Scratching and rubbing the eye area can cause the skin to redden and swell. Some people with atopic dermatitis develop an extra fold of skin under their eyes. Patchy loss of eyebrows and eyelashes may also result from scratching or rubbing.

Researchers have noted differences in the skin of people with atopic dermatitis that may contribute to the symptoms of the disease. The outer layer of skin, called the epidermis, is divided into two parts: an inner part containing moist, living cells, and an outer part, known as the horny layer or stratum corneum, containing dry, flattened, dead cells. Under normal conditions the stratum corneum acts as a barrier, keeping the rest of the skin from drying out and protecting other layers of skin from damage caused by irritants and infections.

When this barrier is damaged, irritants act more intensely on the skin. The skin of a person with atopic dermatitis loses moisture from the epidermal layer, allowing the skin to become very dry and reducing its protective abilities. Thus, when combined with the abnormal skin immune system, the person's skin is more likely to become infected by bacteria (for example, *Staphylococcus* and *Streptococcus*) or viruses, such as those that cause warts and cold sores.

Stages of Atopic Dermatitis

When atopic dermatitis occurs during infancy and childhood, it affects each child differently in terms of both onset and severity of symptoms. In infants, atopic dermatitis typically begins around 6 to 12 weeks of age. It may first appear around the cheeks and chin as a patchy facial rash, which can progress to red, scaling, oozing skin. The skin may become infected. Once the infant becomes more mobile and begins crawling, exposed areas, such as the inner and outer parts of the arms and legs, may also be affected. An infant with atopic dermatitis may be restless and irritable because of the itching and discomfort of the disease.

In childhood, the rash tends to occur behind the knees and inside the elbows; on the sides of the neck; around the mouth; and on the wrists, ankles, and hands. Often, the rash begins with papules that become hard and scaly when scratched. The skin around the lips may be inflamed, and constant licking of the area may lead to small, painful cracks in the skin around the mouth.

In some children, the disease goes into remission for a long time, only to come back at the onset of puberty when hormones, stress, and the use of irritating skin care products or cosmetics may cause the disease to flare.

Although a number of people who developed atopic dermatitis as children also experience symptoms as adults, it is also possible for the disease to show up first in adulthood. The pattern in adults is similar to that seen in children; that is, the disease may be widespread or limited to only a few parts of the body. For example, only the hands or feet may be affected and become dry, itchy, red, and cracked. Sleep patterns and work performance may be affected, and long-term use of medications to treat the atopic dermatitis may cause complications. Adults with atopic dermatitis also have a predisposition toward irritant contact dermatitis, where the skin becomes red and inflamed from contact with detergents, wool, friction from clothing, or other potential irritants. It is more likely to occur in occupations involving frequent hand washing or exposure to chemicals. Some people develop a rash around their nipples. These localized symptoms are difficult to treat. Because adults may also develop cataracts, the doctor may recommend regular eye exams.

Diagnosing Atopic Dermatitis

Each person experiences a unique combination of symptoms, which may vary in severity over time. The doctor will base a diagnosis on the symptoms the patient experiences and may need to see the patient several times to make an accurate diagnosis and to rule out other diseases and conditions that might cause skin irritation. In some cases, the family doctor or pediatrician may refer the patient to a dermatologist (doctor specializing in skin disorders) or allergist (allergy specialist) for further evaluation.

A medical history may help the doctor better understand the nature of a patient's symptoms, when they occur, and their possible causes. The doctor may ask about family history of allergic disease; whether the patient also has diseases such as hay fever or asthma; and about exposure to irritants, sleep disturbances, any foods that seem to be related to skin flares, previous treatments for skin-related symptoms, and use of steroids or other medications. A preliminary diagnosis of atopic dermatitis can be made if the patient has three or more features from each of two categories: major features and minor features.

Currently, there is no single test to diagnose atopic dermatitis. However, there are some tests that can give the doctor an indication of allergic sensitivity.

Pricking the skin with a needle that contains a small amount of a suspected allergen may be helpful in identifying factors that trigger flares of atopic dermatitis. Negative results on skin tests may help rule out the possibility that certain substances cause skin inflammation. Positive skin prick test results are difficult to interpret in people with atopic dermatitis because the skin is very sensitive to many substances, and there can be many positive test sites that are not meaningful to a person's disease at the time. Positive results simply indicate that the individual has IgE (allergic) antibodies to the substance tested. IgE (immunoglobulin E) controls the immune system's allergic response and is often high in atopic dermatitis.

If the quantity of IgE antibodies to a food in the blood is above a certain level, it is indicative of a food allergy. If a food allergy is suspected, a person might be asked to record everything eaten and note any reactions.

Physician-supervised food challenges (that is, the introduction of a food) following a period of food elimination may be necessary to determine if symptomatic food allergy is present. Identifying the food allergen may be difficult when a person is also being exposed to other possible allergens at the same time or symptoms may be triggered by other factors, such as infection, heat, and humidity.

Factors That Make Atopic Dermatitis Worse

Many factors or conditions can make symptoms of atopic dermatitis worse, further triggering the already overactive immune system, aggravating the itch-scratch cycle, and increasing damage to the skin. These factors can be broken down into two main categories: irritants and allergens. Emotional factors and some infections and illnesses can also influence atopic dermatitis.

Irritants are substances that directly affect the skin and, when present in high enough concentrations with long enough contact, cause the skin to become red and itchy or to burn. Specific irritants affect people with atopic dermatitis to different degrees. Over time, many patients and their family members learn to identify the irritants causing the most trouble. For example, frequent wetting and drying of the skin may affect the skin barrier function. Also, wool or synthetic fibers and rough or poorly fitting clothing can rub the skin, trigger inflammation, and cause the itch-scratch cycle to begin. Soaps and detergents may have a drying effect and worsen itching, and some perfumes and cosmetics may irritate the skin. Exposure to certain substances, such as solvents, dust, or sand, may also make the condition worse. Cigarette smoke may irritate the eyelids. Because the effects of irritants vary from one person to another, each person can best determine what substances or circumstances cause the disease to flare.

Allergens are substances from foods, plants, animals, or the air that inflame the skin because the immune system overreacts to the substance. Inflammation occurs even when the person is exposed to small amounts of the substance for a limited time. Although it is known that allergens in the air, such as dust mites, pollens, molds, and dander from animal hair or skin, may worsen the symptoms of atopic dermatitis in some people, scientists aren't certain whether inhaling these allergens or their actual penetration of the skin causes the problems. When people with atopic dermatitis come into contact with an irritant or allergen they are sensitive to, inflammation producing cells become active. These cells release chemicals that cause itching and redness. As the person responds by scratching and rubbing the skin, further damage occurs.

Children with atopic disease tend to have a higher prevalence of food allergy than those in the general population. An allergic reaction to food can cause skin inflammation (generally an itchy red rash), gastrointestinal symptoms (abdominal pain, vomiting, diarrhea), and/or upper respiratory tract symptoms (congestion, sneezing, and wheezing). The most common allergenic (allergy-causing) foods are eggs, milk, peanuts, wheat, soy, tree nuts, shellfish, and fish. A recent analysis of a large number of studies on allergies and breastfeeding indicated that breastfeeding an infant, although preferable for many reasons, has little effect on protecting the infant from developing atopic dermatitis.

In addition to irritants and allergens, emotional factors, skin infections, and temperature and climate play a role in atopic dermatitis. Although the disease itself is not caused by emotional factors, it can be made worse by stress, anger, and frustration. Interpersonal problems or major life changes, such as divorce, job changes, or the death of a loved one, can also make the disease worse.

Bathing without proper moisturizing afterward is a common factor that triggers a flare of atopic dermatitis. The low humidity of winter or the dry year-round climate of some geographic areas can make the disease worse, as can overheated indoor areas and long or hot baths and showers. Alternately sweating and chilling can trigger a flare in some people. Bacterial infections can also trigger or increase the severity of atopic dermatitis. If a patient experiences a sudden flare of illness, the doctor may check for infection.

Treatment of Atopic Dermatitis

Treatment is more effective when a partnership develops that includes the patient, family members, and doctor. The doctor will suggest a treatment plan based on the patient's age, symptoms, and general health.

The patient or family member providing care plays a large role in the success of the treatment plan by carefully following the doctor's instructions and paying attention to what is or is not helpful. Most patients will notice improvement with proper skin care and lifestyle changes.

The doctor has two main goals in treating atopic dermatitis: healing the skin and preventing flares. These may be assisted by developing skin care routines and avoiding substances that lead to skin irritation and trigger the immune system and the itch-scratch cycle. It is important for the patient and family members to note any changes in the skin's condition in response to treatment, and to be persistent in identifying the treatment that seems to work best.

Medications: New medications known as immunomodulators have been developed that help control inflammation and reduce immune system reactions when applied to the skin. They can be used in patients older than 2 years of age and have few side effects (burning or itching the first few days of application). They not only reduce flares, but also maintain skin texture and reduce the need for long-term use of corticosteroids.

Corticosteroid creams and ointments have been used for many years to treat atopic dermatitis and other autoimmune diseases affecting the skin. Sometimes over-the-counter preparations are used, but in many cases the doctor will prescribe a stronger corticosteroid cream or ointment. When prescribing a medication, the doctor will take into account the patient's age, location of the skin to be treated, severity of the symptoms, and type of preparation (cream or ointment) that will be most effective. Sometimes the base used in certain brands of corticosteroid creams and ointments irritates the skin of a particular patient. Side effects of repeated or long-term use of topical corticosteroids can include thinning of the skin, infections, growth suppression (in children), and stretch marks on the skin.

When topical corticosteroids are not effective, the doctor may prescribe a systemic corticosteroid, which is taken by mouth or injected instead of being applied directly to the skin. Typically, these medications are used only in resistant cases and only given for short periods of time. The side effects of systemic corticosteroids can include skin damage, thinned or weakened bones, high blood pressure, high blood sugar, infections, and cataracts.

It can be dangerous to suddenly stop taking corticosteroids, so it is very important that the doctor and patient work together in changing the corticosteroid dose.

Antibiotics to treat skin infections may be applied directly to the skin in an ointment, but are usually more effective when taken by mouth. If viral or fungal infections are present, the doctor may also prescribe specific medications to treat those infections.

Certain antihistamines that cause drowsiness can reduce night-time scratching and allow more restful sleep when taken at bedtime. This effect can be particularly helpful for patients whose nighttime scratching makes the disease worse.

In adults, drugs that suppress the immune system may be prescribed to treat severe cases of atopic dermatitis that have failed to respond to other forms of therapy. These drugs block the production of some immune cells and curb the action of others. The side effects of drugs like these can include high blood pressure, nausea, vomiting, kidney problems, headaches, tingling or numbness, and a possible increased risk of cancer and infections. There is also a risk of relapse after the drug is stopped. Because of their toxic side effects, systemic corticosteroids and immunosuppressive drugs are used only in severe cases and then for as short a period of time as possible. Patients requiring systemic corticosteroids should be referred to dermatologists or allergists specializing in the care of atopic dermatitis to help identify trigger factors and alternative therapies.

In rare cases, when home-based treatments have been unsuccessful, a patient may need a few days in the hospital for intense treatment.

Phototherapy: Use of ultraviolet A or B light waves, alone or combined, can be an effective treatment for mild to moderate dermatitis in older children (over 12 years old) and adults. A combination of ultraviolet light therapy and a drug called psoralen can also be used in cases that are resistant to ultraviolet light alone. Possible long-term side effects of this treatment include premature skin aging and skin cancer. If the doctor thinks that phototherapy may be useful to treat the symptoms of atopic dermatitis, he or she will use the minimum exposure necessary and monitor the skin carefully.

Skin care: Healing the skin and keeping it healthy are important to prevent further damage and enhance quality of life. Developing and sticking with a daily skin care routine is critical to preventing flares.

A lukewarm bath helps to cleanse and moisturize the skin without drying it excessively. Because soaps can be drying to the skin, the doctor may recommend use of a mild bar soap or nonsoap cleanser. Bath oils are not usually helpful.

After bathing, a person should air-dry the skin, or pat it dry gently (avoiding rubbing or brisk drying), and then apply a lubricant to seal in the water that has been absorbed into the skin during bathing. A lubricant increases the rate of healing and establishes a barrier against further drying and irritation. Lotions that have a high water or alcohol content evaporate more quickly, and alcohol may cause stinging. Therefore, they generally are not the best choice. Creams and ointments work better at healing the skin.

Another key to protecting and restoring the skin is taking steps to avoid repeated skin infections. Signs of skin infection include tiny pustules (pus-filled bumps), oozing cracks or sores, or crusty yellow blisters. If symptoms of a skin infection develop, the doctor should be consulted and treatment should begin as soon as possible.

Protection from allergen exposure: The doctor may suggest reducing exposure to a suspected allergen. For example, the presence of the house dust mite can be limited by encasing mattresses and pillows in special dust-proof covers, frequently washing bedding in hot water, and removing carpeting. However, there is no way to completely rid the environment of airborne allergens.

Changing the diet may not always relieve symptoms of atopic dermatitis. A change may be helpful, however, when the medical history, laboratory studies, and specific symptoms strongly suggest a food allergy. It is up to the patient and his or her family and physician to decide whether the dietary restrictions are appropriate. Unless properly monitored by a physician or dietitian, diets with many restrictions can contribute to serious nutritional problems, especially in children.

Atopic Dermatitis and Quality of Life

Despite the symptoms caused by atopic dermatitis, it is possible for people with the disorder to maintain a good quality of life. The keys to quality of life lie in being well-informed; awareness of symptoms and their possible cause; and developing a partnership involving the patient or caregiving family member, medical doctor, and other health professionals. Good communication is essential.

When a child has atopic dermatitis, the entire family may be affected. It is helpful if families have additional support to help them cope with the stress and frustration associated with the disease. A child may be fussy and difficult and unable to keep from scratching and rubbing the skin. Distracting the child and providing activities that keep the hands busy are helpful but require much effort on the part of the parents or caregivers. Another issue families face is the social and emotional stress associated with changes in appearance caused by atopic dermatitis. The child may face difficulty in school or with social relationships and may need additional support and encouragement from family members.

Adults with atopic dermatitis can enhance their quality of life by caring regularly for their skin and being mindful of the effects of the disease and how to treat them. Adults should develop a skin care regimen as part of their daily routine, which can be adapted as circumstances and skin conditions change. Stress management and relaxation techniques may help decrease the likelihood of flares. Developing a network of support that includes family, friends, health professionals, and support groups or organizations can be beneficial. Chronic anxiety and depression may be relieved by short-term psychological therapy.

Recognizing the situations when scratching is most likely to occur may also help. For example, many patients find that they scratch more when they are idle, and they do better when engaged in activities that keep the hands occupied. Counseling also may be helpful to identify or change career goals if a job involves contact with irritants or involves frequent hand washing, such as work in a kitchen or auto machine shop.

Atopic Dermatitis and Vaccination against Smallpox

Although scientists are working to develop safer vaccines, individuals diagnosed with atopic dermatitis (or eczema) should not receive the current smallpox vaccine. According to the Centers for Disease Control and Prevention (CDC), a U.S. Government organization, individuals who have ever been diagnosed with atopic dermatitis, even if the condition is mild or not presently active, are more likely to develop a serious complication if they are exposed to the virus from the smallpox vaccine.

People with atopic dermatitis should exercise caution when coming into close physical contact with a person who has been recently vaccinated, and make certain the vaccinated person has covered the vaccination site or taken other precautions until the scab falls off (about 3 weeks). Those who have had physical contact with a vaccinated person's unhealed vaccination site or to their bedding or other items that might have touched that site should notify their doctor, particularly if they develop a new or unusual rash.

During a smallpox outbreak, these vaccination recommendations may change. People with atopic dermatitis who have been exposed to smallpox should consult their doctor about vaccination.

Current Research

Researchers supported by the National Institute of Arthritis and Musculoskeletal and Skin Diseases and other institutes of the National Institutes of Health are gaining a better understanding of what causes atopic dermatitis and how it can be managed, treated, and, ultimately, prevented.

Genetics: Although atopic dermatitis runs in families, the role of genetics (inheritance) remains unclear. It does appear that more than one gene is involved in the disease.

Research has helped shed light on the way atopic dermatitis is inherited. Studies show that children are at increased risk for developing the disorder if there is a family history of other atopic disease, such as hay fever or asthma. The risk is significantly higher if both parents have an atopic disease. In addition, studies of identical twins (who have the same genes) show that a person whose identical twin has atopic dermatitis is seven times more likely to have atopic dermatitis than someone in the general population. A person whose fraternal (nonidentical) twin has atopic dermatitis is three times more likely to have atopic dermatitis than someone in the general population. These findings suggest that genes play an important role in determining who gets the disease.

Also, scientists have discovered mutations in a certain gene that plays a role in the production of a protein called filaggrin. The filaggrin protein is normally found in the outermost layer of the skin and functions as a component of the skin barrier. The gene mutation disrupts filaggrin's ability to maintain a normal skin barrier and appears to be a genetic factor that predisposes people to develop atopic dermatitis and other diseases in which the skin barrier is compromised.

Biochemical abnormalities: Scientists suspect that changes in the skin's protective barrier make people with atopic dermatitis more sensitive to irritants. Such people have lower levels of fatty acids (substances that provide moisture and elasticity) in their skin, which causes dryness and reduces the skin's ability to control inflammation. Researchers continue to search for treatments that help keep the skin intact and prevent flares.

Other research points to a possible defect in a type of white blood cell called a monocyte. In people with atopic dermatitis, monocytes appear to play a role in the decreased production of an immune system hormone called interferon gamma, which helps regulate allergic reactions. This defect may cause exaggerated immune and inflammatory responses in the blood and tissues of people with atopic dermatitis.

Faulty regulation of immunoglobulin E (IgE): As already described in the section on diagnosis, IgE is a type of antibody that controls the immune system's allergic response. An antibody is a special protein produced by the immune system that recognizes and helps fight and destroy viruses, bacteria, and other foreign substances that invade the body. Normally, IgE is present in very small amounts, but levels are high in about 80 percent of people with atopic dermatitis.

In allergic diseases, IgE antibodies are produced in response to different allergens. When an allergen comes into contact with IgE on specialized immune cells, the cells release various chemicals, including histamine. These chemicals cause the symptoms of an allergic reaction, such as wheezing, sneezing, runny eyes, and itching. The release of histamine and other chemicals alone cannot explain the typical long-term symptoms of the disease. Research is underway to identify factors that may explain why too much IgE is produced and how it plays a role in the disease.

Immune system imbalance: Researchers also think that an imbalance in the immune system may contribute to the development of atopic dermatitis. It appears that the part of the immune system responsible for stimulating IgE is overactive, and the part that handles skin viral and fungal infections is underactive. Indeed, the skin of people with atopic dermatitis shows increased susceptibility to skin infections. This imbalance appears to result in the skin's inability to prevent inflammation, even in areas of skin that appear normal. In one project, scientists are studying the role of the infectious bacterium *Staphylococcus aureus* (*S. aureus*) in atopic dermatitis.

Researchers believe that one type of immune cell in the skin, called a Langerhans cell, may be involved in atopic dermatitis. Langerhans cells pick up viruses, bacteria, allergens, and other foreign substances that invade the body and deliver them to other cells in the immune defense system. Langerhans cells appear to be hyperactive in the skin of people with atopic diseases. Certain Langerhans cells are particularly potent at activating white blood cells called T cells in atopic skin, which produce proteins that promote allergic response. This function results in an exaggerated response of the skin to tiny amounts of allergens.

Scientists have also developed mouse models to study step-by-step changes in the immune system in atopic dermatitis, which may eventually lead to a treatment that effectively targets the immune system.

Drug research: Some researchers are focusing on new treatments for atopic dermatitis, including biologic agents, fatty acid supplements, and phototherapy. For example, they are studying how ultraviolet light affects the skin's immune system in healthy and diseased skin. They are also investigating biologic response modifiers, or biologics, which are a new family of genetically engineered drugs that block specific molecular pathways of the immune system that are involved in the inflammatory process. A clinical trial is underway to test a drug to see if it can help control the itching associated with atopic dermatitis.

Researchers also continue to look for drugs that suppress the immune system. Also, anti-inflammatory drugs have been developed that affect multiple cells and cell functions, and may prove to be an effective alternative to corticosteroids in the treatment of atopic dermatitis.

Other research: Several experimental treatments are being evaluated that attempt to replace substances that are deficient in people with atopic dermatitis.

Evening primrose oil is a substance rich in gamma-linolenic acid, one of the fatty acids that is decreased in the skin of people with atopic dermatitis. Studies to date using evening primrose oil have yielded contradictory results. In addition, dietary fatty acid supplements have not proven highly effective.

There is also a great deal of interest in the use of herbs and plant extracts to treat the disease. Studies to date show some benefit, but not without concerns about toxicity and the risks involved in suppressing the immune system without close medical supervision.

Section 10.2

Taking Care of Your Skin If You Have AD

"Bathing and Moisturizing," © 2009 National Eczema Association. Reprinted with permission. For additional information, visit www.nationaleczema.org or www.easeeczema.org.

What is eczema?

Eczema is a chronic recurring skin disorder that results in dry, easily irritated, itchy skin. There is no cure for eczema, but good daily skin care is essential to controlling the disease.

What are the characteristics of dry skin?

When your skin is dry, it is not because it lacks grease or oil, but because it fails to retain water. For this reason, a good daily skin care regimen focuses on the basics of bathing and moisturizing.

What other factors create dry skin?

Wind, low humidity, cold temperature, excessive washing without use of moisturizers, and use of harsh, drying soaps can all cause dry skin and aggravate eczema.

How do I take care of my dry skin?

The most important treatment for dry skin is to put water back in it. The best way to get water into your skin is to briefly soak in a bath or shower and to moisturize immediately afterwards.

Use of an effective moisturizer several times every day improves skin hydration and barrier function. Moisturizer should be applied to the hands every time they are washed or in contact with water.

The goal of bathing and moisturizing is to help heal the skin. To repair the skin, we need to decrease water loss.

Some dermatologists recommend that you perform your bathing and moisturizing regime at night just before going to bed. You are unlikely to further dry out or irritate your skin while sleeping, so the water can be more thoroughly absorbed into your skin.

If you have hand eczema dermatologists recommend that you soak your hands in water, apply prescription medications and moisturizer (preferably Vaseline), and put on pure cotton gloves before going to sleep.

If I am on prescription drugs for my eczema, do I still need to moisturize?

Basic skin care can enhance the effect of prescription drugs, and it can prevent or minimize the severity of eczema relapse.

What are the basics of bathing and moisturizing?

- Take at least one bath or shower per day. Use warm, not hot, water for at least 5 to 10 minutes. Avoid scrubbing your skin with a washcloth.

- Use a gentle cleansing bar or wash, no soap. During a severe flare, you may choose to limit the use of cleansers to avoid possible irritation.

- While your skin is still wet (within 3 minutes of taking a bath or shower), apply any special skin medications prescribed for you and then liberally apply a moisturizer. This will seal in the water and make the skin less dry and itchy.

- Be sure to apply any special skin medications to areas affected with eczema before moisturizing. The most common skin medications used to treat skin inflammation are prescription and non-prescription topical steroids or prescription topical immunomodulators (TIMS). Used correctly, these medications are safe and effective. (Remember that TIMS can sting if applied to wet skin, so apply a thin coat to affected areas only.)

- Be sure to apply moisturizer on all areas of your skin whether it has or has not been treated with medication. Specific occlusives or moisturizers may be individually recommended for you. Moisturizers are available in many forms. Creams and ointments are more beneficial than lotions. Vaseline® is a good occlusive preparation to seal in the water; however, it contains no water so it only works effectively after a soaking bath.

How does water help my skin?

- Water hydrates the stratum corneum (the top layer of skin).

- Water softens skin so the topical medications and moisturizers can be absorbed.
- Water removes allergens and irritants.
- Water cleanses, debrides, and removes crusted tissue.
- Water is relaxing and reduces stress.

Is water an irritant or a treatment?

Water irritates skin if:

- skin is frequently wet without the immediate application of an effective moisturizer;
- moisture evaporates, causing the skin barrier to become dry and irritated.

Water hydrates skin if:

- after skin is wet, an effective moisturizer is applied within 3 minutes;
- hydration is retained, keeping the skin barrier intact and flexible.

What are some cleansing tips?

- Gently cleanse your skin each day.
- Use mild, non-soap cleansers.
- Use fragrance-free, dye-free, neutral-pH (pH lower than 5.5) soaps.
- Moisturize immediately after cleansing while your skin is still wet.
- Avoid scrubbing with a washcloth or towel; pat instead.

What soap should I use?

Our skin is not nearly as alkaline as most soap is: Our skin's normal pH is about 4 to 5.5 and the average pH of soap is 9 to 10.5. So, you see, soap is actually not recommended.

Following are a few non-soap cleanser suggestions:

- Aquaphor® Gentle Wash
- AVEENO® Advanced Care Wash

- Basis® Sensitive Skin Bar
- CeraVe™ Hydrating Cleanser
- Cetaphil® Gentle Cleansing Bar
- Dove® Sensitive Skin Unscented Beauty Bar
- Mustela® Stelatopia Cream Cleanser
- Oilatum® Cleansing Bar

What are some cleansing pitfalls?

- Aggressive scrubbing
- Use of astringents
- Cleansing without moisturizing
- Use of harsh soap-based cleansers

Harsh surfactants can damage epidermal barrier
Soaps with an alkaline pH can further disrupt skin barrier proteins and lipids.

What does cleansing remove?

- Sebum (an oily substance produced by certain glands in the skin)
- Apocrine and eccrine secretions (skin gland secretions, discarded cells)
- Environmental dirt
- Bacteria, fungus, yeast, and other microorganisms
- Desquamated keratinocytes (dead skin cells that are the normal product of skin maturation)
- Cosmetics, skin care products, medications

What is preferable, a bath or a shower? For how long? How often?

Short baths or showers (no more than 5 to10 minutes) keep the skin from drying out.
Keep the water comfortably warm, not hot or cold. Hot water dries skin quickly, so be sure to use lukewarm water.
Do not rub your skin.

Do not completely dry your skin after your bath or shower. Instead, pat yourself lightly with a towel if needed.

What type of bath should I take?

A soak in a tub of lukewarm water for 10 minutes will help the skin absorb water. You may wish to try one of the following for specific treatment:

- **Bleach baths:** Bleach baths make the tub into a swimming pool. Soak for about 10 minutes and rinse off. Soak for about 10 minutes and rinse off. Use 2–3 times per week. Bleach baths decrease the bacteria on the skin and decrease bacterial skin infections. Use 1/2 cup household bleach for a full bathtub, 1/4 for a half bath.

- **Vinegar baths:** Referred to as the "pickle the patient" treatment. Add 1 cup to 1 pint of vinegar to the bath. Can be used as a wet dressing too as it kills bacteria.

- **Bath oil baths:** Oils in the bath are a favorite of some providers and patients. Bath oils can leave the tub slippery—be careful. They can also leave a hard-to-clean film. See if they work for you.

- **Salt baths:** When there is a significant flare the bath water may sting or be uncomfortable. Add one cup of table salt to the bath water to decrease this side effect.

- **Baking soda baths:** Added to a bath or made into a paste it can be used to relieve the itching.

- **Tar baths:** Tar baths can sooth inflammation and itch. Tar bath oil or tar shampoo can be used. Warning: If the skin is open or excoriated the tar baths can sting.

- **Oatmeal baths:** Added to a bath or made into a paste it can be used to relieve the itching.

What does moisturizing do?

Moisturizing improves skin hydration and barrier function. Moisturizers are more effective when applied to skin that has been soaked in water.

What are the different kinds of moisturizers?

There are three basic classes of moisturizers:

- **Ointments** are semi-solid greases that help to hydrate the skin by preventing water loss. Petroleum jelly has no additional ingredients, whereas other ointments contain a small proportion of water or other ingredients to make the ointment more spreadable. Ointments are very good at helping the skin retain moisture but they are often disliked because of their greasiness.

- **Creams** are thick mixtures of greases in water or another liquid. They contain a lower proportion of grease than ointments, making them less greasy and more liked. A warning: Creams often contain stabilizers and preservatives to prevent separation of their main ingredients, and these additives can cause skin irritation for some people.

- **Lotions** are mixtures of oil and water, with water being the main ingredient. Most lotions do not function well as moisturizers for people with dry skin conditions because the water in the lotion evaporates quickly.

What moisturizer should I use?

Following are a few suggestions:

- Aquaphor® Healing Ointment
- AVEENO® Advanced Care Cream
- Crisco Regular Shortening
- CeraVe™ Moisturizing Cream
- Cetaphil® Moisturizing Cream
- Eucerin® Original Creme
- Moisturel® Therapeutic Cream
- Mustela® Stelatopia Moisturizing Cream
- Vanicream™ Moisturizing Skin Cream
- Vaseline® Petroleum Jelly

Apply moisturizer to your skin immediately after your bath or shower and throughout the day whenever your skin feels dry or itchy. Some people prefer to use creams and lotions during the day and ointments and creams at night. All of these moisturizers should be available through your local pharmacy or grocery store. If you don't see one on the shelf, ask the pharmacist to order it for you in the largest container

155

available. Buying your moisturizers in large containers like 1-pound jars may save you a great deal of money.

What are proper moisturizing techniques?

Just as it is important to use proper bathing techniques, it is important to properly apply moisturizers to your skin within 3 minutes of showering or bathing.

While your skin is still wet, apply prescription medications, and then apply a moisturizer to all your skin.

A thick bland product is best.

Take a glob of moisturizer from the jar, soften it by rubbing it between your hands, and apply it using the palm of your hand stroking in a downward direction.

Do **not** rub by stroking up and down or around in circles.

Leave a tacky film of moisturizer on your skin; it will be absorbed in a few minutes.

Everyone has different preferences concerning how products feel on their skin, so try different products until you find one that feels comfortable. Continue use of the moisturizer(s) even after the affected area heals to prevent recurrence.

How can I reduce skin irritation?

After bathing and moisturizing, the next important step is to attempt to reduce skin irritation.

- Don't scratch or rub the skin. These actions can worsen any itch. Instead, apply a moisturizer whenever the skin feels dry or itchy. A cool gel pack can provide some relief from itch.

- Wash all new clothes before wearing them. This removes formaldehyde and other potentially irritating chemicals which are used during production and packing.

- Add a second rinse cycle to ensure the removal of soap if you are concerned. Use a mild soap that is dye-free and fragrance-free.

- Wear garments that allow air to pass freely to your skin. Open-weave, loose-fitting, cotton-blend clothing may be most comfortable. Avoid wearing wool.

- Wet wrap therapy can effectively rehydrate and calm the skin. Soak in a bath, and then apply moisturizer. Medication should also be applied if currently prescribed. The bandages, moistened in warm water until they are slightly damp, are then wrapped around the area. Dry bandages are wrapped over the wet bandages. In place of bandages, moistened pajamas worn underneath a set of dry pajamas can be used with children and infants.

- Work and sleep in comfortable surroundings with a fairly constant temperature and humidity level. Cooler temperatures are preferred but not so cool as to initiate chilling.

- Keep fingernails very short and smooth by filing them daily to help prevent damage due to scratching.

- Make appropriate use of sedating antihistamines, which may reduce itching to some degree through their tranquilizing and sedative effects.

- Use sunscreen on a regular basis and always avoid getting sunburned. Use a sunscreen with an SPF of 15 or higher. Sunscreens made for the face are often less irritating than regular sunscreens. Zinc oxide or titanium dioxide–based products are less irritating.

- Go for a swim, which can provide good hydration. Chlorine can also decrease bacteria on the skin that can cause itching or develop into an infection. Of course, residual chlorine or bromine left on the skin after swimming in a pool or hot tub may be irritating, so take a quick shower or bath immediately after swimming, washing with a mild cleanser from head to toe, and then apply an appropriate moisturizer while still wet.

The National Eczema Association (NEA) thanks Anna L. Bruckner, MD, Sarah Chamlin, MD, and Sandra Oehlke, CPNP, for their editorial contributions.

This information sets forth current opinions from recognized authorities, but it does not dictate an exclusive treatment course. Persons with questions about a medical condition should consult a physician who is knowledgeable about that condition.

Chapter 11

Allergic Contact Dermatitis

Chapter Contents

Section 11.1

Overview of Contact Dermatitis

"Contact Dermatitis," © 2010 A.D.A.M., Inc. Reprinted with permission.

Causes

Contact dermatitis is an inflammation of the skin caused by direct contact with an irritating or allergy-causing substance (irritant or allergen). Reactions may vary in the same person over time. A history of any type of allergies increases the risk for this condition.

Irritant dermatitis, the most common type of contact dermatitis, involves inflammation resulting from contact with acids, alkaline materials such as soaps and detergents, solvents, or other chemicals. The reaction usually resembles a burn.

Allergic contact dermatitis, the second most common type of contact dermatitis, is caused by exposure to a substance or material to which you have become extra sensitive or allergic. The allergic reaction is often delayed, with the rash appearing 24–48 hours after exposure. The skin inflammation varies from mild irritation and redness to open sores, depending on the type of irritant, the body part affected, and your sensitivity.

Overtreatment dermatitis is a form of contact dermatitis that occurs when treatment for another skin disorder causes irritation.

Common allergens associated with contact dermatitis include:

- poison ivy, poison oak, poison sumac;
- other plants;
- nickel or other metals;
- medications:
  - antibiotics, especially those applied to the surface of the skin (topical);
  - topical anesthetics;
  - other medications;
- rubber or latex;

- cosmetics;
- fabrics and clothing;
- detergents;
- solvents;
- adhesives;
- fragrances, perfumes;
- other chemicals and substances.

Contact dermatitis may involve a reaction to a substance that you are exposed to, or use repeatedly. Although there may be no initial reaction, regular use (for example, nail polish remover, preservatives in contact lens solutions, or repeated contact with metals in earring posts and the metal backs of watches) can eventually cause sensitivity and reaction to the product.

Some products cause a reaction only when they contact the skin and are exposed to sunlight (photosensitivity). These include shaving lotions, sunscreens, sulfa ointments, some perfumes, coal tar products, and oil from the skin of a lime. A few airborne allergens, such as ragweed or insecticide spray, can cause contact dermatitis.

Symptoms

- Itching (pruritus) of the skin in exposed areas
- Skin redness or inflammation in the exposed area
- Tenderness of the skin in the exposed area
- Localized swelling of the skin
- Warmth of the exposed area (may occur)
- Skin lesion or rash at the site of exposure
  - Lesions of any type: redness, rash, papules (pimple-like), vesicles, and bullae (blisters)
  - May involve oozing, draining, or crusting
  - May become scaly, raw, or thickened

Exams and Tests

The diagnosis is primarily based on the skin appearance and a history of exposure to an irritant or an allergen.

According to the American Academy of Allergy, Asthma, and Immunology, "patch testing is the gold standard for contact allergen identification." Allergy testing with skin patches may isolate the suspected allergen that is causing the reaction.

Patch testing is used for patients who have chronic, recurring contact dermatitis. It requires three office visits and must be done by a clinician with detailed experience in the procedures and interpretation of results. On the first visit, small patches of potential allergens are applied to the skin. These patches are removed 48 hours later to see if a reaction has occurred. A third visit approximately 2 days later is to evaluate for any delayed reaction. You should bring suspected materials with you, especially if you have already tested those materials on a small area of your skin and noticed a reaction.

Other tests may be used to rule out other possible causes, including skin lesion biopsy or culture of the skin lesion.

Treatment

Initial treatment includes thorough washing with lots of water to remove any trace of the irritant that may remain on the skin. You should avoid further exposure to known irritants or allergens.

In some cases, the best treatment is to do nothing to the area.

Corticosteroid skin creams or ointments may reduce inflammation. Carefully follow the instructions when using these creams, because overuse, even of low-strength over-the-counter products, may cause a troublesome skin condition. In severe cases, systemic corticosteroids may be needed to reduce inflammation. These are usually tapered gradually over about 12 days to prevent recurrence of the rash. In addition to or instead of corticosteroid skin treatment, your doctor may prescribe tacrolimus ointment or pimecrolimus cream.

Wet dressings and soothing anti-itch (antipruritic) or drying lotions may be recommended to reduce other symptoms.

Outlook (Prognosis)

Contact dermatitis usually clears up without complications within 2 or 3 weeks, but may return if the substance or material that caused it cannot be identified or avoided. A change of occupation or occupational habits may be necessary if the disorder is caused by occupational exposure.

Possible Complications

Secondary bacterial skin infections may occur.

When to Contact a Medical Professional

Call your health care provider if symptoms indicate contact dermatitis and it is severe or there is no improvement after treatment.

Prevention

Avoid contact with known allergens. Use protective gloves or other barriers if contact with substances is likely or unavoidable. Wash skin surfaces thoroughly after contact with substances. Avoid overtreating skin disorders.

Alternative Names

Dermatitis—contact; Allergic dermatitis; Dermatitis—allergic

References

Gober MD, DeCapite TJ, Gaspari AA. Contact dermatitis. In: Adkinson NF Jr, ed. *Middleton's Allergy: Principles and Practice*. 7th ed. Philadelphia, Pa: Mosby Elsevier; 2008:chap 63.

Habif TP. Contact dermatitis and patch testing. In: Habif TP, ed. *Clinical Dermatology*. 5th ed. Philadelphia, Pa: Mosby Elsevier; 2009:chap 4.

Section 11.2

Outsmarting Poison Ivy and Other Poisonous Plants

From "Outsmarting Poison Ivy and Other Poisonous Plants," by the U.S. Food and Drug Administration (FDA, www.fda.gov), September 2, 2008.

First comes the itching, then a red rash, and then blisters. These symptoms of poison ivy, poison oak, and poison sumac can start from a few hours to several days after exposure to the plant oil found in the sap of these poisonous plants.

Poison Ivy

This plant (see Figure 11.1, right) is found throughout the United States except Alaska, Hawaii, and parts of the West Coast. It can grow as a vine or shrub. Each leaf has three glossy leaflets, with smooth or toothed edges. Leaves are reddish in spring, green in summer, and yellow, orange, or red in fall. It may have white berries.

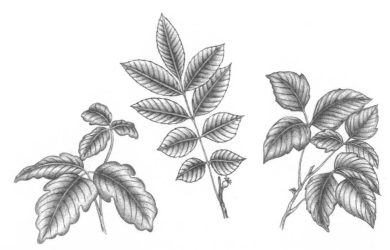

Figure 11.1. *Poison Oak, left; Poison Sumac, middle; and Poison Ivy, right (drawing by Alison DeKlein).*

Poison Oak

This plant (see Figure 11.1, left) grows as a low shrub in the eastern United States, and in tall clumps or long vines on Pacific Coast. Fuzzy green leaves in clusters of three are lobed or deeply toothed with rounded tips. It may have yellow-white berries.

Poison Sumac

This plant (see Figure 11.1, middle) grows as a tall shrub or small tree in bogs or swamps in Northeast, Midwest, and parts of the Southeast. Each leaf has clusters of seven to 13 smooth-edged leaflets. Leaves are orange in spring, green in summer, and yellow, orange, or red in fall. It may have yellow-white berries.

Not Contagious

Poison ivy and other poison plant rashes can't be spread from person to person. But it is possible to pick up the rash from plant oil that may have stuck to clothing, pets, garden tools, and other items that have come in contact with these plants. The plant oil lingers (sometimes for years) on virtually any surface until it's washed off with water or rubbing alcohol.

The rash will only occur where the plant oil has touched the skin, so a person with poison ivy can't spread it on the body by scratching. It may seem like the rash is spreading if it appears over time instead of all at once. But this is either because the plant oil is absorbed at different rates in different parts of the body or because of repeated exposure to contaminated objects or plant oil trapped under the fingernails. Even if blisters break, the fluid in the blisters is not plant oil and cannot further spread the rash.

Tips for Prevention

- Learn what poison ivy, oak, and sumac plants look like so you can avoid them.

- Wash your garden tools and gloves regularly. If you think you may be working around poison ivy, wear long sleeves, long pants tucked into boots, and gloves.

- Wash your pet if it may have brushed up against poison ivy, oak, or sumac. Use pet shampoo and water while wearing rubber gloves, such as dishwashing gloves. Most pets are not sensitive to poison ivy, but the oil can stick to their fur and cause a reaction in someone who pets them.

- Wash your skin in cool water as soon as possible if you come in contact with a poisonous plant. The sooner you cleanse the skin, the greater the chance that you can remove the plant oil or help prevent further spread.

- Use the topical product Ivy Block if you know you will come into contact with the poisonous plants. This FDA-approved product is available over the counter (OTC).

Tips for Treatment

Don't scratch the blisters. Bacteria from under your fingernails can get into the blisters and cause an infection. The rash, blisters, and itch normally disappear in several weeks without any treatment. But you can relieve the itch by:

- using wet compresses or soaking in cool water;

- applying over-the-counter (OTC) topical corticosteroid preparations or taking prescription oral corticosteroids;

- applying topical OTC skin protectants, such as calamine, labeled to dry oozing and weeping or to relieve itching and irritation caused by poison ivy, poison oak, and poison sumac.

See a doctor:

- if you have a temperature over 100 degrees Fahrenheit;

- if there is pus, soft yellow scabs, or tenderness on the rash;

- if the itching gets worse or keeps you awake at night;

- if the rash spreads to your eyes, mouth, genital area, or covers more than one fourth of your skin area;

- if the rash is not improving within a few days.

Section 11.3

Allergic Contact Rashes

Allergic contact dermatitis is an itchy skin condition caused by an allergic reaction to material in contact with the skin. It arises some hours after contact with the responsible material, and settles down over some days providing the skin is no longer in contact with it.

Contact dermatitis should be distinguished from contact urticaria, in which a rash appears within minutes of exposure and fades away within minutes to hours. The allergic reaction to latex is the best known example of allergic contact urticaria.

Allergic contact dermatitis is also distinct from irritant contact dermatitis, in which a similar skin condition is caused by excessive contact with irritants. Irritants include water, soaps, detergents, solvents, acids, alkalis, and friction. Irritant contact dermatitis may affect anyone, providing they have had enough exposure to the irritant, but those with atopic dermatitis are particularly sensitive. Most cases of hand dermatitis are due to contact with irritants.

Allergy is the term given to a reaction by a small number of people to a substance (known as the allergen) which is harmless to those who are not allergic to it. Only small quantities of allergen are necessary to induce the reaction. Contact allergy occurs predominantly from the allergen on the skin rather than from internal sources or food. The first contact does not result in allergy; often the person has been able to touch the material for many years without adverse reaction.

Clinical Features

The dermatitis is generally confined to the site of contact with the allergen, although severe cases may extend outside the contact area or it may become generalized. Sometimes the allergen is transmitted from the fingers so unexpected sites can be affected, e.g. the eyelids and genitals. Dermatitis is unlikely to be due to a specific allergen if the area of skin most in contact with that allergen is unaffected. The affected skin may be red, swollen and blistered, or dry and bumpy.

Some typical examples of allergic contact dermatitis include:

- an eczema of the wrist underlying a watch strap due to contact allergy to nickel;

- an eczema of the lower leg when ankle strapping has been removed due to contact allergy to rosin in the adhesive plaster;

- hand dermatitis caused by thiuram, an antioxidant chemical used in the manufacture of rubber gloves;

- itchy red face due to contact allergy with Kathon CG, a preservative in a moisturizer.

Some substances are particularly prone to cause contact allergy. In New Zealand, contact with plants related to the Japanese Wax Tree (*Toxicodendron succedaneum*) results in allergic dermatitis in the majority of people, characteristically resulting in severe blisters and swelling.

Other common allergies are to nickel (jewelry), fragrances, preservatives, rubber (gloves), dye (hair colorants), adhesives of various kinds, and topical medications such as antibiotics. There is a very long list of materials that have caused contact allergy in a small number of individuals.

Photoallergy

Sometimes contact allergy arises only after the skin has been exposed to ultraviolet light. The rash is confined to sun exposed areas even though the allergen may have been in contact with covered areas. This is called photocontact dermatitis.

Examples include:

- dermatitis due to a sunscreen chemical, affecting the top but not the under surface of the arm;

- dermatitis of face, neck, arms and hands due to antiseptic in soap.

Testing for Contact Allergy

Sometimes it is easy to recognize contact allergy and no specific tests are necessary. The rash usually (but not always) completely clears up if the allergen is no longer in contact with the skin, but recurs even with slight contact with it again.

The open user test is used to confirm contact allergy to a cosmetic such as a moisturizer. The product under suspicion is applied several times daily for several days to a small area of sensitive skin. The inner aspect of the upper arm is suitable. Contact allergy is likely if dermatitis arises in the treated area.

If you think you may have a contact allergy, consult a dermatologist to have patch tests performed.

Treatment

It is important to recognize how you are in contact with the responsible substance so that, where possible, you can avoid it.

- Find out precisely what you are allergic to by having comprehensive patch tests.

- Identify where the allergen is found.

- Carefully study your environment to locate the allergen. Note: Many chemicals have several names, and cross-reactions to similar chemicals with different names are common.

- Ask your dermatologist to help.

Active dermatitis is usually treated with the following:

- Emollient creams

- Topical steroids

- Topical or oral antibiotics for secondary infection

- Oral steroids, usually short courses, for severe cases

- Photochemotherapy

- Azathioprine, ciclosporin, or other immunosuppressive agent

- Tacrolimus ointment and pimecrolimus cream are immune modulating drugs that inhibit calcineurin and may prove helpful for allergic contact dermatitis. Pimecrolimus has recently become available in New Zealand.

Contact allergy may disappear but often persists indefinitely.

Chapter 12

Other Allergic Skin Reactions

Chapter Contents

Section 12.1

Urticaria (Hives)

What are hives?

Hives, or urticaria, are raised swellings of the skin or mucous membranes. The raised swelling is called a wheal, or a welt. A red ring surrounds the wheal. This is called the flair. The size of each hive may vary greatly, from a tiny spot to a swollen, red area several inches in diameter. The hives may cover just one small area or cover large area of the body. In infants and young children, hives may cause swelling of the arms and legs. Hives may come, go, and then come back again on another area of the body. Hives can be very itchy. Most hives occur suddenly and then go away completely.

Hives are usually not serious and go away with minimal treatment. Sometimes, the reaction may be more severe.

If the face, lips, tongue or throat swell, there may be wheezing or difficulty breathing. This can be life-threatening. If it happens, call 911 for transportation to a hospital.

What causes them?

The most common cause of hives is an allergy to foods and drugs. Other causes are infections, immunizations, insect bites, or inhaled allergens. Heat, cold, or stress can cause hives. In some children, pressure on the skin, sunlight, or sweating during exercise can cause hives. The exact cause of hives cannot be identified in most children. Write down everything that was eaten (food, liquids, medicines, candy, etc.) in the past 24 to 48 hours. This may help find a cause if the hives come back at another time.

How long do they last?

A single hive rarely lasts more than 12 to 48 hours. Hives caused by a food or drug reaction generally last a few days to several weeks.

Some children have chronic hives, which means the hives have lasted for more than 6 weeks. Chronic hives may occur on and off from several months to several years. Hives caused by viral illnesses normally come and go for 3 or 4 days, then disappear. Some hives may come and go for as long as several weeks to months.

How are hives treated?

Treatment works better if the cause of the hives is found and eliminated. Treatment may include:

- Antihistamines such as Benadryl® relieve the hives and itching for most children. To prevent the return of hives, antihistamines are often continued for 1 to 2 weeks after the hives are gone.

- Corticosteroids may be given if your child does not get relief from antihistamines.

- Epinephrine may be given as a shot to give fast relief of acute, severe hives or problems breathing.

- For hives possibly caused by pollens, animal contact, or playing in the grass or weeds, give your child a shower or bath. Wash all clothing your child was wearing at the time.

Alert: Call your child's doctor, nurse, or clinic if you have any questions or concerns or if your child has special health care needs that were not covered by this information.

This information is meant to provide you with additional information about your child's care. Diagnosis, treatment, and follow-up should be provided by your health care professional.

Section 12.2

Photosensitivity: Exposure to Light Can Cause Allergic Reactions

Some people are sensitive to sunlight; this is known as photosensitivity. Photosensitivity may produce a rash, which is known by the general term, photodermatosis.

Patients may not associate their skin complaint with exposure to light. It is not always the bright summer sun which is responsible; some people also react to sunlight in winter, and very sensitive subjects may even be affected by fluorescent lamps indoors.

Ultraviolet Radiation

Sunlight contains both ordinary visible light and shorter invisible light rays called ultraviolet radiation (UVR). UVR can produce tanning but also causes burning and skin cancer.

UVR is divided into UVB (short wavelength rays that cause sunburn and tan) and UVA (longer wavelength tanning rays). Patients can be sensitive to one kind of sunlight (i.e. only to UVB, UVA, or visible light) or to a wider range of radiation. The most common photosensitivity is to UVA.

Cause of Photosensitivity and Photodermatoses

Photosensitivity occurs for a variety of reasons. These can be classified into the following groups.

Idiopathic Photodermatoses

Cause is unknown but exposure to UV light produces a clearly defined disease entity. These include:

- polymorphic light eruption;
- juvenile spring eruption;
- actinic prurigo;
- solar urticaria;
- chronic actinic dermatitis;
- hydroa vacciniforme;
- pseudoporphyria.

Exogenous Photodermatoses

Photosensitivity is caused by the introduction of an external agent that is applied topically or administered internally. These agents are called photosensitizers and include:

- medicines, e.g. amiodarone, tetracyclines;
- contact with plant, vegetable, fruit, chemicals, fragrances, dyes, disinfectants.

Metabolic Photodermatoses

Photosensitivity is caused by a metabolic defect or imbalance of a body chemical. The most common disorders of this type are porphyrias, in which there are increased porphyrins in the skin.

- Porphyria cutanea tarda
- Erythropoietic protoporphyria
- Variegate porphyria
- Erythropoietic porphyria (Günther's disease)

Photoexacerbated Dermatoses

Photosensitivity is caused by a pre-existing disease or skin. These include conditions such as:

- lupus erythematosus (especially subacute and systemic forms);
- dermatomyositis;
- Darier's disease;
- rosacea;
- pemphigus;
- atopic dermatitis;
- psoriasis.

Genetic Photodermatoses

Photosensitivity is caused by a pre-existing genetic disorder, e.g.:

- xeroderma pigmentosum;
- Bloom syndrome;
- Rothmund Thomson syndrome.

Although most people with the common skin conditions psoriasis and atopic dermatitis (eczema) find sun exposure or ultraviolet light treatment helpful, about 10% report they cause flare-ups.

How Do You Confirm the Skin Is Photosensitive?

Photosensitivity can be confirmed by phototests—artificial light from various different sources is shone on small areas of the skin to see whether the rash can be reproduced, or if sunburn occurs more easily than expected.

Photosensitivity induced by contact with certain items can be tested by photopatch tests. Adhesive patches containing known photosensitizing materials are applied to the upper back, removed after 2 days, and light is shone on the area. The reaction is observed 2 days later.

Sun Protection

UVR is present in significant quantities in New Zealand between September and April. There is enough UVR to cause a rash on photosensitive skin between 10 a.m. and 5 p.m. even on a cloudy day. Bright surfaces, like snow, concrete, and sand, reflect UVR and can nearly double the amount that gets to the skin.

- Confine summer excursions out of doors to early in the morning or late in the evening.
- Sun protection is needed whatever the weather. It is needed even if you sit in the shade.
- Protect yourself in the car and house, too; UVA can pass through window glass.

There are two basic ways of protecting your skin from the damaging effects of UVR:

- Block out all light with an opaque material such as sun protective clothing. Dark colored and densely woven fabric is the most effective. Wear shirts with high collar and long sleeves, trousers or a long skirt, socks and shoes, a wide-brimmed hat, and if possible gloves. Some clothes are now labeled with UPF, the sun protection factor for fabrics. Choose those with a UPF of 40+.

- Use topical sunscreen agents.

  - Physical blocker/reflectant sunscreens: These are very effective sunscreens as they block out UVA and UVB by reflecting the ultraviolet radiation. Their only drawback is they can be messy to use and cosmetically unappealing.

  - Chemical sunscreens: It is vital that photosensitive individuals select a sunscreen with a very high Sun Protection Factor (SPF 30+), which is a water resistant and broad spectrum product that complies with current Australian and New Zealand Standard for Sunscreens (AS/NZS2604:1998). Ask your dermatologist which products are most suitable for you.

Unfortunately, photosensitive patients often find it difficult to find a sunscreen they can tolerate. Contact allergy or contact photodermatitis to the sunscreening chemicals themselves can occur, although this is uncommon, particularly benzophenone or butyl methoxy dibenzoyl methane, and in the past, PABA [para-aminobenzoic acid]. Patch and photopatch tests will identify which ones are safe for you.

Other Measures

Oral antioxidants may provide some extra protection, particularly *Polypodium leucotomos*.

UVR-absorbing film can be applied to windows at home or in the car (e.g. Bonwyke DermaGard). Masks can be made to cover the face for trips outside too (clear ones are available), but not surprisingly, only the most disabled patients are prepared to wear these.

Unguarded fluorescent daylight lamps can occasionally provoke a rash, because they may produce some ultraviolet radiation (UVA). Ordinary tungsten light bulbs are usually all right. It is perfectly safe to watch television.

For the most severely light sensitive patients, normal activities may be severely curtailed. Some find night work and sleep during the day, others put up with the rash. Nearly always, medications in the form of ointments or tablets can help to a variable extent.

Chapter 13

Anaphylaxis: Life-Threatening Allergies

Chapter Contents

Section 13.1

Signs of Anaphylaxis

Causes

Anaphylaxis is a severe, whole-body allergic reaction. After being exposed to a substance like bee sting venom, the person's immune system becomes sensitized to that allergen. On a later exposure, an allergic reaction may occur. This reaction is sudden, severe, and involves the whole body.

Tissues in different parts of the body release histamine and other substances. This causes the airways to tighten and leads to other symptoms.

Some drugs (polymyxin, morphine, x-ray dye, and others) may cause an anaphylactic-like reaction (anaphylactoid reaction) when people are first exposed to them. This is usually due to a toxic reaction, rather than the immune system response that occurs with "true" anaphylaxis.

The symptoms, risk for complications without treatment, and treatment are the same, however, for both types of reactions.

Anaphylaxis can occur in response to any allergen. Common causes include:

- drug allergies;

- food allergies;

- insect bites/stings.

Pollens and other inhaled allergens rarely cause anaphylaxis. Some people have an anaphylactic reaction with no known cause.

Anaphylaxis rarely occurs. However, it is life-threatening and can occur at any time. Risks include history of any type of allergic reaction.

Symptoms

Symptoms develop rapidly, often within seconds or minutes. They may include the following:

- Abdominal pain or cramping
- Abnormal (high-pitched) breathing sounds
- Anxiety
- Confusion
- Cough
- Diarrhea
- Difficulty breathing
- Fainting, light-headedness, dizziness
- Hives, itchiness
- Nasal congestion
- Nausea, vomiting
- Sensation of feeling the heart beat (palpitations)
- Skin redness
- Slurred speech
- Wheezing

Exams and Tests

Signs include:

- abnormal heart rhythm (arrhythmia);
- fluid in the lungs (pulmonary edema);
- hives;
- low blood pressure;
- mental confusion;
- rapid pulse;
- skin that is blue from lack of oxygen or pale from shock;
- swelling (angioedema) in the throat that may be severe enough to block the airway;
- swelling of the eyes or face;
- weakness;
- wheezing.

The health care provider will wait to test for the specific allergen that caused anaphylaxis (if the cause is not obvious) until after treatment.

Treatment

Anaphylaxis is an emergency condition requiring immediate professional medical attention. Call 911 immediately.

Check the ABCs (airway, breathing, and circulation from Basic Life Support) in all suspected anaphylactic reactions.

CPR should be started, if needed. People with known severe allergic reactions may carry an Epi-Pen or other allergy kit, and should be helped if necessary.

Paramedics or physicians may place a tube through the nose or mouth into the airways (endotracheal intubation) or perform emergency surgery to place a tube directly into the trachea (tracheostomy or cricothyrotomy).

Epinephrine should be given by injection in the thigh muscle right away. This opens the airways and raises the blood pressure by tightening blood vessels.

Treatment for shock includes fluids through a vein (intravenous) and medications that support the actions of the heart and circulatory system.

The person may receive antihistamines, such as diphenhydramine, and corticosteroids, such as prednisone, to further reduce symptoms (after lifesaving measures and epinephrine are administered).

Outlook (Prognosis)

Anaphylaxis is a severe disorder that can be life-threatening without prompt treatment. However, symptoms usually get better with the right therapy, so it is important to act right away.

Possible Complications

- Airway blockage
- Cardiac arrest (no effective heartbeat)
- Respiratory arrest (no breathing)
- Shock

When to Contact a Medical Professional

Call 911 if you develop severe symptoms of anaphylaxis. If you are with another person, he or she may take you to the nearest emergency room.

Prevention

Avoid known allergens. Any person experiencing an allergic reaction should be monitored, although monitoring may be done at home in mild cases.

Occasionally, people who have a history of drug allergies may safely be given the medication they are allergic to after being pretreated with corticosteroids (prednisone) and antihistamines (diphenhydramine).

People who have a history of allergy to insect bites/stings should carry (and use) an emergency kit containing injectable epinephrine and chewable antihistamine. They should also wear a MedicAlert or similar bracelet or necklace stating their allergy.

Alternative Names

Anaphylactic reaction; Anaphylactic shock; Shock—anaphylactic

References

The diagnosis and management of anaphylaxis: An updated practice parameter. *J Allergy Clin Immunol.* 2005;115(3 Suppl):S483–S523.

Sicherer SH, Simons FE, Section on Allergy and Immunology, American Academy of Pediatrics. Self-injectable epinephrine for first-aid management of anaphylaxis. *Pediatrics.* 2007;119:638–646.

Simons FE. Anaphylaxis. *J Allergy Clin Immunol.* 2008;121:S402–S407.

Sampson HA, Muñoz-Furlong A, Campbell RL, Adkinson NF Jr, Bock SA, Branum A, et al. Second symposium on the definition and management of anaphylaxis: Summary report—second National Institute of Allergy and Infectious Disease/Food Allergy and Anaphylaxis Network symposium. *Ann Emerg Med.* 2006;47:373–380.

Section 13.2

Abnormal Immune Cells May Cause Unprovoked Anaphylaxis

Excerpted from "Abnormal Immune Cells May Cause
Unprovoked Anaphylaxis," by the National Institutes of
Health (NIH, www.nih.gov), November 9, 2007.

Two new clinical reports shed light on why some people suffer from recurrent episodes of idiopathic anaphylaxis—a potentially life-threatening condition of unknown cause characterized by a drop in blood pressure, fainting episodes, difficulty in breathing, and wheezing.

In some of these individuals, researchers have found mast cells (a type of immune cell involved in allergic reactions) that have a mutated cell surface receptor that disturbs normal processes within the cell. Scientists supported by the National Institute of Allergy and Infectious Diseases (NIAID), part of the National Institutes of Health (NIH), say the association of this mutation with unprovoked anaphylaxis is striking. The hope is that these individuals may respond to inhibitors targeting the mutated cell surface receptor.

While some people suffer anaphylaxis as part of a serious allergic reaction, in two out of three people, anaphylaxis has no known cause and thus the anaphylactic reaction is called idiopathic.

Anaphylaxis occurs when mast cells release large quantities of chemicals (histamines, prostaglandins, and leukotrienes) that cause blood vessels to leak, bronchial tissues to swell, and blood pressure to drop. Resulting conditions such as shock and unconsciousness usually resolve in most people treated with epinephrine (adrenaline) and first aid measures. In rare cases, however, death may occur.

Abnormally low blood pressure and fainting episodes are also features of mastocytosis—a disease in which people have an excessive number of mast cells.

Several years ago, Dean Metcalfe, MD, chief of the Laboratory of Allergic Diseases at NIAID, Cem Akin, MD, PhD, and their NIAID colleagues decided to find out whether idiopathic anaphylaxis might have a genetic trigger related to that seen in mastocytosis. It is known that systemic mastocytosis in adults often results from a mutation in the Kit receptor found on the surface of mast cells, a discovery first made by Dr. Metcalfe's team in 1995.

The mutation causes an abnormal growth of mast cells, as is observed in bone marrow biopsies of patients with mastocytosis. So the NIAID team asked, if the Kit mutation could make mast cells grow and cause mastocytosis, and this was associated with anaphylactic reactions, could the same mutation predispose mast cells to release chemicals responsible for idiopathic anaphylaxis?

In a 2-year study conducted at the NIH Clinical Center, the researchers examined 48 patients diagnosed with mastocytosis with or without associated anaphylaxis, 12 patients with idiopathic anaphylaxis, and 12 patients with neither disease. Within the group of 12 patients who had idiopathic anaphylaxis, five were found with evidence of a disorder in a line of mast cells (clonal mast cell disorder). The researchers looked for evidence of a Kit mutation in three patients by analyzing bone marrow samples, and all three samples yielded a positive result. The findings demonstrate that some patients with idiopathic anaphylaxis have an aberrant population of mast cells with mutated Kit.

"We believe the mutation may be predisposing people to idiopathic anaphylaxis," says Dr. Metcalfe. "Our findings suggest that in patients with idiopathic anaphylaxis as well as in people with severe allergies, we should look for critical genetic mutations that may change the way a mast cell reacts."

According to the NIAID team, both Kit and the IgE receptor responsible for allergic reactions activate mast cells via a common interior protein of mast cells. They also found that the mutated Kit markedly elevates the activity of that protein, which results in increased cell signaling.

The scientists are now looking to see if artificial mast cells with mutated Kit behave or release chemicals in a manner different from normal mast cells, and also if they respond to inhibitors targeting Kit.

Section 13.3

Medical Identification Critical for People with Life-Threatening Allergies

"Why are medical IDs critical? Who should wear a medical ID?"
© 2010 American Medical ID (www.americanmedical-id.com).
Reprinted with permission.

Why are medical IDs critical?

Perhaps your doctor, nurse, or pharmacist advised you to obtain and always wear a medical ID [identification]. Why is it important?

- In an emergency, when you might not be able to speak for yourself, a medical ID bracelet or necklace speaks for you.

- Symptoms of common ailments can easily be misdiagnosed. Prompt diagnosis is critical to effective treatment. A brief description of vital medical facts engraved on your medical ID ensures appropriate and timely medical care.

- According to a published study, half of all medical errors occur because of mistakes made upon admission or discharge from the hospital. Wearing a medical ID protects against potentially harmful medical errors.

- More than 95 percent of emergency responders look for a medical ID; more than 75 percent check for a medical ID immediately upon assessing the patient. If you're wearing a medical ID, it won't be missed.

- Medical IDs can eliminate trips to the hospital, reduce unnecessary hospital admissions, and prevent minor emergencies from becoming major ones. Medical IDs save lives! One day, a medical ID may save you.

Who should wear a medical ID?

If you have ongoing medical conditions, drug or food allergies, or are taking multiple medicines, you should wear a medical ID alert—we offer medical bracelets for women and medical bracelets for men alike. An engraved medical ID bracelet or necklace presenting a concise overview of your conditions, allergies, and medicines will alert a doctor or medic before starting treatment. Informing medical personnel about your unique medical conditions and needs will greatly aid pre-hospital care.

Below is a partial list of ailments or persons who should wear a medical ID:

- Diabetes

- Heart disease (angina, atrial fibrillation, pacemakers)

- Blood thinners/anticoagulants (Coumadin/Warfarin)/even aspirin

- Drug allergies (such as penicillin)

- Food allergies (such as peanut)

- Insect allergies (such as bee stings)

- Alzheimer's/dementia/memory impairment

- Anemia

- Ankylosing spondylitis

- Arrhythmias

- Asthma

- Autism

- ADD/ADHD [attention deficit disorder/attention deficit hyperactivity disorder]

- Bariatric surgery patients

- Blood disorders

- Breathing disorders

- Cerebral palsy

- Clinical trial patients

- COPD [chronic obstructive pulmonary disease]

- Cystic fibrosis

- Emphysema

- Epilepsy, seizures

- Hearing, sight, or mentally impaired

- Hypertension

- Kidney failure

- Mental health patients

- Multiple sclerosis

- Parkinson's disease

- People taking multiple medications

- Rare diseases

- Special needs children

- Stroke risk

- Surgery, transplant, or cancer patients

- Tourette syndrome

These medical ailments demand a medical ID. In particular, many individuals suffer from allergies or asthma yet do not wear an allergy bracelet or asthma ID. Or for those suffering from epilepsy, an epilepsy bracelet is a must. If you're unsure whether you need to wear a medical ID tag, consult your physician or pharmacist. Or, if you prefer, contact our office for assistance.

Medical IDs are also recommended for family caregivers, in case they are ever in an accident, to ensure their loved one can get the care they need.

Part Three

Foods and Food Additives That Trigger Allergic Reactions

Chapter 14

Food Allergy: An Overview

Food allergy affects up to 6 to 8 percent of children under the age of 3 and close to 4 percent of adults. If you have an unpleasant reaction to something you have eaten, you might wonder if you have a food allergy. One out of three people either believe they have a food allergy or modify their or their family's diet. Thus, while food allergy is commonly suspected, healthcare providers diagnose it less frequently than most people believe.

This text describes allergic reactions to foods and their possible causes as well as the best ways to diagnose and treat allergic reactions to food. It also describes other reactions to foods, known as food intolerances, which can be confused with food allergy, and describes some unproven and controversial food allergy theories.

What Is Food Allergy?

Food allergy is an abnormal response to a food triggered by the body's immune system. In this text, food allergy refers to a particular type of response of the immune system in which the body produces what is called an allergic, or IgE, antibody to a food. (IgE, or immunoglobulin E, is a type of protein that works against a specific food.)

"Food Allergy: An Overview," by the National Institute for Allergy and Infectious Diseases (NIAID, www.niaid.nih.gov), part of the National Institutes of Health, July 2007.

Allergic reactions to food can cause serious illness and, in some cases, death. Therefore, if you have a food allergy, it is extremely important for you to work with your healthcare provider to find out what food(s) causes your allergic reaction.

Sometimes, a reaction to food is not an allergy at all but another type of reaction called "food intolerance."

Food intolerance is more common than food allergy. The immune system does not cause the symptoms of food intolerance, though these symptoms may look and feel like those of a food allergy.

How Do Allergic Reactions Work?

An immediate allergic reaction involves two actions of your immune system:

- Your immune system produces IgE. This protein is called a food-specific antibody, and it circulates through your blood.

- The food-specific IgE then attaches to mast cells and basophils. Basophils are found in blood. Mast cells are found in body tissues, especially in areas of your body that are typical sites of allergic reactions. Those sites include your nose, throat, lungs, skin, and gastrointestinal (GI) tract.

Generally, your immune system will form IgE against a food if you come from a family in which allergies are common—not necessarily food allergies but perhaps other allergic diseases, such as hay fever or asthma. If you have two allergic parents, you are more likely to develop food allergy than someone with one allergic parent.

If your immune system is inclined to form IgE to certain foods, you must be exposed to the food before you can have an allergic reaction.

As this food is digested, it triggers certain cells in your body to produce a food-specific IgE in large amounts. The food-specific IgE is then released and attaches to the surfaces of mast cells and basophils.

- The next time you eat that food, it interacts with food-specific IgE on the surface of the mast cells and basophils and triggers those cells to release chemicals such as histamine.

- Depending on the tissue in which they are released, these chemicals will cause you to have various symptoms of food allergy.

Food allergens are proteins in the food that enter your bloodstream after the food is digested. From there, they go to target organs, such as your skin or nose, and cause allergic reactions.

An allergic reaction to food can take place within a few minutes to an hour. The process of eating and digesting food affects the timing and the location of a reaction.

- If you are allergic to a particular food, you may first feel itching in your mouth as you start to eat the food.

- After the food is digested in your stomach, you may have GI symptoms such as vomiting, diarrhea, or pain.

- When the food allergens enter and travel through your bloodstream, they may cause your blood pressure to drop.

- As the allergens reach your skin, they can cause hives or eczema.

- When the allergens reach your mouth and lungs, they may cause throat tightness and trouble breathing.

Cross-Reactive Food Allergies

If you have a life-threatening reaction to a certain food, your healthcare provider will show you how to avoid similar foods that might trigger this reaction. For example, if you have a history of allergy to shrimp, allergy testing will usually show that you are not only allergic to shrimp but also to crab, lobster, and crayfish. This is called "cross-reactivity."

Another interesting example of cross-reactivity occurs in people who are highly sensitive to ragweed. During ragweed pollen season, they sometimes find that when they try to eat melons, particularly cantaloupe, they experience itching in their mouths and simply cannot eat the melon. Similarly, people who have severe birch pollen allergy also may react to apple peels. This is called the "oral allergy syndrome."

Common Food Allergies

In adults, the foods that most often cause allergic reactions include the following:

- Shellfish such as shrimp, crayfish, lobster, and crab
- Peanuts
- Tree nuts such as walnuts
- Fish
- Eggs

The most common foods that cause problems in children are the following:

- Eggs
- Milk
- Peanuts
- Tree nuts

Peanuts and tree nuts are the leading causes of the potentially deadly food allergy reaction called anaphylaxis.

Adults usually keep their allergies for life, but children sometimes outgrow them. Children are more likely to outgrow allergies to milk, egg, or soy, however, than allergies to peanuts. The foods to which adults or children usually react are those foods they eat often. In Japan, for example, rice allergy is frequent. In Scandinavia, codfish allergy is common.

Food Allergy or Food Intolerance?

If you go to your healthcare provider and say, "I think I have a food allergy," your provider has to consider other possibilities that may cause symptoms and could be confused with food allergy, such as food intolerance. To find out the difference between food allergy and food intolerance, your provider will go through a list of possible causes for your symptoms. This is called a "differential diagnosis." This type of diagnosis helps confirm that you do indeed have a food allergy rather than a food intolerance or other illness.

Types of Food Intolerance

Food Poisoning

One possible cause of symptoms like those of food allergy is food contaminated with microbes, such as bacteria, and bacterial products, such as toxins. Contaminated meat and dairy products sometimes cause symptoms, including GI discomfort, that resemble a food allergy when it is really a type of food poisoning.

Histamine Toxicity

There are substances, such as the powerful chemical histamine, present in certain foods that cause a reaction similar to an allergic reaction. For example, histamine can reach high levels in cheese, some wines, and certain kinds of fish such as tuna and mackerel.

In fish, histamine is believed to come from contamination by bacteria, particularly in fish that are not refrigerated properly. If you eat one of these foods with a high level of histamine, you could have a reaction that strongly resembles an allergic reaction to food. This reaction is called "histamine toxicity."

Lactose Intolerance

Another cause of food intolerance confused with a food allergy is lactose intolerance or lactase deficiency. This common food intolerance affects at least one out of 10 people.

Lactase is an enzyme that is in the lining of your gut. Lactase breaks down or digests lactose, a sugar found in milk and most milk products.

Lactose intolerance, or lactase deficiency, happens when there is not enough lactase in your gut to digest lactose. In that case, bacteria in your gut use lactose to form gas, which causes bloating, abdominal pain, and sometimes diarrhea.

Your healthcare provider can use laboratory tests to find out whether your body can digest lactose.

Food Additives

Another type of food intolerance is a reaction to certain products that are added to food to enhance taste, provide color, or protect against the growth of microbes. Several chemical compounds, such as MSG (monosodium glutamate) and sulfites, are tied to reactions that can be confused with food allergy.

MSG

MSG is a flavor enhancer and, when taken in large amounts, can cause some of the following signs:

- Flushing
- Sensations of warmth
- Headache
- Chest discomfort
- Feelings of detachment

These passing reactions occur rapidly after eating large amounts of food to which MSG has been added.

Sulfites

Sulfites occur naturally in foods or may be added to increase crispness or prevent mold growth. Sulfites in high concentrations sometimes pose problems for people with severe asthma. Sulfites can give off a gas called sulfur dioxide that a person with asthma inhales while eating food containing sulfites. This gas irritates the lungs and can send an asthmatic into severe bronchospasm, a tightening of the lungs.

The Food and Drug Administration (FDA) has banned sulfites as spray-on preservatives in fresh fruits and vegetables. Sulfites are still used in some foods, however, and occur naturally during the fermentation of wine.

Gluten Intolerance

Gluten intolerance is associated with the disease called "gluten-sensitive enteropathy" or "celiac disease." It happens if your immune system responds abnormally to gluten, which is a part of wheat and some other grains. Some researchers include celiac disease as a food allergy. This abnormal immune system response, however, does not involve IgE antibody.

Psychological Causes

Some people may have a food intolerance that has a psychological trigger. If your food intolerance is caused by this type of trigger, a careful psychiatric evaluation may identify an unpleasant event in your life, often during childhood, tied to eating a particular food. Eating that food years later, even as an adult, is associated with a rush of unpleasant sensations.

Other Causes

There are several other conditions, including ulcers and cancers of the GI tract, that cause some of the same symptoms as food allergy. These symptoms include vomiting, diarrhea, and cramping abdominal pain made worse by eating.

Exercise-Induced Food Allergy

At least one situation may require more than simply eating food with allergens to start a reaction: Exercise-induced food allergy. People who have this reaction only experience it after eating a specific food before exercising. Some people get this reaction from many foods, and others get it only after eating a specific food. As exercise increases and body temperature rises, itching and light-headedness start and allergic reactions such as hives may appear and even anaphylaxis may develop.

The management of exercised-induced food allergy is simple—avoid eating for a couple of hours before exercising.

Diagnosis

After ruling out food intolerances and other health problems, your healthcare provider will use several steps to find out if you have an allergy to specific foods.

Detailed History

A detailed history is the most valuable tool for diagnosing food allergy. Your provider will ask you several questions and listen to your history of food reactions to decide if the facts fit a food allergy.

- What was the timing of your reaction?

- Did your reaction come on quickly, usually within an hour after eating the food?

- Did allergy medicines help? Antihistamines should relieve hives, for example.

- Is your reaction always associated with a certain food?

- Did anyone else who ate the same food get sick? For example, if you ate fish contaminated with histamine, everyone who ate the fish should be sick.

- How much did you eat before you had a reaction? The severity of a reaction is sometimes related to the amount of food eaten.

- How was the food prepared? Some people will have a violent allergic reaction only to raw or undercooked fish. Complete cooking of the fish may destroy the allergen, and they can then eat it with no allergic reaction.

- Did you eat other foods at the same time you had the reaction? Some foods may delay digestion and thus delay the start of the allergic reaction.

Diet Diary

Sometimes your healthcare provider can't make a diagnosis solely on the basis of your history. In that case, you may be asked to record what you eat and whether you have a reaction. This diet diary gives more detail from which you and your provider can see if there is a consistent pattern in your reactions.

Elimination Diet

The next step some healthcare providers use is an elimination diet. In this step, which is done under your provider's direction, certain foods are removed from your diet.

- You don't eat a food suspected of causing the allergy, such as eggs.

- You then substitute another food—in the case of eggs, another source of protein.

Your provider can almost always make a diagnosis if the symptoms go away after you remove the food from your diet. The diagnosis is confirmed if you then eat the food and the symptoms come back. You should do this only when the reactions are not significant and only under healthcare provider direction.

Your provider can't use this technique, however, if your reactions are severe or don't happen often. If you have a severe reaction, you should not eat the food again.

Skin Test

If your history, diet diary, or elimination diet suggests a specific food allergy is likely, your healthcare provider will then use either the scratch or the prick skin test to confirm the diagnosis.

During a scratch skin test, your healthcare provider will place an extract of the food on the skin of your lower arm. Your provider will then scratch this portion of your skin with a needle and look for swelling or redness, which would be a sign of a local allergic reaction.

A prick skin test is done by putting a needle just below the surface of your skin of the lower arm. Then, a tiny amount of food extract is placed under the skin.

If the scratch or prick test is positive, it means that there is IgE on the skin's mast cells that is specific to the food being tested. Skin tests are rapid, simple, and relatively safe.

You can have a positive skin test to a food allergen, however, without having an allergic reaction to that food. A healthcare provider diagnoses a food allergy only when someone has a positive skin test to a specific allergen and when the history of reactions suggests an allergy to the same food.

Blood Test

Your healthcare provider can make a diagnosis by doing a blood test as well. Indeed, if you are extremely allergic and have severe anaphylactic reactions, your provider can't use skin testing because causing an allergic reaction to the skin test could be dangerous. Skin testing also can't be done if you have eczema over a large portion of your body.

Your healthcare provider may use blood tests such as the RAST (radioallergosorbent test) and newer ones such as the CAP-RAST. Another blood test is called ELISA (enzyme-linked immunosorbent assay). These blood tests measure the presence of food-specific IgE in your blood. The CAP-RAST can measure how much IgE your blood has to a specific food. As with skin testing, positive tests do not necessarily mean you have a food allergy.

Double-Blind Oral Food Challenge

The final method healthcare providers use to diagnose food allergy is double-blind oral food challenge.

- Your healthcare provider will give you capsules containing individual doses of various foods, some of which are suspected of starting an allergic reaction. Or your provider will mask the suspected food within other foods known not to cause an allergic reaction.

- You swallow the capsules one at a time or swallow the masked food and are watched to see if a reaction occurs.

In a true double-blind test, your healthcare provider is also "blinded" (the capsules having been made up by another medical person). In that case your provider does not know which capsule contains the allergen.

The advantage of such a challenge is that if you react only to suspected foods and not to other foods tested, it confirms the diagnosis. You cannot be tested this way if you have a history of severe allergic reactions.

In addition, this testing is difficult because it takes a lot of time to perform and many food allergies are difficult to evaluate with this procedure. Consequently, many healthcare providers do not perform double-blind food challenges.

This type of testing is most commonly used if a healthcare provider thinks the reaction described is not due to a specific food and wishes to obtain evidence to support this. If your provider finds that your reaction is not due to a specific food, then additional efforts may be used to find the real cause of the reaction.

Treatment

Food allergy is treated by avoiding the foods that trigger the reaction. Once you and your healthcare provider have identified the food(s) to which you are sensitive, you must remove them from your diet. To do this, you must read the detailed ingredient lists on each food you are considering eating.

Many allergy-producing foods such as peanuts, eggs, and milk, appear in foods one normally would not associate them with. Peanuts, for example, may be used as a protein source, and eggs are used in some salad dressings.

Because of a new law in the United States, FDA now requires ingredients in a packaged food to appear on its label. You can avoid most of the things to which you are sensitive if you read food labels carefully and avoid restaurant-prepared foods that might have ingredients to which you are allergic.

Controversial and Unproven Disorders

There are several disorders that are popularly thought by some to be caused by food allergies. Either there is not enough scientific evidence to support those claims, or there is evidence that goes against such claims.

Migraine Headaches

There is controversy about whether migraine headaches can be caused by food allergy. Studies show people who are prone to migraines can have their headaches brought on by histamine and other substances in foods. The more difficult issue is whether food allergies actually cause migraines in such people.

Arthritis

There is virtually no evidence that most rheumatoid arthritis or osteoarthritis can be made worse by foods, despite claims to the contrary.

Allergic Tension Fatigue Syndrome

There is no evidence that food allergies can cause a disorder called the allergic tension fatigue syndrome, in which people are tired, nervous, and may have problems concentrating or have headaches.

Cerebral Allergy

Cerebral allergy is a term that has been given to people who have trouble concentrating and have headaches as well as other complaints. These symptoms are sometimes blamed on mast cells activated in the brain but no other place in the body. Researchers have found no evidence that such a scenario can happen. Most health experts do not recognize cerebral allergy as a disorder.

Environmental Illness

In a seemingly pristine environment, some people have many non-specific complaints such as problems concentrating or depression. Sometimes this is blamed on small amounts of allergens or toxins in the environment. There is no evidence that these problems are due to food allergies.

Childhood Hyperactivity

Some people believe hyperactivity in children is caused by food allergies. Researchers, however, have found that this behavioral disorder in children is only occasionally associated with food additives, and then only when such additives are consumed in large amounts.

There is no evidence that a true food allergy can affect a child's activity except for the possibility that if a child itches and sneezes and wheezes a lot, the child may be uncomfortable and therefore more difficult to guide. Also, children who are on anti-allergy medicines that cause drowsiness may get sleepy in school or at home.

Controversial and Unproven Diagnostic Methods

Cytotoxicity Testing

One controversial diagnostic technique is cytotoxicity testing, in which a food allergen is added to a blood sample. A technician then examines the sample under the microscope to see if white cells in the blood "die." Scientists have evaluated this technique in several studies and have found it does not effectively diagnose food allergy.

Provocative Challenge

Another controversial approach is called sublingual (placed under the tongue) or subcutaneous (injected under the skin) provocative challenge. In this procedure, diluted food allergen is put under your tongue if you feel that your arthritis, for instance, is due to foods. The technician then asks you if the food allergen has made your arthritis symptoms worse. In clinical studies, researchers have not shown that this procedure can effectively diagnose food allergy.

Sublingual provocative challenge is not the same as a potentially new treatment for food allergy called sublingual immunotherapy or SLIT. Researchers are currently evaluating this treatment.

Immune Complex Assay

An immune complex assay is sometimes done on people suspected of having food allergies to see if groups, or complexes, of certain antibodies connect to the food allergen in the bloodstream. Some think that these immune groups link with food allergies. The formation of such immune complexes is a normal offshoot of food digestion, however, and everyone, if tested with a sensitive-enough measurement, has them. To date, no one has conclusively shown that this test links with allergies to foods.

IgG subclass Assay

Another test is the IgG subclass assay, which looks specifically for certain kinds of IgG antibody. Again, there is no evidence that this diagnoses food allergy.

Controversial and Unproven Treatments

One controversial treatment, which sometimes may be used with provocative challenge, includes putting a diluted solution of a particular food under your tongue about a half hour before you eat the food suspected of causing an allergic reaction. This is an attempt to "neutralize" the subsequent exposure to the food you believe is harmful. The results of carefully conducted clinical research show this procedure does not prevent an allergic reaction.

Allergy Shots

Another unproven treatment involves getting allergy shots (immunotherapy) containing small quantities of the food extracts to which you are allergic. These shots are given regularly for a long period of time with the aim of "desensitizing" you to the food allergen. Researchers have not yet proven that allergy shots reliably relieve food allergies.

Research

The National Institute of Allergy and Infectious Diseases conducts research on food allergy and other allergic diseases. This research is focused on understanding what happens to the body during the allergic process—the sequence of events leading to the allergic response and the factors responsible for allergic diseases. This understanding will lead to better methods of diagnosing, preventing, and treating allergic diseases. Researchers also are looking at better ways to study allergic reactions to foods.

Educating people, including patients, healthcare providers, school teachers, and daycare workers, about the importance of food allergy is also an important research focus. The more people know about the disorder, the better equipped they will be to control food allergies.

Several treatment approaches are currently being tested in research settings.

Immunotherapy with Allergen Injections

One potential treatment for food allergy involves getting injections or shots (immunotherapy) subcutaneously (under the skin) that contain small quantities of the food extracts to which a person is allergic. These shots are given regularly for a long period of time with the aim of increasing the ability to tolerate the food allergen. Researchers have not yet found a safe and effective way to give allergens subcutaneously, because people often have allergic reactions to these injections.

Immunotherapy with Allergen under the Tongue

Another potential treatment for food allergy involves putting allergens under the tongue, called sublingual immunotherapy (SLIT). Researchers think this is safer than giving under the skin. As of mid-2007, however, this treatment was only in very early stages.

Anti-IgE Therapy

One published study suggested that some (but not all) people with peanut allergy might be partially protected against allergic reactions to low doses of peanut by taking regular subcutaneous injections of one particular form of a medicine called anti-IgE. Because the FDA-approved anti-IgE medicine has not yet been tested for peanut allergy, this treatment is not currently available for peanut allergy. Scientists need to do further research to determine the value of anti-IgE.

Chapter 15

Food Allergy or Food Intolerance: How Do You Tell the Difference?

The statement "I'm allergic to milk" is used quite often in normal conversation; however, true milk allergies in adults are not common. Instead of a milk allergy, a person making this comment is likely to be lactose intolerant. This confusion between food allergies and food intolerance is a frequent misconception; yet there are clear differences between the two.

Food allergies involve an immune response, while food intolerances do not. Only about two to four percent of adults and six to eight percent of children under the age of 3 have true food allergies. Others reacting to foods most likely have food intolerance.

What Is a Food Allergy?

A food allergy involves an abnormal immune response to a protein in a food. Over 170 foods have been documented as causing food allergies. Yet the eight major food allergens—cow's milk, eggs, fish, crustaceans, peanuts, soybeans, tree nuts, and wheat—account for over 90 percent of allergic reactions. After an initial exposure to the food allergen, the body assumes that the food is a harmful substance; thus antibodies to the food are created. Second and subsequent exposures cause the body to release chemicals into the bloodstream that cause adverse reactions.

Reactions to food allergens range from mild to severe. Symptoms can occur within minutes to hours in an immediate reaction, while delayed reactions may not appear for 24 hours or more. Symptoms can affect the GI [gastrointestinal] tract (nausea, vomiting, diarrhea, and cramping), skin (rashes, hives, and eczema), and the cardiovascular system.

Life-threatening allergic reactions, known as anaphylaxis, occur rapidly and involve several body parts. Anaphylaxis symptoms can range from mild to severe and include itching, hives, swelling of the throat, difficulty breathing, hypotension, unconsciousness, and even death. The Food Allergy and Anaphylaxis Network (FAAN) estimates that between 150 and 200 people die annually from food-related anaphylaxis; therefore, immediate medical treatment is needed in the event that a person with a life-threatening allergy is exposed to the food allergen.

Do I Have a Food Allergy?

If you suspect you have a food allergy, seek a board-certified allergist for diagnosis. A variety of methods such as a food diary, elimination diet, or a skin or blood test may be used by an allergist to safely evaluate whether you have a true food allergy.

Food Allergy Management

Management of food allergies starts simply by not consuming food containing the allergen. In some circumstances the allergen may not be apparent, such as peanuts in Pad Thai, or anchovies and/or sardines in Worcestershire sauce. Because allergens can be difficult to identify, individuals with food allergies must be well aware of what they are eating. In restaurants, individuals should explain their allergies thoroughly to restaurant staff, and ask them to check with the chef if they don't know what ingredients are in a dish. At home and at the grocery store, individuals must pay attention to food labels—manufacturers of packaged foods are now required, by the Food Allergen Labeling and Consumer Protection Act (FALCPA), to list the eight major food allergens in plain English.

What Is Food Intolerance?

A food intolerance is any form of food sensitivity or abnormal reaction that does not involve the immune system; consequently, symptoms are less severe and generally are not life threatening.

There are three accepted types of food intolerances—anaphylactoid, metabolic, and idiosyncratic reactions. Anaphylactoid reactions result from the ingestion of a substance that causes the release of histamine, such as an abnormal reaction to strawberries. Metabolic reactions arise when a food or component of a food cannot be metabolized normally. Lactose intolerance, caused by deficiencies of the enzyme lactase, is the most common example of a metabolic reaction. Idiosyncratic reactions, like sulfite-induced asthma, occur via unknown mechanisms.

Symptoms of food intolerances typically involve the gastrointestinal tract and include nausea, bloating, gas, cramps, vomiting, and diarrhea. Other reactions can occur such as headaches, irritability, or nervousness. Symptoms arise from the body's inability to properly digest the food, as in lactose intolerance, or the food itself irritating the digestive system.

Do I Have Food Intolerance?

Since symptoms of food intolerance are similar to the flu and other common ailments, food intolerances can be difficult to identify. If food intolerance is suspected, assessment with trial and error can be used to determine the cause of the adverse reaction.

Food Intolerance Management

Unlike a true food allergy where the food must be avoided, individuals with food intolerance can ingest small amounts of the afflicting food. Reactions are usually related to frequency and amount of the food ingested; thus, small amounts are not likely to cause a significant reaction. Individuals with food intolerance can also choose to manage less severe symptoms instead of reducing the amount of food ingested.

What Do I Need to Know about Food Allergies and Intolerance?

If you have a food allergy, avoid the food. There is more flexibility with food intolerances—you can choose to eat small amounts only, or manage your symptoms. In either case, you should always be aware of what is in the foods you eat—whether from a grocer, restaurant, or your own kitchen. Awareness is the key to management.

Chapter 16

Milk Allergy

About Milk Allergy

Almost all infants are fussy at times. But some are excessively fussy because they have an allergy to the protein in cow's milk, which is the basis for most commercial baby formulas.

A person of any age can have a milk allergy, but it's more common among infants (about 2% to 3% of babies), though most outgrow it.

If you think that your child has a milk allergy, talk with your doctor about testing and alternatives to milk-based formulas and dairy products.

A milk allergy occurs when the immune system mistakenly sees the milk protein as something the body should fight off. This starts an allergic reaction, which can cause an infant to be fussy and irritable, and cause an upset stomach and other symptoms. Most kids who are allergic to cow's milk also react to goat's milk and sheep's milk, and some of them are also allergic to the protein in soy milk.

Infants who are breastfed have a lower risk of developing a milk allergy than those who are formula fed. But researchers don't fully understand why some develop a milk allergy and others don't, though it's believed that in many cases, the allergy is genetic.

Typically, a milk allergy goes away on its own by the time a child is 3 to 5 years old, but some kids never outgrow it.

A milk allergy is not the same thing as lactose intolerance, the inability to digest the sugar lactose, which is rare in infants and more common among older kids and adults.

Symptoms of a Milk Allergy

Symptoms of cow's milk protein allergy will generally appear within the first few months of life. An infant can experience symptoms either very quickly after feeding (rapid onset) or not until 7 to 10 days after consuming the cow's milk protein (slower onset).

The slower-onset reaction is more common. Symptoms may include loose stools (possibly containing blood), vomiting, gagging, refusing food, irritability or colic, and skin rashes. This type of reaction is more difficult to diagnose because the same symptoms may occur with other health conditions. Most children will outgrow this form of allergy by 2 years of age.

Rapid-onset reactions come on suddenly with symptoms that can include irritability, vomiting, wheezing, swelling, hives, other itchy bumps on the skin, and bloody diarrhea. In rare cases, a potentially severe allergic reaction (anaphylaxis) can occur and affect the baby's skin, stomach, breathing, and blood pressure. Anaphylaxis is more common with other food allergies than with milk allergy.

Diagnosing a Milk Allergy

If you suspect that your infant is allergic to milk, call your doctor, who'll ask about any family history of allergies or food intolerance and then do a physical exam. There's no single lab test to accurately diagnose a milk allergy, so your doctor might order several tests to make the diagnosis and rule out any other health problems.

In addition to a stool test and a blood test, the doctor may order an allergy skin test, in which a small amount of the milk protein is inserted just under the surface of the child's skin with a needle. If a raised spot called a wheal emerges, the child may have a milk allergy.

The doctor may also request an oral challenge test. After you stop feeding your baby milk for about a week, the doctor will have the infant consume milk, then wait for a few hours to watch for any allergic reaction. Sometimes doctors repeat this test to reconfirm the diagnosis.

Treating a Milk Allergy

If your infant has a milk allergy and you are breastfeeding, it's important to restrict the amount of dairy products that you ingest because the milk protein that's causing the allergic reaction can cross into your breast milk. You may want to talk to a dietician about finding alternative sources of calcium and other vital nutrients to replace what you were getting from dairy products.

All food makers must clearly state on package labels whether the foods contain milk or milk-based products, indicating this in or next to the ingredient list on the packaging. This law applies only to foods packaged after the start of 2006, so some foods packaged before then may not have any information about food allergens.

If you're formula-feeding, your doctor may advise you to switch to a soy protein-based formula. If your infant can't tolerate soy, the doctor may have you switch to a hypoallergenic formula, one in which the proteins are broken down into particles so that the formula is less likely to trigger an allergic reaction.

Two major types of hypoallergenic formulas are available:

- Extensively hydrolyzed formulas have cow's milk proteins that are broken down into small particles so they're less allergenic than the whole proteins in regular formulas. Most infants who have a milk allergy can tolerate these formulas, but in some cases, they still provoke allergic reactions.

- Amino acid-based infant formulas contain protein in its simplest form (amino acids are the building blocks of proteins). This may be recommended if your baby's condition doesn't improve even after a switch to a hydrolyzed formula.

Unsafe Formulas

"Partially hydrolyzed" formulas also are on the market, but aren't considered truly hypoallergenic and can still provoke a significant allergic reaction.

The formulas available in the market today are approved by the U.S. Food and Drug Administration (FDA) and created through a very specialized process that cannot be duplicated at home. Goat's milk, rice milk, or almond milks are not safe and are not recommended for infants.

Switching Formulas

Once you switch your baby to another formula, the symptoms of the allergy should go away in 2 to 4 weeks. Your doctor will probably recommend that you continue with a hypoallergenic formula up until the baby's first birthday, then gradually introduce cow's milk into his or her diet.

If you have any questions or concerns, talk with your doctor.

Chapter 17

Egg Allergy

Chapter Contents

Section 17.1

Understanding Egg Allergy

Helping a child manage an egg allergy means being aware of what the child eats and reading food labels carefully. It's work, but it's important.

About Egg Allergy

Eggs in themselves aren't bad, but when someone is allergic to them, the body thinks they are. When a person is allergic to eggs, the body's immune system overreacts to proteins in the egg. So every time something made with eggs enters the digestive system, the body thinks that these proteins are harmful invaders.

The immune system responds by creating specific antibodies to that food, which are designed to fight off the "invader." These antibodies—called immunoglobulin E (IgE)—trigger the release of certain chemicals into the body, one of which is histamine.

So when a child with an egg allergy eats a food that contains eggs, the immune system unleashes an army of chemicals to protect the body. The release of these chemicals can affect the respiratory system, gastrointestinal tract, skin, and the cardiovascular system—causing allergy symptoms like wheezing, nausea, headache, stomachache, and itchy hives.

Most people who are allergic react to the proteins in egg whites, but some can't tolerate proteins in the yolk. Egg allergy usually first appears when kids are very young, and most kids outgrow it by the time they're 5 years old.

Egg allergy is like most food allergy reactions: It usually happens within minutes to hours after eating eggs. Most reactions last less than a day and may affect these three body systems:

1. **The skin:** In the form of red, bumpy rashes (hives), eczema, or redness and swelling around the mouth

2. **The gastrointestinal tract:** In the form of belly cramps, diarrhea, nausea, or vomiting

3. **The respiratory tract:** Symptoms can range from a runny nose, itchy, watery eyes, and sneezing to the triggering of asthma with coughing and wheezing

Most kids with egg allergy have some of the reactions listed above, but a few may have a very strong reaction called anaphylaxis. This severe allergic reaction causes swelling of the mouth, throat, and airways leading to the lungs, resulting in breathing difficulty. In addition, there is a dangerous drop in blood pressure, which can make a child dizzy or pass out, and may quickly lead to shock.

For kids who are especially sensitive to eggs, even egg fumes or getting egg on the skin can cause an anaphylactic reaction, so eggs should be kept out of the house completely.

Diagnosing an Egg Allergy

If your doctor suspects your child might have an egg allergy, he or she will probably refer you to an allergist or allergy specialist for further testing. The allergy specialist will ask things like how often your child has the reaction, the time it takes between eating a particular food and the start of the symptoms, and whether any other family members have allergies or conditions like eczema and asthma.

The allergy specialist may perform a skin test. This test involves placing liquid extracts of egg protein on a child's forearm or back, pricking the skin a tiny bit, and waiting to see if a reddish, raised spot forms, indicating an allergic reaction.

Your child may need to stop taking anti-allergy medications (such as over-the-counter antihistamines) 2 to 3 days before the skin test because they can interfere with the results. Most cold medications as well as some antidepressants may also affect skin testing. Check with the allergist's office if you're unsure about what medications need to be stopped and for how long.

Some doctors may also take a blood sample and send it to a lab where it will be mixed with some of the suspected allergen and checked for IgE antibodies.

In some cases, however, positive results of skin and blood tests aren't enough to prove that symptoms are definitely being caused by eggs. So doctors may use what's called a food challenge to help diagnose the allergy.

With a food challenge, the person is told to not eat eggs or anything made with egg proteins for a certain period of time—usually a few weeks. After that, the person will eat foods that contain eggs only under close supervision from a doctor. If symptoms come back after eating egg products, it's likely the person has an egg allergy.

Treatment

Treating egg allergy might seem simple—just make sure your child doesn't eat eggs. But so many foods are made with eggs and egg products that it can be really hard to know what's OK and not OK to eat. Consider working with a registered dietitian to develop an eating plan that provides all the nutrients your child needs while avoiding things made with eggs.

If your child has a severe egg allergy—or any kind of serious allergy—your doctor may want you to carry a shot of epinephrine with you in case of an emergency. Epinephrine comes in an easy-to-carry container about the size of a large marker. It's easy to use—the doctor will show you how to give a shot to your child should you ever need to.

If your child accidentally eats something with egg in it and starts having serious allergic symptoms, like swelling inside the mouth, chest pain, or difficulty breathing, give the shot right away to counteract the reaction while you wait for medical help. Always call for emergency help (911) if your child has needed to use epinephrine. Besides keeping epinephrine in your home, briefcase, or purse, also be sure it's at relatives' homes and your child's day care or school.

Also carry an over-the-counter antihistamine as this can help alleviate allergy symptoms in some kids. Antihistamines should be used in addition to the epinephrine and not as a replacement for the shot.

If your child has had to have an epinephrine shot because of an allergic reaction, go immediately to a medical facility or hospital emergency room so they can provide additional treatment if needed. Up to one third of anaphylactic reactions can have a second wave of symptoms several hours following the initial attack. So your child might need to be observed in a clinic or hospital for 4 to 8 hours following the reaction.

Living with an Egg Allergy

The best way to be sure a food is egg free is to read the label. Manufacturers of foods sold in the United States must list on their labels whether a food contains any of the most common allergens. So look for statements like these somewhere on the label: "contains egg ingredients," "made using egg ingredients," or "made in a facility that also processes eggs."

This label requirement makes things a little easier than reading the ingredients list—instead of needing to know that the ingredient "ovoglobulin" comes from egg protein, you should be able to tell at a glance which foods to avoid. Still, to make sure the foods your child eats are egg free, you'll need to be on the lookout for any ingredients that might come from eggs. That means asking questions when eating out at restaurants or others' homes and carefully reading food labels.

Try to find out how foods are cooked and what's in them. In some cases, you may want to bring your child's own food with you. When you're shopping, look for egg-free alternatives to foods that usually contain eggs, such as pasta.

When preparing food, use one of these egg alternatives in recipes. Each of these replaces one egg (these substitutes may not work as well in recipes that call for more than three eggs):

- 1 teaspoon baking powder + 1 tablespoon liquid + 1 tablespoon vinegar

- 1 teaspoon yeast dissolved in 1/4 cup warm water

- 1 1/2 tablespoons water + 1 1/2 tablespoons oil + 1 teaspoon baking powder

- 1 packet gelatin + 2 tablespoons warm water (don't mix until ready to use)

- 1 tablespoon pureed fruit such as apricots or bananas

When cooking at home, always carefully scrub the utensils you're using in case they have been used on egg products.

Although the number of people in the United States with food allergies is low (just over 1% of the total population), there's a growing awareness about food allergies. This means that everyone—from the waitstaff at a restaurant to food manufacturers—is more understanding and willing to accommodate a child's food needs.

Section 17.2

Flu Vaccine and Egg Allergy

"Vaccines and Egg Allergies," © 2009 Children's Hospital of Philadelphia—
Vaccine Education Center (www.chop.edu/service/vaccine-education-center).
Reprinted with permission.

Egg Allergy

Egg allergy is one of the more common pediatric food allergies. It typically affects just 0.5 percent of the pediatric population (less than one of every 100 children) and five of every 100 children with allergies. Reactions to egg can vary from life-threatening anaphylaxis to atopic dermatitis (eczema) to hives.

Food allergies are diagnosed by physical examination, previous experience, and allergy testing. There are two types of allergy testing: skin testing and blood testing for specific antibodies to eggs (commonly called RAST [radioallergosorbent test] testing). Each test has advantages and disadvantages. In general, if you are negative on either test, you do not have an allergy to egg; however, the blood test can be negative in about five of every 100 children who actually have an egg allergy. A positive blood or skin test indicates a potential to react to egg, and the larger the skin or blood test, the more likely it is that a reaction will occur. However, the size of the skin or blood test does not correlate with how severe a reaction will be.

Egg Allergies and Vaccines

Because influenza and yellow fever vaccines are both made in eggs, egg proteins (primarily ovalbumin) are present in the final products and are in sufficient quantities to cause allergic reactions in susceptible patients.

For patients who are at a high risk of getting these diseases, there is concern if they can't get the vaccine; however, the good news is that protocols exist to give the vaccines to egg-allergic patients. The most common protocol involves skin testing the individual to the vaccine, administration of the vaccine in the same visit, and observing the patient for 30 minutes to monitor for an allergic reaction. The vaccine is typically administered in partial doses (up to four doses) that together make the whole dose. The entire protocol takes about one to four hours to complete and is usually done in a single visit. Reactions, if any, are usually mild, such as hives near the site of administration. At The Children's Hospital of Philadelphia, we have done this type of testing in over 900 egg-allergic patients and have not seen any significant reactions.

Getting the Testing

If you or your child is allergic to eggs and you are interested in getting the vaccine, you should make an appointment with an allergist. Most allergists are aware of and comfortable performing this type of vaccine testing and administration.

What about Future Doses of the Vaccine?

Current protocols require that people with egg allergies repeat the process with an allergist each time they get the vaccine because the protocols do not prevent the allergy, they simply provide a way to get around the allergic response in the short term, so that the vaccine can be given safely.

References

Erlewyn-Lajeunesse et al, *BMJ* 2009.

Piquer-Gibert M, *Allergol Immunopathol* (Madr). 2007 Sep-Oct;35(5):209–12.

James et al, *J Pediatr.* 1998 Nov;133(5):624–8.

Saltzman, et al. *J Aller Clinical Immuno* 2009; 123 (2):S175.

Chapter 18

Fish and Shellfish Allergy

Chapter Contents

Section 18.1

Fish Allergy

"Fish Allergy," © 2010 Food Allergy Initiative
(www.faiusa.org). Reprinted with permission.

Finned fish can cause severe allergic reactions. This allergy is usually life-long. The protein in the flesh of fish most commonly causes the allergic reaction; however, it is also possible to have a reaction to fish gelatin, made from the skin and bones of fish. Although fish oil does not contain protein from the fish from which it was extracted, it is likely to be contaminated with small molecules of protein and therefore should be avoided.

More than half of all people who are allergic to one type of fish also are allergic to other fish, so allergists often advise their patients to avoid all fish. However, many people with fish allergies are able to eat canned tuna or salmon, which are less allergenic than fresh fish. Finned fish and shellfish do not come from related families of foods, so being allergic to one does not mean that you will not be able to tolerate the other. Be sure to talk to your doctor about which kinds of fish you can eat and which to avoid.

When eating out, people with fish allergies should be particularly alert to cross-contamination. Always check with the chef to make sure that the fish is not cooked on the same skillet or in the same oil as other food. You also should make sure that your dishes are not prepared with the same utensils or on the same work surfaces as fish.

How to Avoid Fish

The federal Food Allergen Labeling and Consumer Protection Act (FALCPA) requires that any packaged food product that contains fish as an ingredient must list the name of the specific fish on the label. Please be sure to read all product labels carefully before purchasing and consuming any item. Remember, also, that ingredients change from time to time, so check labels every time you shop. If you are still not sure whether or not a product contains fish, call the manufacturer. Always take extra precaution when dining in restaurants or eating foods prepared by others. If you are ever in doubt about any product or dish, don't eat it.

The term "fish" encompasses all species of finned fish, including (but not limited to): anchovies; bass; catfish; cod; flounder; grouper; haddock; hake; herring; mahi mahi; perch; pike; pollock; salmon; scrod; sole; snapper; swordfish; tilapia; trout; and tuna.

- Some sensitive individuals may react to aerosolized fish protein through cooking vapors.

- Seafood restaurants are considered high risk due to the possibility of cross-contamination, even if you do not order fish.

- Ethnic restaurants (e.g., Chinese, African, Indonesian, Thai, and Vietnamese) are considered high-risk because of the common use of fish and fish ingredients and the possibility of cross-contamination, even if you do not order fish.

- Worcestershire sauce, Caesar salad, and Caesar dressing usually contain fish ingredients (anchovies).

- Caponata, a Sicilian eggplant relish, may contain anchovies.

- Surimi, an artificial crab meat (also known as "sea legs" or "sea sticks"), is made from fish.

- Carrageen is a marine algae, not a fish, and is considered safe for those avoiding fish and shellfish.

Section 18.2

Shellfish Allergy

"Shellfish Allergy," © 2010 Food Allergy Initiative
(www.faiusa.org). Reprinted with permission.

Shellfish allergy usually develops in young adults. In fact, it is the most common significant food allergy reported by adults and is considered life-long. Along with peanuts and tree nuts, shellfish are the most frequent triggers of anaphylactic reactions.

There are two kinds of shellfish: crustacea (such as shrimp, crab, and lobster) and mollusks (such as clams, mussels, oysters, and scallops). Reactions to crustacean shellfish tend to be particularly severe. If you are allergic to one group of shellfish, you might be able to eat some varieties from the other group. Since most people who are allergic to one kind of shellfish usually are allergic to other types, however, allergists usually advise their patients to avoid all varieties. If you have been diagnosed with a shellfish allergy, never eat any kind of shellfish without consulting your doctor first.

When eating out, people with shellfish allergies should be particularly alert to cross-contamination. Always check with the chef to make sure that shellfish are not cooked on the same skillet or in the same oil as other food. You also should make sure that your dishes are not prepared with the same utensils or on the same work surfaces as shellfish.

How to Avoid Shellfish

The federal Food Allergen Labeling and Consumer Protection Act (FALCPA) requires that any packaged food product that contains shellfish as an ingredient must list the name of the specific shellfish on the label. Please be sure to read all product labels carefully before purchasing and consuming any item. Remember, also, that ingredients change from time to time, so check labels every time you shop. If you are still not sure whether or not a product contains shellfish, call the manufacturer. Always take extra precaution when dining in restaurants or eating foods prepared by others. If you are ever in doubt about any product or dish, don't eat it.

- Crustaceans
- Shrimp (prawns, crevette)
- Crab
- Crawfish (crayfish, ecrevisse)
- Lobster (langouste, langoustine, scampo, coral, tomalley)
- Mollusks
- Abalone
- Clam
- Cockle
- Mussel
- Oyster
- Octopus
- Scallop
- Snail (escargot)
- Squid (calamari)

The following ingredients may indicate the presence of a shellfish protein:

- Bouillabaisse
- Fish stock
- Flavoring
- Seafood flavoring
- Surimi

Some sensitive individuals may react to aerosolized shellfish protein through cooking vapors. It is wise to stay away from steam tables or stovetops when shellfish are being cooked.

Seafood restaurants are considered high-risk due to the possibility of cross-contamination, even if a non-shellfish item is ordered.

Carrageen is a marine algae, not a fish, and is considered safe for those avoiding fish and shellfish.

Chapter 19

Peanut and Tree Nut Allergy

Chapter Contents

Section 19.1

Peanut Allergy

Amy Altizer will never forget January 3, 2007. Not because it was her baby boy's 3-month birthday. It was the day he had a life-threatening allergic reaction.

Amy left baby James at home with a sitter while she took 3-year-old Mary Grace for a checkup at the pediatrician's office. "The doctor was running late, so I told the sitter to give James a bottle rather than wait for me to breastfeed him," Amy remembers. "I'd given him formula once before without any problems."

When Amy got home, James was about 2 ounces into his bottle. Amy decided to switch him over to breast milk and pulled the bottle out of James' mouth. "The skin around his mouth was very red. My first thought was that the bottle nipple had irritated his skin. But before I could really look at it, Mary Grace announced she needed help in the potty." By the time Amy came back, "James was covered head to toe with hives—even the bottoms of his feet!"

Amy immediately called the pediatrician's office. The nurse told her to give James half a teaspoon of Benadryl®, but James' lips and tongue were so swollen he couldn't swallow. "I put some in his mouth and it just dribbled back out." By then James' hands, feet, head, and ears were also swollen. Amy called 911.

During the ride to the hospital, James was coughing but still getting in some air. The emergency medical technicians didn't want to give James a shot of epinephrine because they only had premeasured doses and James was far below the weight range. At the hospital, James received a weight-adjusted shot of epinephrine and an IV with prednisone. Thirty minutes later James needed another shot of epinephrine because he started wheezing. James stayed overnight at Children's Memorial Hospital for treatment and observation.

Gooey Clues

Jennifer Kim, MD, an allergy/immunology specialist on staff at Northwestern Memorial Hospital, came to see the Altizers the next day. Based on Amy's description of what happened, Dr. Kim thought James had reacted to the milk in the baby formula. Amy wasn't so sure. James had suffered terrible gas and stomach pains since he'd been born, and cutting dairy from Amy's diet the first few months of breastfeeding had not made a difference. Dr. Kim asked Amy to keep milk out of her diet while she was breastfeeding—at least until Dr. Kim could confirm James' diagnosis with allergy testing.

The plot got stickier at a Valentine's Day party for Mary Grace and her friends. Amy was searching for something dairy-free to eat. The chicken salad was out. So was grilled cheese. Then Amy spied a peanut butter and jelly sandwich. "I was holding James in one hand and eating the PB&J with the other hand, and James started to break out around the mouth—just from being that close to peanut butter!" Could James have had a peanut allergy all along?

Big Allergies for Little People

If peanut allergy was the source of James' symptoms, he'd have lots of company—recent studies put the rate of peanut allergy among children at 1 in 100. Unlike some other food allergies, peanut allergy is usually permanent. Only 20 percent of children outgrow peanut allergy by school age, and 8 percent of these children will have a recurrence. A child's first allergic reaction to peanuts usually happens between the ages of 10 and 20 months. Peanut allergy is less common in very young infants, particularly a severe reaction like James had, but not unheard of.

Risk factors for peanut allergy include a family history of any allergy—especially other types of food allergies—atopic dermatitis (eczema) or asthma. Common symptoms in children include skin problems like hives or eczema (itchy, dry patches) and intestinal distress such as nausea, vomiting, diarrhea, and stomach pain. Respiratory symptoms, including wheezing, nasal congestion, and mucus, are less common but can be severe.

James had several of these symptoms and risk factors. In addition to his unresolved tummy trouble, James developed eczema when he was just 6 weeks old. "At first we thought it was just baby acne," says Amy. "But it never cleared up and went beyond his face to his knees, wrists, and thumbs. We thought, 'Lots of people have allergies. It will be fine.' Food allergy causes eczema symptoms in about 40 percent of children with moderate to severe eczema. James also had a family history of allergic diseases: Big sister Mary Grace has asthma and James' aunt developed egg allergy as a child and never outgrew it.

Top Test Scores

When James was 6 months old, Dr. Kim performed skin tests for milk and peanut. James tested negative for milk but had a huge reaction to peanut! Amy thought about the baby formula incident months earlier to see if she could link it to peanut exposure. Amy's husband Jay used to snack on peanut butter every night. Did he have peanut butter on his hands while unloading bottles from the dishwasher? At this point they couldn't be sure, but Dr. Kim recommended that Amy continued a nut- and dairy-free diet while nursing.

At 11 months old, James underwent blood tests for milk, egg, and peanut allergy. (They added egg based on Amy's family history.) James' milk test came back negative again, but he tested positive for peanut—much higher than usually seen in babies his age—and egg.

Hide and Seek

In light of the test results and the family's experiences, James' physician agreed that he had a serious peanut allergy and recommended the whole family steer clear of peanuts and keep auto-injectable epinephrine on hand at all times. Peanut butter was out and reading food labels was in!

Although new food labeling laws make finding peanuts in food much easier, some not-so-obvious places peanuts may be hiding include:

- arachis oil—another name for peanut oil;
- artificial tree nuts—sometimes peanuts are flavored to taste like other nuts;
- chocolate candies—some chocolates are produced on equipment used for processing peanuts or foods that contain peanuts;
- nut butters—some alternatives to peanut butter are processed on the same equipment used to make peanut butter;
- sunflower seeds—many brands are processed on equipment used to process peanuts.

Grain breads, salad dressings, energy bars, and marzipan also can contain peanuts. Peanut butter may be used to thicken sauces—even spaghetti sauce. With so many uses for peanuts, it's easy for children with peanut allergy to accidentally eat peanuts: A 2006 study of school-children in Quebec, Canada, found an annual incidence rate of more than 14 percent!

Everyday Life

"We're learning as we go and try to stay vigilant," says Amy, "but we want James to be a rough and tough boy with as normal a life as possible." Amy makes sure their house is a safe haven where James can just be a kid. Even Mary Grace pitches in to keep her baby brother safe, keeping foods that could contain peanut or were made in a plant that processes peanuts out of the house and car. But Mary Grace does get one special treat. "We go out for PB&J dates!" Every Thursday, Amy takes Mary Grace out to a restaurant for a peanut butter and jelly sandwich. "We wash her hands carefully after lunch, and after that Mary Grace goes to preschool for several hours. We wash her hands again when she comes home and we haven't had any problems."

Amy's strategy for family harmony—and safety—is a good one. A study published in the *Journal of Allergy and Clinical Immunology* (*JACI*) (2004; 113:973–4) found that washing with soap and water or using commercial wipes was sufficient to remove peanut proteins from your hands. Researchers in another study took saliva samples to figure out how long peanut proteins stay in your mouth after eating peanuts (*JACI* 2006; 118:719–24). They found that several hours and another meal later, 90 percent of people who ate peanut butter would not have peanut protein left in their saliva. But Amy and her husband Jay don't eat or touch peanuts or peanut butter at all, just to be safe.

If there can be a silver lining to the Altizer family's story, it's that "James' eczema is actually the best that it's ever been!" Now that they've eliminated foods that James is allergic to, his eczema has cleared up.

Section 19.2

Animal Model Helps Researchers Understand Peanut Allergy

From "Of Mice and Peanuts: A New Mouse Model for Peanut Allergy," by the National Institute of Allergy and Infectious Diseases (NIAID, www.niaid .nih.gov), part of the National Institutes of Health, January 12, 2009.

Researchers report the development of a new mouse model for food allergy that mimics symptoms generated during a human allergic reaction to peanuts. The animal model provides a new research tool that will be invaluable in furthering the understanding of the causes of peanut and other food allergies and in finding new ways to treat and prevent their occurrence, according to experts at the National Institute of Allergy and Infectious Diseases (NIAID), the component of the National Institutes of Health (NIH) that funded the research. Peanut allergy is of great public health interest because this food allergy is the one most often associated with life-threatening allergic reactions, resulting in up to 100 deaths in the United States each year.

The findings of the research team, led by Paul Bryce, PhD, of the Feinberg School of Medicine at Northwestern University, appear in the January 2009 issue of the Journal of Allergy and Clinical Immunology. The development of new animal models for food allergy was identified as a critical need by the 2006 NIH Expert Panel on Food Allergy Research.

"Food allergies affect the health and quality of life of many Americans, particularly young children," says NIAID Director Anthony S. Fauci, MD. "Finding an animal model that mimics a severe human allergic reaction to peanuts will help us better understand peanut allergy and develop new and improved treatment and prevention strategies."

Allergic reactions to food can range from mild hives to vomiting to difficulty breathing to anaphylaxis, the most severe reaction. Anaphylaxis may result from a whole-body allergic reaction to the release of the chemical histamine, causing muscles to contract, blood vessels to dilate and fluid to leak from the bloodstream into the tissues. These effects can result in narrowing of the upper or lower airways, low blood pressure, shock or a combination of these symptoms, and also can lead to a loss of consciousness and even death.

The most significant obstacle to developing an animal model of food allergy is that animals are not normally allergic to food. Scientists must add a strong immune stimulant to foods to elicit a reaction in animals that resembles food allergy in humans. Because of this requirement, useful animal models have been developed only in the last few years, and such animal models have until now used cholera toxin as the immune stimulant.

Dr. Bryce's team took the novel approach of feeding mice a mixture of whole peanut extract (WPE) and a toxin from the bacteria *Staphylococcus aureus*, called staphylococcal enterotoxin B (SEB) to simulate the human anaphylactic reaction to peanuts in mice.

"Persistent *S. aureus* colonization is commonly found on the skin of people with eczema and in the nasal cavities of people with sinusitis," says Dr. Bryce. "The history between *S. aureus* and allergic diseases led us to use staphylococcal toxins to stimulate food allergy in animals."

According to Dr. Bryce, the results using the SEB/WPE mixture were considerably better than those seen with previous animal models, which failed to mimic many features of food allergy. They showed that the SEB/WPE mixture stimulated severe symptoms in mice that closely resemble those found in human anaphylaxis, including swelling around the eyes and mouth, reduced movement, and significant problems breathing. Additionally, mice given the SEB/WPE mixture had high blood levels of histamine, which indicates a severe allergic reaction.

The researchers also observed that the blood and tissues of mice in the SEB/WPE group had higher-than-normal numbers of eosinophils, which are white blood cells often associated with allergy-related inflammation. Future studies will be needed to determine if eosinophils play an important role in human food allergy.

These results, say Dr. Bryce, suggest that this animal model of food allergy will be useful for many types of future research studies.

Approximately 4 percent of Americans have food allergies. For reasons that are not well understood, the prevalence in children increased by 18 percent between 1997 and 2007. The most common causes of food allergies are milk, eggs, shellfish, peanuts, tree nuts, wheat, and soy.

Each year there are between 15,000 and 30,000 episodes of food-induced anaphylaxis, which are associated with 100 to 200 deaths in the United States.

References

K Ganeshan et al. Impairing oral tolerance promotes allergy and anaphylaxis: a new murine food allergy model. *Journal of Allergy and Clinical Immunology*. (2008).

Section 19.3

How to Avoid Peanut

"Peanut Allergy,"
© 2010 Food Allergy Initiative
(www.faiusa.org). Reprinted with permission.

Peanut allergy is one of the most common food allergies. Unfortunately, it also is one of the most dangerous, since peanuts tend to cause particularly severe reactions (anaphylaxis). Some people are very sensitive and have reactions from eating trace amounts of peanut. Non-ingestion contact (touching peanuts or inhaling airborne peanut allergens, such as dust from the shells) is less likely to trigger a severe reaction.

Peanut allergies seem to be on the rise in children. In the United States, the number of children with peanut allergy doubled between 1997 and 2002. Subsequent studies in the United Kingdom and Canada also showed a high prevalence of peanut allergy in schoolchildren. Unlike egg and cow's milk allergies, which most children outgrow, peanut allergies tend to be life-long. Recent studies, however, indicate that approximately 20% of peanut-allergic children do eventually outgrow their allergy.

The peanut (*Arachis hypogaea*) is not really a nut, but a kind of legume. It is related to other beans, such as peas, lentils, and soybeans. People with peanut allergy are not necessarily allergic to other legumes (even soy, another of the "big eight" food allergens), so be sure to speak with your doctor before assuming that you have to avoid these protein-rich foods. A person with a peanut allergy may also be allergic to tree nuts (almonds, walnuts, hazelnuts, cashews, etc.). In fact, some 30–40% of people who have peanut allergy also are allergic to tree nuts. Not surprisingly, allergists usually tell their peanut-allergic patients to avoid tree nuts.

Researchers have isolated three major peanut allergens. They are trying to learn why peanuts cause such severe reactions and why the number of people who suffer from peanut allergy is increasing. Investigators also are trying to develop therapies that would prevent anaphylaxis in people with peanut allergies.

How to Avoid Peanuts

The federal Food Allergen Labeling and Consumer Protection Act (FALCPA) requires that any packaged food product that contains peanuts as an ingredient must list the word "Peanut" on the label. Please be sure to read all product labels carefully before purchasing and consuming any item. Remember, also, that ingredients change from time to time, so check labels every time you shop. If you are still not sure whether or not a product contains peanuts, call the manufacturer. Always take extra precaution when dining in restaurants or eating foods prepared by others. If you are in doubt about any product or dish, don't eat it.

- The following ingredients indicate the presence of peanut protein: Beer nuts, ground nuts, mixed nuts, and peanut (including peanut flour and peanut butter).

- Peanut protein is found in Arachis oil, and in cold pressed, expressed, expelled, and extruded peanut oils. Highly processed peanut oil has been shown to be safe for the vast majority of people allergic to peanut. As the degree of processing of commercial peanut oil may be difficult to determine, avoidance is prudent.

- Nu-Nuts® and other artificial flavored nuts contain peanut protein.

- Ethnic restaurants (such as Chinese, African, Indonesian, Thai, and Vietnamese), bakeries, and ice cream parlors are considered high-risk for individuals with peanut allergy due to the common use of peanut and the risk of cross contamination—even if you order a peanut-free item.

- Peanut butter and/or peanut flour have been used in chili and spaghetti sauce as thickeners. Always ask if peanut was in the recipe.

- Many candies and chocolates contain peanut or run the risk of cross contact with peanut protein.

- Lupine or lupin is a legume that may cause an allergic reaction in those with peanut allergy. Lupine is used in this country in many gluten-free and high-protein products. In many European countries, particularly Italy and France, lupine flour and/or peanut flour may be mixed with wheat flour in baked goods.

- Many tree nuts are processed with peanuts and therefore may contain trace amounts of peanut protein. Extreme caution is advised.

Section 19.4

Tree Nut Allergy

"Tree Nut Allergy," © 2010 Food Allergy Initiative
(www.faiusa.org). Reprinted with permission.

Tree nut allergy is one of the most common food allergies in children
and adults. Like peanuts, tree nuts (almonds, cashews, walnuts, etc.)
tend to cause particularly severe reactions, even if a person is exposed
to only a tiny amount.

In a registry of 5,149 people who had peanut or tree nut allergy, the
median age of reaction to tree nuts was 36 months. Sixty-eight percent
of the tree nut-allergic participants were not aware of any previous
exposure to tree nuts before their first reaction. This allergy tends to
be life-long; recent studies have shown that approximately 9% of tree
nut-allergic children eventually outgrow their allergy.

People seldom are allergic to just one type of tree nut, so allergists
usually will tell patients to avoid all tree nuts.

How to Avoid Tree Nuts

The federal Food Allergen Labeling and Consumer Protection Act
(FALCPA) requires that any packaged food product that contains tree
nuts as an ingredient must list the specific tree nut on the label. Please
be sure to read all product labels carefully before purchasing and consuming any item. Remember, also, that ingredients change from time
to time, so check labels every time you shop. If you are still not sure
whether or not a product contains tree nuts, call the manufacturer.
Always take extra precaution when dining in restaurants or eating
foods prepared by others. If you are in doubt about any product or
dish, don't eat it.

The following common nuts are considered tree nuts under U.S. law:
almond; Brazil nut; cashew; chestnut; filbert/hazelnut; macadamia nut;
pecan; pine nut (pignolia nut); pistachio; walnut.

The following are uncommon, additional tree nuts that require disclo-
sure by U.S. law. However, the risk of an allergic reaction to these nuts
is unknown: beechnut; ginkgo; shea nut; butternut; hickory; chinquapin;

lychee nut; pili nut; coconut. The American Academy of Allergy, Asthma and Immunology (AAAAI) states: "There is conflicting information on whether or not coconut must be avoided by tree nut allergic individuals. In the past, coconut has not been considered a tree nut and typically has not been restricted in the diets of people with a tree nut allergy. Coconut is in the palm family and it is actually the seed of a drupaceous fruit, not a tree nut. It does not cross-react with tree nuts. However, in October 2006, the FDA began to define coconut as a tree nut. There are a small number of documented cases of allergic reactions to coconut. However, most occurred in individuals who were not allergic to other tree nuts. Thus, it is possible to be allergic to coconut, although coconut does not cross-react with tree nuts. It is important to discuss this issue with your allergist/immunologist who can instruct you on whether or not you need to avoid coconut if you are tree nut allergic."

- Tree nut proteins may be found in cereals, crackers, cookies, candy, chocolates, energy bars, flavored coffee, frozen desserts, marinades, barbecue sauces, and some cold cuts, such as mortadella.

- Tree nut protein will be found in foods such as gianduja (a creamy mixture of chocolate and chopped almonds and hazelnuts, although other nuts may be used); marzipan (almond paste); nougat; Nu-Nuts® artificial nuts; pesto; and nut meal.

- Tree nut oils may contain nut protein and should be avoided.

- Ethnic restaurants (e.g., Chinese, African, Indian, Thai, and Vietnamese), ice cream parlors, and bakeries are considered high risk for people with tree nut allergy due to the common use of nuts and the possibility of cross contamination, even if you order a tree-nut-free item.

- Avoid natural extracts, such as pure almond extract and natural wintergreen extract (for the filbert/hazelnut allergy). Imitation or artificially flavored extracts generally are safe.

- The following are not considered nuts: nutmeg, water chestnuts, and butternut squash.

- Tree nut oils are sometimes used in lotions and soaps. Shea nut, although not usually found in food products, is often used in lotions.

- Some alcoholic beverages may contain nut flavoring and should be avoided. Since these beverages are not currently regulated by FALCPA, you may need to call the manufacturer to determine the safety of ingredients such as natural flavoring.

Chapter 20

Wheat Allergy

Chapter Contents

Section 20.1

What Is Wheat Allergy?

"Wheat Allergy," © 2010 Food Allergy Initiative
(www.faiusa.org). Reprinted with permission.

Wheat allergy most commonly affects children and often is outgrown by age 3. Wheat, a type of grain, contains four major proteins that can cause an allergy: albumin, globulin, gliadin, and gluten. Gluten is also found in barley, rye, and oats. You or your child may not necessarily have to avoid foods that contain grains other than wheat. However, about 20% of wheat-allergic children also are allergic to other grains. Be sure to ask your doctor whether foods containing barley, rye, or oats are safe for you or your child to eat.

A wheat allergy should not be confused with "gluten intolerance" or celiac disease. Celiac disease (also known as celiac sprue), which affects the small intestine, is caused by an abnormal immune reaction to gluten. Usually diagnosed by a gastroenterologist, it is a digestive disease that can cause serious complications, including malnutrition and intestinal damage, if left untreated.

How to Avoid Wheat

The federal Food Allergen Labeling and Consumer Protection Act (FALCPA) requires that any packaged food product that contains wheat as an ingredient must list the word "Wheat" on the label. The law states that any species in the genus Triticum is considered wheat. Please be sure to read all product labels carefully before purchasing and consuming any item. Remember, also, that ingredients change from time to time, so check labels every time you shop. If you are still not sure whether or not a product contains wheat, call the manufacturer. Always take extra precaution when dining in restaurants or eating foods prepared by others. If you are ever in doubt about any product or dish, don't eat it.

The following ingredients indicate the presence of wheat protein:

- Bread crumbs

- Bulgur

- Cereal extract

- Couscous

- Durum, durum flour, durum wheat

- Emmer

- Einkorn

- Farina

- Flour (all wheat types, such as all-purpose, cake, enriched, graham, high protein or high gluten, pastry)

- Kamut

- Semolina

- Spelt

- Sprouted wheat

- Triticale

- Vital wheat gluten

- Wheat (bran, germ, gluten, grass, malt, starch)

- Whole-wheat berries

Wheat may be found in ale, baking mixes, baked products, batter-fried foods, beer, breaded foods, breakfast cereals, candy, crackers, frankfurters and processed meats, ice cream products, salad dressings, sauces, soups, soy sauce, and surimi.

The following flour substitutes are available and may be used by people with wheat allergies if tolerated: amaranth, arrowroot, buckwheat, corn, millet, oat, potato, rice, soybean, tapioca, and quinoa flour. Please check with your doctor before including these in your diet.

Section 20.2

Wheat Allergy Often Confused with Celiac Disease

Celiac disease has been known by many different names in the medical literature over the years, including gluten-sensitive enteropathy and celiac sprue (to differentiate it from tropical sprue). Celiac disease can be defined as a permanent intolerance to the gliadin fraction of wheat protein and related alcohol-soluble proteins (called prolamines) found in rye and barley. Celiac disease occurs in genetically susceptible individuals who eat these proteins, leading to an autoimmune disease, where the body's immune system starts attacking normal tissue. This condition continues as long as these food products are in the diet.

The resulting inflammation and atrophy of the intestinal villi (small, finger-like projections in the small intestine) results in the malabsorption of critical vitamins, minerals, and calories. Signs and symptoms of the disease classically include diarrhea, short stature, iron-deficiency anemia, and lactose intolerance. However, many patients will also present with non-classical symptoms, such as abdominal pain, irritable bowel, and osteoporosis. Patients may also be screened for celiac disease because of the presence of another autoimmune disease, such as type I diabetes or thyroid disease, or a family history of celiac disease, without having any obvious symptoms. Serum antibodies can be utilized to screen for celiac disease. However, the key to confirming the diagnosis remains a small intestinal biopsy, and the patient's subsequent clinical response to a gluten-free diet. Clinicians in the United States must maintain a high index of suspicion for this disease, as it is significantly underdiagnosed in this country.

What is a wheat allergy?

People can also have other medical problems, besides celiac disease, when they eat wheat and related proteins. Wheat allergy is one of the top eight food allergies in the United States. Allergic reactions after eating wheat may include reactions in the skin, mouth, lungs, and even the GI [gastrointestinal] tract. Symptoms of wheat allergy can include rash, wheezing, lip swelling, abdominal pain, and diarrhea. The branch of the immune system activated in allergic reactions is different from the branch thought to be responsible for the autoimmune reactions of celiac disease.

What is gluten intolerance?

People can also experience intolerance to gluten. Food intolerances are not thought to be immune mediated. GI symptoms with wheat or gluten intolerance may include gassiness, abdominal pain, abdominal distension, and diarrhea. These symptoms are usually transient, and are thought not to cause permanent damage.

Patients with lactose intolerance, where the lactose sugar in diary products is not digested well, may also experience gassiness, abdominal pain, abdominal distension, and diarrhea. Like gluten or wheat intolerance, these symptoms will pass once the lactose is out of the person's system, and will not cause permanent damage.

Why is it important to know if you have celiac disease, versus wheat allergy or gluten intolerance?

Celiac disease, wheat allergy, and gluten intolerance are treated similarly, in that patients with these conditions must remove wheat from their diet. It is important to note, however, that there is a difference between these three medical problems. Celiac disease is an autoimmune condition, where the body's immune system starts attacking normal tissue, such as intestinal tissue, in response to eating gluten. Because of this, people with celiac disease are at risk for malabsorption of food in the GI tract, causing nutritional deficiencies. This can lead to conditions such as iron deficiency anemia and osteoporosis. Since a person with wheat allergy or gluten intolerance usually does not have severe intestinal damage, he or she is not at risk for these nutritional deficiencies. Celiac disease is an autoimmune condition, putting the patient at risk for other autoimmune conditions, such as thyroid disease, type I diabetes, joint diseases, and liver diseases. Since wheat allergy and gluten intolerance are not autoimmune conditions, people who have food allergies and intolerances are not at increased risk to develop an autoimmune condition over the general population's risk. And finally, celiac disease involves the activation of a particular type of white blood cell, the T lymphocyte, as well as other parts of the immune system. Because of this, patients with celiac disease are at increased risk to develop GI cancers, in particular lymphomas. Because food allergies and intolerances do not involve this particular immune system pathway, and do not cause severe GI tract damage, these patients are not at increased risk for these cancers.

Thus, while celiac disease, wheat allergy, and gluten intolerance may be treated with similar diets, they are not the same conditions. It is very important for a person to know which condition they have, as the person with celiac disease needs to monitor himself or herself for nutritional deficiencies, other autoimmune diseases, and GI cancers. In general, the symptoms from food allergies and intolerances resolve when the offending foods are removed from the diet and do not cause permanent organ damage.

Chapter 21

Soy Allergy

Soy

Soy, a plant in the pea family, has been common in Asian diets for thousands of years. It is found in modern American diets as a food or food additive. Soybeans, the high-protein seeds of the soy plant, contain isoflavones—compounds similar to the female hormone estrogen. The following information highlights what is known about soy when used by adults for health purposes.

What Soy Is Used For

People use soy products to prevent or treat a variety of health conditions, including high cholesterol levels, menopausal symptoms such as hot flashes, osteoporosis, memory problems, high blood pressure, breast cancer, and prostate cancer.

How Soy Is Used

Soy is available in dietary supplements, in forms such as tablets and capsules. Soy supplements may contain isoflavones or soy protein or both.

This chapter contains text from "Soy," by the National Center for Complementary and Alternative Medicine (NCCAM, www.nccam.nih.gov), part of the National Institutes of Health, March 2008, and excerpted from "Guidance on the Labeling of Certain Uses of Lecithin Derived from Soy Under Section 403(w) of the Federal Food, Drug, and Cosmetic Act," by the U.S. Food and Drug Administration (FDA, www.fda.gov), April 2006.

Soybeans can be cooked and eaten or used to make tofu, soy milk, and other foods. Also, soy is sometimes used as an additive in various processed foods, including baked goods, cheese, and pasta.

What the Science Says

Research suggests that daily intake of soy protein may slightly lower levels of LDL ("bad") cholesterol.

Some studies suggest that soy isoflavone supplements may reduce hot flashes in women after menopause. However, the results have been inconsistent.

There is not enough scientific evidence to determine whether soy supplements are effective for any other health uses.

NCCAM supports studies on soy, including its effects on cardiovascular disease and breast cancer and on menopause-related symptoms and bone loss.

Side Effects and Cautions

Soy is considered safe for most people when used as a food or when taken for short periods as a dietary supplement. Minor stomach and bowel problems such as nausea, bloating, and constipation are possible.

Allergic reactions such as breathing problems and rash can occur in rare cases.

The safety of long-term use of soy isoflavones has not been established.

Evidence is mixed on whether using isoflavone supplements over time can increase the risk of endometrial hyperplasia (a thickening of the lining of the uterus that can lead to cancer). Studies show no effect of dietary soy on risk for endometrial hyperplasia.

Soy's possible role in breast cancer risk is uncertain. Until more is known about soy's effect on estrogen levels, women who have or who are at increased risk of developing breast cancer or other hormone-sensitive conditions (such as ovarian or uterine cancer) should be particularly careful about using soy and should discuss it with their health care providers.

Tell all your health care providers about any complementary and alternative practices you use. Give them a full picture of what you do to manage your health. This will help ensure coordinated and safe care.

Guidance on the Labeling of Certain Uses of Lecithin Derived from Soy Under Section 403(w) of the Federal Food, Drug, and Cosmetic Act

Soy is recognized as one of the eight most common food allergens. Although definitive studies assessing the prevalence of soy allergy are lacking, it is currently estimated that 0.2% of children and adults in the United States are allergic to soy. Based on this estimate, soy allergy appears to be less prevalent than allergies to other major food allergens.

As with most common food allergens, allergic reactions to soy may result in life-threatening symptoms, such as anaphylaxis. Furthermore, even low levels of soy protein may cause adverse effects in some sensitive individuals. FDA considers an "adverse effect" to be any objective sign of an allergic reaction. Currently, due to limited data, there is no consensus on the minimal dose of soy protein that will elicit an adverse effect (also referred to as the lowest observed adverse effect level, or LOAEL). At least some researchers have suggested, however, that the LOAEL for soy protein appears to be higher than the LOAELs reported for other major allergens, such as milk, egg, and peanuts.

Lecithin Derived from Soy

Lecithin is a food ingredient that is derived from plant sources, including soy. Lecithin is isolated following hydration of solvent-extracted soy, sunflower, or corn oil. Lecithin is affirmed as generally recognized as safe (GRAS) with no limitation other than current good manufacturing practice. Common food applications of lecithin include use as an emulsifier, a stabilizer, a dispersing aid, and an incidental additive, such as a release agent for baked goods. Regardless of its food application, lecithin is generally used in small amounts, with the result that it is, according to one lecithin manufacturer, present in finished foods at levels rarely exceeding 1% by weight of the final food product.

During manufacture of lecithin derived from soy, most, but not all, of the soy protein is removed. Soy allergens, to the extent they are present in lecithin, would be found in the protein fraction of the ingredient. Accurately measuring lecithin's protein content presents challenges to current analytical methodology due to the ingredient's oily matrix and low levels of protein. The GRAS affirmation regulation specifies that the ingredient meet the specifications of the Food Chemicals Codex (FCC). The FCC monograph stipulates that food grade lecithin contain not more than 0.3% hexane-insoluble matter. Because the protein fraction of lecithin would reside in such insoluble material, this specification would limit the amount of protein in food grade lecithin to 0.3% or 300 mg/ 100 g lecithin. At least one major U.S. producer has stated that its manufacturing standard for lecithin derived from soy is set at 0.05% hexane-insoluble material or 50 mg/100g lecithin.

Allergic Potential of Lecithin Derived from Soy

As noted, lecithin derived from soy contains very small amounts of soy protein and it is generally used in small amounts, whether for a functional or technical effect in the finished food or as an incidental additive. The proteins in soy lecithin have been found, in some cases, to be soy allergens, and there are a few case reports in the medical literature of allergic reactions to lecithin derived from soy. However, allergy to lecithin derived from soy has been neither definitively established nor definitively negated by oral food challenge studies. Despite its widespread use in the food supply, FDA is aware of only a few allergen-related complaints about FDA-regulated products containing lecithin derived from soy. Also, FDA is aware that some clinicians believe that foods containing lecithin derived from soy present little or no allergic risk to soy-sensitive consumers, and these physicians do not advise their soy allergic patients to avoid lecithin derived from soy.

Labeling of Lecithin Derived from Soy

Whether intended to have a technical or functional effect in the finished food or used as an incidental additive (such as a release agent), lecithin derived from soy must be declared as an ingredient, using its common or usual name, and with the food source ("soy," "soya", or "soybeans") declared as required by food labeling laws.

Chapter 22

Ingredients and Food Additives That Trigger Reactions

Chapter Contents

Section 22.1

Seed Allergy

"Seed Allergy," © 2010 Food Allergy Initiative
(www.faiusa.org). Reprinted with permission.

Sesame seed allergy appears to be on the rise in many countries, including the United States. These seeds are capable of causing severe allergic reactions. Canada and the European Commission have added sesame to the list of ingredients that must be reported on food labels, although the United States has not yet done so.

The more widely an allergenic food is consumed in a particular country, the more likely the population is to report an allergy to that food. In the Middle East, where sesame seeds and oil are dietary staples, the incidence of sesame seed allergy is very high. In fact, sesame is the third most common allergy in Israeli children, after cow's milk allergy and egg allergy. Researchers theorize that the growing popularity of snacks and ethnic foods that contain sesame in Europe, North America, Australia, and New Zealand accounts for the increase in sesame seed allergy in these parts of the world.

Allergies to other seeds (e.g., poppy, sunflower, pumpkin, rapeseed, and flaxseed, also known as linseed) are much less common, so they are not discussed in detail in this text. People who are allergic to one type of seed don't necessarily have to avoid all others, so you should discuss this matter with your doctor.

How to Avoid Seeds

The federal Food Allergen Labeling and Consumer Protection Act (FALCPA) currently does not require that manufacturers list sesame or any other type of seed on ingredient labels. That means that if you have a seed allergy, you will have to be especially vigilant. Always read all product labels carefully before purchasing and consuming any item. Be on the lookout for vague language (e.g., "spices") and call the manufacturer to find out whether or not the product contains sesame. Remember, also, that ingredients change from time to time, so check labels every time you shop. Sesame and other seeds are found in a wide array of foods, so always take extra precaution when dining in restaurants or eating foods prepared by others. If you are ever in doubt about any product or dish, don't eat it.

The following ingredients and foods indicate the presence of sesame seed protein:

- Benne/benne seed/benniseed

- Gomasio (sesame salt)

- Halvah

- Hummus

- Tahini

- Seeds

- Sesame oil (also known as gingelly or til oil)

- Sesamol/sesamolina

- Sesamum indicum

- Sim sim

- Vegetable oil

Baked goods (breads, buns, rolls, crackers, cookies, pastries, bagels, etc.) and certain cereals (e.g., muesli) often contain sesame and other seeds (e.g., poppy, sunflower).

Many snack foods (e.g., trail mix, granola bars, protein bars, candy, rice cakes, pretzels, bagel chips or pita chips) contain sesame seeds.

Sesame seeds may be found in a wide variety of other foods, including margarine, sauces, dips, soups, salad dressing, processed meats, and vegetarian burgers.

Bakeries and ethnic restaurants (such as Middle Eastern and Asian) are considered high-risk for people with sesame allergy due to the common use of sesame and the risk of cross-contamination, even if a sesame-free item is ordered.

Non-food sources of sesame seeds include health and beauty aids (cosmetics, soaps, hair care products, etc.), certain drugs and ointments, pet food, and livestock feed.

Section 22.2

Sulfite Sensitivity

Sensitivity to sulfites can develop at any time during a person's lifespan, with some initial reactions not showing up until a person has reached their forties or fifties. The manifestations of sulfite sensitivity include a large array of dermatological, pulmonary, gastrointestinal, and cardiovascular symptoms. Asthmatics that are steroid-dependent or have a great degree of airway hyperreactivity may be at an increased risk of having a reaction to a sulfite containing food. Varying degrees of bronchospasm, angioedema, urticaria, nausea, abdominal cramping, and diarrhea are commonly reported. Adverse reactions to sulfites in nonasthmatics are extremely rare.

Although literature lists a range of figures as to what percent of the population is affected, the Food and Drug Administration (FDA) estimates that one out of a hundred people is sulfite-sensitive, and of that group 5% have asthma. Another source states that 5% of asthmatics are sulfite sensitive, compared to only 1% of the nonasthmatic population, while another source estimates that up to 500,000 (or less than .05% of the population) sulfite-sensitive individuals live in the United States.

Symptoms of sulfite intolerance can occur within 5 minutes following parenteral exposure and within 15–30 minutes following oral exposure. Sensitive individuals vary in their degree of intolerance towards sulfites, with each having a specific threshold of exposure needed to elicit a reaction. While the majority of reactions are mild, severe nonspecific signs and symptoms do occur on occasion. Although the precise mechanisms of the sensitivity responses to sulfites have not been completely elucidated, three have been implicated: inhalation of sulfur dioxide (SO_2) generated in the stomach proceeding ingestion of sulfite-containing foods or beverages; deficiency in a mitochondrial enzyme; or an IgE [immunoglobulin E]-mediated immune response.

Recommendations for Sulfite-Sensitive Individuals

The following are measures those with sensitivity to sulfites should take when buying unlabeled foods at a deli, supermarket, or food service establishment:

- If the food is being sold loose or by portion, ask the store manager or waiter to check the ingredient list on the product's original bulk size packaging.

- Avoid processed foods that contain sulfites, such as dried fruits, canned vegetables, maraschino cherries, and guacamole.

- When ordering a potato, opt for a baked potato over any kind that involves peeling of the vegetable during preparation.

If you have asthma, don't go out to eat without your inhaler. If you've experienced a reaction to sulfites in the past, carry an antihistamine with you, and make sure you have self-injectable epinephrine in order to stabilize your condition until you can reach an emergency room.

Section 22.3

Histamine Intolerance

"Dietary Management of Histamine Intolerance," by Janice Vickerstaff
Joneja, PhD, RD. © Vickerstaff Health Services Inc. Reprinted with permission. For additional information, visit www.allergynutrition.com. The
text that follows this document under the heading *"Health Reference Series
Medical Advisor's Notes and Updates"* was provided to Omnigraphics, Inc.
by David A. Cooke, MD, FACP, August 10, 2010. Dr. Cooke is not affiliated
with Vickerstaff Health Services Inc.

What Is Histamine?

Histamine is an extremely important bioactive chemical that is
indispensable in the efficient functioning of many body systems. It is
a neurotransmitter (a chemical that conveys messages between cells
of the nervous system) and is involved in the regulation of stomach
(gastric) acid, the permeability of blood vessels, muscle contraction,
and brain function. Histamine appears in various concentrations in
a range of mammalian tissues. In humans, the highest histamine
concentrations are found in the skin, lung, and stomach, with smaller
amounts in the brain and heart.

Histamine is also essential in defending the body against invasion
by potentially disease-causing agents such as bacteria, viruses, and
other foreign invaders. Histamine is made and stored within white
blood cells (leukocytes) such as mast cells in tissues and basophils that
circulate in blood. When the immune system is activated in response
to foreign material entering the body, histamine is the first "defense
chemical," or more correctly, inflammatory mediator, released in the
process called inflammation. Inflammation is the clinical evidence that
the immune system is responding.

In addition to its role in controlling vital body processes and defending against foreign invaders, histamine is a key mediator in the
symptoms of an allergic reaction. Since allergy is essentially an inflammatory reaction, histamine, together with other protective inflammatory mediators is released in response to the allergen. Allergens are
components of living cells that in themselves are harmless, such as
plant pollens, animal dander, mold spores, dust particles, dust mites,

and foods. An allergic reaction to these "foreign but harmless" substances occurs when the immune system mistakes these innocuous materials for a potential threat.

Where Does Histamine Come From?

Body Cells and Systems (Intrinsic Histamine)

Histamine is a biogenic amine (sometimes referred to as a vasoactive amine) that, in mammals, is produced primarily by the action of the enzyme histidine decarboxylase on the amino acid histidine. Histidine is one of the 20 or so amino acids that combine together to make a protein. Histidine decarboxylase is present in large quantities in leukocytes known as granulocytes (granule-containing cells), especially tissue mast cells and blood basophils. In these cells it converts histidine to histamine. The newly formed histamine is then stored in structures within the cell (called intracellular granules) in readiness for release in response to signals from a variety of body systems. In inflammation, whether produced in defending the body from injury or infection, or as a result of an allergic reaction, these signals come from lymphocytes, cytokines, and antibodies. However, this is not the only source of histamine in our bodies.

Microorganisms in the Large Bowel

There are a large number of microorganisms that are capable of producing histamine. Many of the bacteria that live in the human large bowel produce histidine decarboxylase and are capable of converting the histidine in any protein that enters the bowel into histamine. Therefore, the more microorganisms that produce histidine decarboxylase that are present in the colon, and the greater the amount of protein material that enters the bowel, the higher the level of histamine in the digestive tract. From here, histamine can be conveyed through the bowel wall to various sites in the body.

Histamine in Natural Foods (Extrinsic Histamine)

Another source of histamine is the food we eat. Microorganisms capable of converting histidine to histamine exist ubiquitously in nature, so histamine can arise from various sources. For example, histidine decarboxylase-producing bacteria colonize the gut of fish. As soon as a fish dies, the gut bacteria start to break down the tissue proteins, releasing histidine, which is then rapidly converted to histamine. Since bacteria multiply rapidly, it is possible that the level of histamine in the ungutted fish can double every 20 minutes. The longer a fish remains ungutted after it dies, the higher the level of histamine in its tissues. Furthermore, since shellfish are not gutted after harvesting, the bacteria in their gut will produce histamine as long as the fish remain uncooked. Many a reaction to fish or shellfish has been blamed on allergy, when in reality it was a reaction to an exceedingly high level of histamine in an incorrectly processed fish.

Histamine in Manufactured Foods

There are a number of food manufacturing processes that depend on the production of amines and similar chemicals for the flavor and nature of the food. Any process that requires microbial fermentation will result in the production of relatively high levels of amines, especially histamine. Cheese of all types, alcoholic beverages, vinegar, fermented vegetables such as sauerkraut, fermented soy products such as soy sauce, and processed meats such as pepperoni, bologna, and salami that are produced by a process of fermentation all contain substantial levels of histamine.

Other Food Sources of Histamine

Certain foods seem to contain high levels of histamine in conditions where microbial fermentation is an unlikely event. Histamine has been consistently detected in fruits such as citrus fruits, berries such as strawberry and raspberry, tomatoes, several types of tree fruits such as apricot, cherry, and plums, and some vegetables, particularly eggplant (aubergine) and pumpkin. Some preliminary research studies have indicated that histamine may be produced during ripening in tomatoes, and it may be that some, if not all fruits that go through a similar process produce histamine in the course of ripening. It remains for future research to explain this phenomenon.

Histamine Derived from Foods by Unknown Mechanisms

Traditionally, certain foods have been said to have "histamine-releasing" properties because ingestion of the food tends to result in symptoms of histamine. For example, egg white is a food that is frequently referred to as "histamine-releasing," separate and distinct from its activity as an allergen. Strawberries, raspberries, and shellfish were previously similarly designated, but more recent research has uncovered evidence of physiological and biochemical processes as the origin of histamine from these foods. However, a non-allergic mechanism of histamine release by egg white remains to be determined.

Another mode of histamine release associated with food materials is suggested by research into the mechanisms of intolerance associated with food additives. Azo (nitrogen-containing) food dyes such as tartrazine, and preservatives such as benzoates, sorbates, and possibly sulfites have been suggested to release histamine by as yet undisclosed processes. Clinical experiments have demonstrated that persons sensitive to these chemicals experience an increase in plasma histamine that remains elevated long after histamine levels in the non-reactive person have returned to normal. Again, an understanding of the way in which histamine is released in such reactions will depend on future research.

How Much Histamine Is Excessive?

Pre-formed histamine ingested from a food at a level of more than 2.7 mg/kg body weight will induce symptoms of histamine intolerance or even "histamine poisoning," but if ingested at lower concentrations only a few sensitive individuals will experience an adverse reaction. It has been speculated that the differences between people in the level of histamine that they can tolerate may be of genetic origin. In addition, disease, various abnormal physiological conditions, and medications can reduce the tolerance threshold of any individual.

It has been suggested that certain abnormal physiological conditions may lead to histamine intolerance, in particular a defect in the process of histamine breakdown (catabolism). Under normal physiological conditions dietary histamine is degraded by two enzyme systems: histamine N-methyl transferase, and in the intestine by the mucosal enzyme diamine oxidase (DAO). Of the two systems, it is deficiency in the DAO enzyme system that has received most attention as the probable cause of "histamine intolerance." Under normal physiological conditions, when histamine levels from any source rise above a certain level, these enzymes rapidly degrade the excess. However, when the rate of breakdown of excess histamine is insufficient to deal with the excess, the total level of histamine in the body rises. At a certain critical level, signs and symptoms occur that are the result of histamine coupling with histamine receptors on specific cells, producing a clinical picture that is often indistinguishable from allergy.

Symptoms of Histamine Excess

Whatever the source of histamine, when the total body level exceeds the catabolic enzymes' capacity to break it down, symptoms of histamine excess occur. Histamine intolerance manifests itself in a variety of signs and symptoms such as:

- pruritus (itching especially of the skin, eyes, ears, and nose);
- urticaria (hives);
- tissue swelling (angioedema) especially of facial and oral tissues;
- hypotension (drop in blood pressure);
- tachycardia (increased pulse rate, "heart racing");
- symptoms resembling a panic attack;
- chest pain;
- nasal congestion and runny nose;
- conjunctivitis (irritated, watery, reddened eyes);
- some types of headaches not believed to be migraine;
- fatigue, confusion, irritability;
- digestive tract upset, especially heartburn, indigestion, and reflux.

Not all of these symptoms occur in any single individual, but the pattern of symptoms seems to be consistent for each person.

How Can Diet Help in Reducing Excess Histamine?

Because the appearance and severity of symptoms depends on the level of excess histamine in the body, histamine intolerance, in contrast to allergy, is a dose-related phenomenon. In other words, symptoms of histamine excess depend on the sum total of histamine from all sources. It is often possible to reduce or eliminate the symptoms of histamine excess by reducing exposure to histamine-releasing events (such as airborne and food allergens), and avoiding consumption of histamine-containing and histamine releasing foods and food additives.

The degree of improvement or resolution of the symptoms of histamine excess that can be achieved by diet alone will depend on whether the food sources of histamine can be reduced below a person's limit of tolerance. An analogy can be drawn to a bucket being filled with water. When the water rises above the top of the bucket it overflows. If the top of the bucket is likened to the limit of tolerance, overflowing the bucket would be analogous to the appearance of symptoms. By reducing a person's total level of histamine to below the symptom range (i.e., below the top of the bucket), it should be possible to achieve relief of their symptoms. The diet in my book *Dealing with Food Allergies* is designed to exclude all known sources of histamine. However, some people will not achieve relief by diet alone because even by excluding all of the histamine-rich foods, their total level of histamine is still above the top of the bucket.

Identifying the Culprit Foods

When symptomatic relief is achieved on the diet, each food component can be reintroduced in a process of incremental dose challenge that should clearly identify a person's limit of tolerance to it. However, because histamine intolerance is dose-related, a person's limit of tolerance can be exceeded by eating several histamine-associated foods at the same meal, or within a short span of time, thus reaching a total level of histamine that will result in symptoms.

Because a person's total histamine level varies as a result of many circumstances, especially allergy, there will be a constant fluctuation in the signs and symptoms of histamine excess in response to changing conditions. For example, when a person is experiencing allergy to airborne allergens such as seasonal pollens, the histamine released in the allergic response alone might put them into the symptom range. In such a case, avoiding histamine-associated foods will no longer relieve their symptoms because their total level of histamine will remain above their limit of tolerance. This explains the observation that during their "pollen allergy season" many people find themselves reacting to foods (usually histamine-rich foods) that they could normally eat with impunity.

As a result of the multiple factors contributing to excess histamine, combined with each individual's capacity to deal with histamine excess, symptoms of histamine intolerance are constantly changing in incidence and severity. Unlike IgE-mediated allergy (type 1 hypersensitivity) in which the presence of the antigen results in an immediate immunological response and development of typical symptoms, histamine intolerance is frequently baffling because a certain food does not always result in clinical symptoms. Therefore, it is not possible to eliminate just those foods that cause a reaction on challenge. It is necessary to restrict a person's intake of histamine-associated foods to a total that remains below their personal limit of tolerance. That is why it is important that a person not only records their reactions to specific foods, but also obtains an idea of the quantity of the food that results in symptoms. This is built into the protocol for testing each food component known as incremental dose challenge (SIDC).

More information on histamine intolerance can be found in the article: Joneja JMV and Carmona Silva C. Outcome of a histamine-restricted diet based on chart audit. *Journal of Nutritional and Environmental Medicine* 2001;11(4):249–262.

Histamine Function References

1. Lessof MH, Gant V, Hinuma K, Murphy GM, Dowling RH. Recurrent urticaria and reduced diamune oxidase activity. *Clin Exper Allergy* 1990 20:373–376.

2. Rangachari PK. Histamine: mercurial messenger in the gut. *Amer J Physiology* 1992 262:G1–G13.

3. Wantke F, Proud D, Siekierski E, Kagey-Sobotka A. Daily variations of serum diamine oxidase and the influence of H1 and H2 blockers: A critical approach to routine diamine oxidase assessment. *Inflammation Research* 1998 47:396–400.

4. Picton S, Gray JE, Payton S, Barton SL, Lowe A, Grierson D. A histidine decarboxylase-like mRNA is involved in tomato fruit ripening. *Plant Molecular Biology* 1993 23:627–631.

5. Chin KW, Garriga MM, Metcalfe DD. The histamine content of oriental foods. *Food Chem Toxic* 1989 27(5):283–287.

6. Halasz A, Barath A, Simon-Sarkadi L, Holzapfel W. Biogenic amines and their production by microorganisms in food. *Trends in Food Science and Technology* 1994 5:42–49.

7. Diel E, Bayas N, Stibbe A, Muller S, Bott A, Schrimpf D, Diel F. Histamine containing food: Establishment of a German food intolerance databank (NFID). *Inflammation Research* 1997 46(Suppl 1):S87–S88.

8. Beljaars PR, Van Dijk R, Jonker KM, Schout LJ. Liquid chromatographic determination of histamine in fish, sauerkraut, and wine: Interlaboratory study. *Journal of AOAC International* 1998 81(5):991–998.

9. Soares VFM, and Gloria MBA. Histamine levels in canned fish available in Belo Horizonte, Minas Gerais, Brazil. *Journal of Food Composition and Analysis* 1994 7:102–109.

10. Vidal-Carou MC, Isla-Gavin MJ, Marine-Font A, Codony-Salcedo R. Histamine and tyramine in natural sparkling wine, vermouth, cider, and vinegar. *Journal of Food Composition and Analysis* 1989 2:210–218.

11. Izquierdo-Pulido ML, Vidal-Carou MC, Marine-Font A. Histamine and tyramine in beers: contents and relationships with other analytical data. *J Food Comp Anal* 1989 2:219–227.

12. Wantke F, Gotz M, Jarisch R. Histamine-free diet: treatment of choice for histamine induced food intolerance and supporting treatment for chronical headaches. *Clin Exper Allergy* 1993 23:982–985.

13. Wantke F, Gotz M, Jarisch R. Histamine-free diet: Treatment of choice for histamine-induced food intolerance and supporting treatment for chronic headaches. *Clinical and Experimental Allergy* 1993 23:982–985.

14. Jarisch R, Beringer K, Hemmer W. Role of food allergy and food intolerance in recurrent urticaria. In: Wuthrich B. (ed). *Food Allergy The Atopy Syndrome in the Third Millennium. Curr Probl Dermatol* 1999 28:64–73.

15. Jarisch R and Wantke F. Wine and headache. *Int Arch Allergy Immunol* 1996 110:7–12.

16. Befani O, Shiozaki TS, Turini P, Gerosa P, Mondovi B. Inhibition of diamine oxidase activity by metronidazole. Biochemical and Biophysical Research Communications 1995 212(2):589–594.

17. Joosten HMLJ. Conditions allowing the formation of biogenic amines in cheese III Factors influencing the amounts formed. *Netherlands Milk and Dairy Journal* 1987 41(4):329–357.

18. Freed DLJ. Dietary lectins and disease. In Brostoff J and Challacombe SJ (eds) *Food Allergy and Intolerance* Bailliere Tindall, London 1987 375–400.

19. Moneret-Vautrin DA. Food intolerance masquerading as food allergy. In Brostoff J and Challacombe SJ (eds) *Food Allergy and Intolerance* Bailliere Tindall, London 1987 836–849.

20. Sampson HA and Burks AW. Mechanisms of food allergy. *Ann Rev Nutr* 1996; 16:161–177.

21. Dannaeus A, Inganas M. A follow-up study of children with food allergy. Clinical course in relation to serum IgE- and IgG-antibody levels to milk, egg, and fish. *Clin Allergy* 1981; 11:533–539.

22. Drasar BS, and Hill MJ. *Human intestinal flora.* Academic Press, London 1974.

23. Mertz HR. New concepts of irritable bowel syndrome. *Current Gastroenterology Reports* 1999 1:433–440.

24. Gue M, Del Rio-Lacheze C, Eutamene H, et al. Stress induced visceral hypersensitivity to rectal distension in rats: Role of CRF and mast cells. *Neurogastroenterol Motil* 1997 9:271–279.

Health Reference Series Medical Advisor's Notes and Updates

The concept of histamine intolerance as a disease remains quite controversial. While some researchers believe it is a common and underdiagnosed condition, other experts question whether there is sufficient evidence to prove it exists. This article is in keeping with the arguments of proponents of the condition, but the reader should understand that not all experts will agree with the statements presented here.

Chapter 23

Other Health Problems Related to Food Allergic Reactions

Chapter Contents

Section 23.1

Eosinophilic Esophagitis

What is eosinophilic esophagitis (EE)?

EE is an inflammation in the tube that connects the throat to the
stomach (esophagus). It is also called "EoE" or "allergic esophagitis."
Eosinophils (also called "eos") are white blood cells. They are connected
with the body's allergic response. The exact cause of EE is not always
known. Diet is a factor. Long-term diet changes and/or medicine will
often control the disease.

What are the symptoms?

- Feeding problems and vomiting in infants and young children

- Vomiting or stomach pain in school age children

- Swallowing problems (dysphagia) or food getting stuck in the
  esophagus (food impaction) in older children and teens

Who tends to get it?

Anyone can have it, but it happens more often in:

- school-age children;

- boys;

- a child whose family has allergies. Allergy problems are asthma,
  hay fever, food allergy, and eczema.

How is it diagnosed?

A small piece of tissue is taken (called a biopsy) from the esophagus.
The procedure is called an endoscopy. More endoscopies will be needed
to see if the treatments are working. This is the only way to check on
the status of the disease.

How is EE treated?

Care is given by a team of health care providers. They include [the following]:

- Gastroenterologist (GI): The GI doctor does the endoscopy and talks with a pathologist about the biopsies.

- Allergist: This doctor does allergy testing to find foods in the diet that are a problem. They may also treat other allergy problems such as asthma and hay fever.

- Nurse: The nurse coordinates care and answers questions between clinic visits.

- Dietitian: The dietitian talks about taking certain foods out of the diet and your child's nutrition.

Your child's care will be based on:

- how severe the disease is;

- your child's allergies;

- your ability to follow the plan.

Treatment includes taking foods out of the diet, taking medicine, or both. In general, the treatment should not be worse than the disease.

Severe disease will need an aggressive treatment plan. It may take trying several things before finding the best treatment for your child.

Regular visits are needed and may include:

- an endoscopy (this is needed to see if the treatment is working);

- allergy tests;

- dietitian visits to check growth, nutrition, and issues with the diet.

Diet: Diet changes are the best treatment. They are the only long-term control for EE. Foods that cause an allergic response or discomfort when eaten need to be taken out of your child's diet. This is called food elimination. It can be done in three ways.

- **Guided food elimination:** Allergy tests of foods that cause reactions are done by blood, skin prick, or skin patch testing. After the allergy tests are done, the foods that are found to cause a reaction may be removed from the diet.

- **Non-guided food elimination:** Foods known to cause EE are removed from the diet. Sometimes even when allergy testing is

negative they are removed. They include milk, soy, egg, peanut/
tree nut, wheat, and seafood.

- **Complete food elimination (Elemental Diet):** This is the final option. It is used for those who are very allergic to foods and/or already have feeding tubes. Age-appropriate liquid formula will replace food. These formulas are pre-digested and invisible to the immune system. The formula has all the nutrition needed for growth and development. Often a large amount must be given. A feeding tube may be needed to help your child meet their nutrition needs.

Medicine: Medicines may be added if changes in the diet do not help. They do not cure the disease. Stopping the medicine may cause the symptoms to come back.

Medicines may be needed to quickly help the symptoms while they look for allergies.

Oral steroids (prednisone) will often help. A steroid affects all of the body and has side effects. They include weight gain, high blood pressure, bloating, and/or mood changes. If these side effects can be managed, the medicine is often very useful.

Local steroids such as those used for asthma can also be used. They work directly on the inflamed area. This limits the side effects of the steroids. Examples of this are swallowing Flovent® from an inhaler or drinking thickened Pulmicort® flavored with Splenda®.

What happens in the long run?

Most often, EE will not go away on its own. Without treatment it may cause scarring and more severe problems later on. Without treatment, adults may end up on a mostly liquid diet. Regular stretching (dilatation) of the esophagus during endoscopy may also be needed. At this time there is no known increased risk for patients with EE having esophageal cancer.

Where can I get more information?

Information about your child's specific case should come from your child's health care team.

General information about eosinophilic esophagitis and /or food allergy may be found at:

- The American Partnership for Eosinophilic Disorders (APFED, www.apfed.org)

- The Food Allergy and Anaphylaxis Network (FAAN, www.food allergy.org)

- The Food Allergy Project (www.foodallergyproject.org)

- Wisconsin Partners of Eosinophilic Patients (WI-PEP) Support group (For more information e-mail wisconsinpep@gmail.com)

Alert: Call your child's doctor, nurse, or clinic if you have any questions or concerns or if your child has special health care needs that were not covered by this information.

This information is meant to help you care for your child. It does not take the place of medical care. Talk with your healthcare provider for diagnosis, treatment, and follow-up.

Section 23.2

Food Protein-Induced Enterocolitis Syndrome

"FPIES: Food Protein Induced Enterocolitis Syndrome,"
© 2008 Kids With Food Allergies, Inc. (www.kidswithfoodallergies.org).
Reprinted with permission.

What does FPIES stand for?

FPIES is food protein-induced enterocolitis syndrome. It is commonly pronounced "F-Pies," as in "apple pies," though some physicians may refer to it as FIES (pronounced "fees," considering food-protein as one word). Enterocolitis is inflammation involving both the small intestine and the colon (large intestine).

What is FPIES?

FPIES is a non-IgE [immunoglobulin E] mediated immune reaction in the gastrointestinal system to one or more specific foods, commonly characterized by profuse vomiting and diarrhea. FPIES is presumed to be cell mediated. Poor growth may occur with continual ingestion.

Upon removing the problem food(s), all FPIES symptoms subside. (Note: Having FPIES does not preclude one from having other allergies/intolerances with the food.) The most common FPIES triggers are cow's milk (dairy) and soy. However, any food can cause an FPIES reaction, even those not commonly considered allergens, such as rice, oat, and barley.

A child with FPIES may experience what appears to be a severe stomach bug, but the "bug" only starts a couple hours after the offending food is given. Many FPIES parents have rushed their children to the ER, limp from extreme, repeated projectile vomiting, only to be told, "It's the stomach flu." However, the next time they feed their children the same solids, the dramatic symptoms return.

What does IgE vs cell mediated mean?

IgE stands for Immunoglobulin E. It is a type of antibody, formed to protect the body from infection, that functions in allergic reactions. IgE-mediated reactions are considered immediate hypersensitivity immune system reactions, while cell mediated reactions are considered delayed hypersensitivity. Antibodies are not involved in cell mediated reactions. For the purpose of understanding FPIES, you can disregard all you know about IgE-mediated reactions.

When do FPIES reactions occur?

FPIES reactions often show up in the first weeks or months of life, or at an older age for the exclusively breastfed child. Reactions usually occur upon introducing first solid foods, such as infant cereals or formulas, which are typically made with dairy or soy. (Infant formulas are considered solids for FPIES purposes.) While a child may have allergies and intolerances to food proteins they are exposed to through breast milk, FPIES reactions usually don't occur from breast milk, regardless of the mother's diet. An FPIES reaction typically takes place when the child has directly ingested the trigger food(s).

What is a typical FPIES reaction?

As with all things, each child is different, and the range, severity, and duration of symptoms may vary from reaction to reaction. Unlike traditional IgE-mediated allergies, FPIES reactions do not manifest with itching, hives, swelling, coughing, or wheezing, etc. Symptoms typically only involve the gastrointestinal system, and other body organs are not involved. FPIES reactions almost always begin with delayed onset vomiting (usually 2 hours after ingestion, sometimes as late as 8 hours after). Symptoms can range from mild (an increase in reflux and several days of runny stools) to life threatening (shock). In severe cases, after repeatedly vomiting, children often begin vomiting bile. Commonly, diarrhea follows and can last up to several days. In the worst reactions (about 20% of the time), the child has such severe vomiting and diarrhea that s/he rapidly becomes seriously dehydrated and may go into shock.

What is shock and what are the symptoms?

Shock is a life-threatening condition. Shock may develop as the result of sudden illness, injury, or bleeding. When the body cannot get enough blood to the vital organs, it goes into shock.

Signs of shock include:

- weakness, dizziness, and fainting;
- cool, pale, clammy skin;
- weak, fast pulse;
- shallow, fast breathing;
- low blood pressure;
- extreme thirst, nausea, or vomiting;
- confusion or anxiety.

How do you treat an FPIES reaction?

Always follow your doctor's emergency plan pertaining to your specific situation. Rapid dehydration and shock are medical emergencies. If your child is experiencing symptoms of FPIES or shock, immediately contact your local emergency services (911). If you are uncertain if your child is in need of emergency services, contact 911 or your physician for guidance.

The most critical treatment during an FPIES reaction is intravenous (IV) fluids, because of the risk and prevalence of dehydration. Children experiencing more severe symptoms may also need steroids and in-hospital monitoring. Mild reactions may be able to be treated at home with oral electrolyte rehydration (e.g., Pedialyte®).

Does FPIES require epinephrine?

Not usually, because epinephrine reverses IgE-mediated symptoms, and FPIES is not IgE-mediated. Based on the patient's history, some doctors might prescribe epinephrine to reverse specific symptoms of shock (e.g., low blood pressure). However, this is only prescribed in specific cases.

What are some common FPIES triggers?

The most common FPIES triggers are traditional first foods, such as dairy and soy. Other common triggers are rice, oat, barley, green beans, peas, sweet potatoes, squash, chicken, and turkey. A reaction to one common food does not mean that all of the common foods will be an issue, but patients are often advised to proceed with caution with those foods. Note that while the above foods are the most prevalent, they are not exclusive triggers. Any food has the potential to trigger an FPIES reaction. Even trace amounts can cause a reaction.

How is FPIES diagnosed?

FPIES is difficult to diagnose, unless the reaction has happened more than once, as it is diagnosed by symptom presentation. Typically, foods that trigger FPIES reactions are negative with standard skin and blood allergy tests (SPT [skin prick test], RAST [radioallergosorbent test]) because they look for IgE-mediated responses. However, as stated before, FPIES is not IgE-mediated.

Atopy patch testing (APT) is being studied for its effectiveness in diagnosing FPIES, as well as predicting if the problem food is no longer a trigger. Thus, the outcome of APT may determine if the child is a potential candidate for an oral food challenge (OFC). APT involves placing the trigger food in a metal cap, which is left on the skin for 48 hours. The skin is then watched for symptoms in the following days after removal. Please consult your child's doctor to discuss if APT is indicated in your situation.

How do you care for a child with FPIES?

Treatment varies, depending on the patient and his/her specific reactions. Often, infants who have reacted to both dairy and soy formulas will be placed on hypoallergenic or elemental formula. Some children do well breastfeeding. Other children who have fewer triggers may just strictly avoid the offending food(s).

New foods are usually introduced very slowly, one food at a time, for an extended period of time per food. Some doctors recommend trialing a single food for up to 3 weeks before introducing another.

Because it's a rare, but serious condition, in the event of an emergency, it is vital to get the correct treatment. Some doctors provide their patients with a letter containing a brief description of FPIES and its proper treatment. In the event of a reaction, this letter can be taken to the ER with the child.

Is FPIES a lifelong condition?

Typically, no. Many children outgrow FPIES by about age 3. Note, however, that the time varies per individual and the offending food, so statistics are a guide, but not an absolute. In one study, 100% of children with FPIES reactions to barley had outgrown and were tolerating barley by age 3. However, only 40% of those with FPIES to rice, and 60% to dairy tolerated it by the same age.

How do I know if my child has outgrown FPIES?

Together with your child's doctor, you should determine if/when it is likely that your child may have outgrown any triggers. Obviously, determining if a child has outgrown a trigger is something that needs to be evaluated on a food-by-food basis. As stated earlier, APT testing may be an option to assess oral challenge readiness. Another factor for you and your doctor to consider is if your child would physically be able to handle a possible failed challenge.

When the time comes to orally challenge an FPIES trigger, most doctors familiar with FPIES will want to schedule an in-office food challenge. Some doctors (especially those not practicing in a hospital clinic setting) may choose to challenge in the hospital, with an IV already in place, in case of emergency. Each doctor may have his or her own protocol, but an FPIES trigger is something you should definitely **not** challenge without discussing thoroughly with your doctor.

Be aware that if a child passes the in-office portion of the challenge, it does not mean this food is automatically guaranteed "safe." If a child's delay in reaction is fairly short, a child may fail an FPIES food challenge while still at the office/hospital. For those with longer reaction times, it may not be until later that day that symptoms manifest. Some may react up to 3 days later. Delay times may vary by food as well. If a child has FPIES to multiple foods, one food may trigger symptoms within 4 hours; a different food may not trigger symptoms until 6 or 8 hours after ingestion.

How is FPIES different from MSPI, MSPIES, MPIES, etc.?

MPIES (milk-protein induced enterocolitis syndrome) is FPIES to cow's milk only. MSPIES (milk- and soy-protein induced enterocolitis syndrome) is FPIES to milk and soy. Some doctors do create these subdivisions, while others declare that milk and soy are simply the two most common FPIES triggers and give the diagnosis of "FPIES to milk and/or soy."

MSPI is milk and soy protein intolerance. Symptoms are those of allergic colitis and can include colic, vomiting, diarrhea, and blood in stools. These reactions are not as severe or immediate as an FPIES reaction.

Section 23.3

Oral Allergy Syndrome

Do you ever get an itchy mouth when eating watermelon or cantaloupe? What about that luscious peach that left your gums raw and irritated?

Could be you're one of millions whose pollen allergy also sets them up to react to certain foods.

It's called oral allergy syndrome (OAS) and what's behind it are similarities among some pollen-producing plants and related fruits and vegetables. For instance, a person who gets a runny nose or drippy eyes when exposed to ragweed pollen in the air might develop an itchy, tingling mouth or lips when eating foods with similar proteins.

For ragweed, that includes banana, chamomile, cucumber, echinacea, melon (watermelon, cantaloupe, honeydew), sunflower seed, and zucchini.

New York allergist Clifford Bassett, MD, says as many as one out of every three people with seasonal allergies may experience oral allergy syndrome. The exact number is unclear because the condition often goes undiagnosed. Symptoms can be mild and go away quickly, making it less likely that people will see a doctor for diagnosis. Or parents might not associate a child's dislike of a vegetable with an allergic reaction.

Symptoms can also seem quite random. For instance, many people are only bothered during pollen season; the rest of the year they can eat pollen-related foods with no problem. So if you're allergic to ragweed, a melon in February (when ragweed is dormant) may not bother you at all, while one in September (when ragweed pollen counts are high) could set off symptoms with the first bite.

Dr. Bassett says some people with OAS will react to fresh foods but not cooked or canned varieties. If you have grass allergy, for instance, you may be able to eat tomato sauce on pizza but develop itchy mouth from fresh tomato in a salad. Others may find they can eat certain varieties of a fruit (Macintosh apples versus Granny Smith, for instance) or fruits without their skins.

In addition to itchiness and irritation, OAS symptoms can include mild swelling or hives in or around the mouth. While most will go away when you stop eating the food, Dr. Bassett says it's a good idea to see an allergist for an individual consultation any time you experience allergy symptoms related to food.

Food-related symptoms can sometimes alert you to a more dangerous allergy, such as latex. A board-certified allergist can give you an accurate diagnosis, advise you which foods to avoid and recommend treatments to relieve symptoms.

Oral allergy syndrome is particularly common among people allergic to ragweed—some 36 million people in the United States—but it also affects people with other allergies. Researchers have identified specific foods that relate to birch, grasses and ragweed.

- Birch pollen: Almond, apple, carrot, celery, cherry, hazelnut, kiwi, peach, pear, plum, potato, pumpkin seed

- Grass pollen: Kiwi, melon, peach, tomato

- Ragweed pollen: Banana, chamomile, cucumber, echinacea, melon (watermelon, cantaloupe, honeydew), sunflower seed, zucchini

Chapter 24

What You Should Know about Living with Food Allergy

Checklist for Managing a Food Allergy Lifestyle

This is a must-have checklist for parents of children with food allergies. By adding these habits into your lifestyle, you can effectively manage food allergies.

Make Sure Food Is Free of Allergens Your Child Needs to Avoid

- Totally avoid all foods containing allergens—even traces of those allergens—to prevent allergic reactions.

- Educate yourself about food allergy management and then educate your child, friends, school, and community about food allergies.

- Focus on what your child can have; not what he cannot.

- Read labels every time and become familiar with the names for hidden ingredients in foods your child needs to avoid.

- Prepare and choose foods that are not cross contaminated with allergens your child needs to avoid.

- Don't ever assume that a food item is allergen-free without reading the label or verifying its safety with whoever prepared it.

This chapter begins with "Checklist for managing a food allergy lifestyle," © 2009 Kids With Food Allergies, Inc. (www.kidswithfoodallergies.org). Reprinted with permission. Additional text under the heading "Questions and Answers about Living with Food Allergies," from the National Institute of Allergy and Infectious Diseases, is cited separately within the chapter.

Take Charge of Your Child's Health Care

- Find a board-certified allergist or pediatric allergist for diagnosis and management of your child's food allergies.

- Work with your child's doctors to develop a food allergy action plan to treat an allergic reaction.

- Work with your schools, daycares, preschools, and other places that care for your child to develop a plan to reduce exposure to your child's allergens.

- Have emergency medicines available at all times.

- Consider having your child wear an emergency medical identification bracelet.

- Work closely with your doctors and don't hesitate to seek guidance from a registered dietitian to help maintain your child's nutritionally balanced diet—removing foods from a child's diet can result in nutritional deficiencies.

- Work with your pharmacist to help select medications and health products that do not include your child's allergens.

Empower Your Child

- Teach your child, in an age-appropriate way, how to be responsible for his food allergies. Involve him in meal preparation, grocery shopping, and label reading—and teach him how to refuse food that a parent or responsible caregiver hasn't approved in advance.

- Make sure your child understands why she can't eat the same things as her siblings/friends/family.

Questions and Answers about Living with Food Allergies

The information that follows is excerpted and adapted from "Food Allergy: An Overview," by the National Institute for Allergy and Infectious Diseases (NIAID, www.niaid.nih.gov), part of the National Institutes of Health, July 2007.

How do I avoid unintentional exposures to an allergen?

If you are highly allergic, even the tiniest amounts of a food allergen (for example, a small portion of a peanut kernel) can prompt an allergic reaction.

If you have food allergies, you must be prepared to treat unintentional exposure. Even people who know a lot about what they are sensitive to occasionally make a mistake. To protect yourself if you have had allergic reactions to a food, you should do the following:

- Wear a medical alert bracelet or necklace stating that you have a food allergy and are subject to severe reactions.

- Carry an auto-injector device containing epinephrine (adrenaline), such as an EpiPen or Twinject, that you can get by prescription and give to yourself if you think you are getting a food allergic reaction.

- Seek medical help immediately, even if you have already given yourself epinephrine, by either calling the rescue squad or by getting transported to an emergency room.

Anaphylactic allergic reactions can be fatal even when they start off with mild symptoms such as a tingling in the mouth and throat or GI discomfort.

Are there medicines I can take to relieve symptoms of allergic reaction?

There are several medicines you can take to relieve food allergy symptoms that are not part of an anaphylactic reaction. These include:

- antihistamines to relieve GI symptoms, hives, or sneezing and a runny nose;

- bronchodilators to relieve asthma symptoms.

It is not easy to determine if a reaction to food is anaphylactic, however. It is important to develop a plan with a healthcare provider as to what reactions you should treat with epinephrine first, rather than antihistamines or bronchodilators.

What about food allergies in infants or children?

Allergy to cow's milk is particularly common in infants and young children. It causes hives and asthma in some children. In others, it can lead to colic and sleeplessness, and perhaps blood in the stool or poor growth. Infants are thought to be particularly susceptible to this allergic syndrome because their immune and digestive systems are immature. Milk allergy can develop within days to months of birth.

If your baby is on cow's milk formula, your healthcare provider may suggest a change to soy formula or an elemental formula if possible. Elemental formulas are produced from processed proteins with supplements added (basically sugars and amino acids). There are few if any allergens within these materials.

Healthcare providers sometimes prescribe glucocorticosteroid medicines to treat infants with very severe GI reactions to milk formulas. Fortunately, this food allergy tends to go away within the first few years of life.

Breast feeding often helps babies avoid feeding problems related to allergic reactions. Therefore, health experts often suggest that mothers feed their baby only breast milk for the first months of life to avoid milk allergy from developing within that timeframe.

Some babies are very sensitive to a certain food. If you are nursing and eat that food, sufficient amounts can enter your breast milk to cause a food reaction in your baby. To keep possible food allergens out of your breast milk, you might try not eating those foods, such as peanuts, that could cause an allergic reaction in your baby.

There is no conclusive evidence that breastfeeding prevents allergies from developing later in your child's life. It does, however, delay the start of food allergies by delaying your infant's exposure to those foods that can prompt allergies. Plus, it may avoid altogether food allergy problems sometimes seen in infants.

By delaying the introduction of solid foods until your baby is 6 months old or older, you can also prolong your baby's allergy-free period. Speak to your healthcare provider for specific instructions on when to add specific food groups to your child's diet.

How do I protect my child at school or daycare?

Schools and daycare centers must have plans in place to address any food allergy emergency. Parents and caregivers should take special care with children and learn how to:

- protect children from foods to which they are allergic;

- manage children if they eat a food to which they are allergic;

- give children epinephrine.

Simply washing your hands with soap and water will remove peanut allergens. Also, most household cleaners will remove them from surfaces such as food preparation areas at home as well as daycare facilities and schools. These easy-to-do measures will help prevent peanut allergy reactions in children and adults.

Chapter 25

Advice for Consumers about Food Labels

Chapter Contents

Section 25.1

Questions and Answers about Food Labels

Excerpted from "Food Allergen Labeling and Consumer Protection
Act of 2004 Questions and Answers," by the U.S. Food and Drug
Administration (FDA), July 18, 2006.

The Food Allergen Labeling and Consumer Protection Act (FALCPA)
improves food labeling information for the millions of consumers who
suffer from food allergies. The Act will be especially helpful to children
who must learn to recognize the allergens they must avoid.

What is the Food Allergen Labeling and Consumer Protection Act (FALCPA) of 2004?

FALCPA is an amendment to the Federal Food, Drug, and Cosmetic
Act and requires that the label of a food that contains an ingredient
that is or contains protein from a "major food allergen" declare the
presence of the allergen in the manner described by the law.

Why did Congress pass this Act?

Congress passed this Act to make it easier for food allergic consumers and their caregivers to identify and avoid foods that contain major
food allergens. In fact, in a review of the foods of randomly selected
manufacturers of baked goods, ice cream, and candy in Minnesota and
Wisconsin in 1999, FDA found that 25 percent of sampled foods failed
to list peanuts or eggs as ingredients on the food labels although the
foods contained these allergens.

What is a "major food allergen?"

FALCPA identifies eight foods or food groups as the major food allergens. They are milk, eggs, fish (e.g., bass, flounder, cod), Crustacean
shellfish (e.g., crab, lobster, shrimp), tree nuts (e.g., almonds, walnuts,
pecans), peanuts, wheat, and soybeans.

FALCPA identifies only eight allergens. Aren't there more foods consumers are allergic to?

Yes. More than 160 foods have been identified to cause food allergies in sensitive individuals. However, the eight major food allergens identified by FALCPA account for over 90 percent of all documented food allergies in the United States and represent the foods most likely to result in severe or life-threatening reactions.

Does FALCPA apply to imported foods as well?

FALCPA applies to both domestically manufactured and imported packaged foods that are subject to FDA regulation.

How have food labels changed as a result of FALCPA?

FALCPA required food manufacturers to label food products that contain an ingredient that is or contains protein from a major food allergen in one of two ways.

The first option for food manufacturers is to include the name of the food source in parenthesis following the common or usual name of the major food allergen in the list of ingredients in instances when the name of the food source of the major allergen does not appear elsewhere in the ingredient statement. For example: Ingredients: Enriched flour (wheat flour, malted barley, niacin, reduced iron, thiamin mononitrate, riboflavin, folic acid), sugar, partially hydrogenated soybean oil, and/or cottonseed oil, high fructose corn syrup, whey (milk), eggs, vanilla, natural and artificial flavoring) salt, leavening (sodium acid pyrophosphate, monocalcium phosphate), lecithin (soy), mono- and diglycerides (emulsifier).

The second option is to place the word "Contains" followed by the name of the food source from which the major food allergen is derived, immediately after or adjacent to the list of ingredients, in type size that is no smaller than the type size used for the list of ingredients. For example: Contains Wheat, Milk, Egg, and Soy.

Is the ingredient list specific about what type of tree nut, fish, or shellfish is in the product?

FALCPA requires the type of tree nut (e.g., almonds, pecans, walnuts); the type of fish (e.g., bass, flounder, cod); and the type of Crustacean shellfish (e.g., crab, lobster, shrimp) to be declared.

281

Does FALCPA require the use of a "may contain" statement in any circumstance?

No. Advisory statements are not required by FALCPA.

Are flavors, colors, and food additives subject to the allergen labeling requirements?

Yes. FALCPA requires that food manufacturers label food products that contain ingredients, including a flavoring, coloring, or incidental additive that are, or contain, a major food allergen using plain English to identify the allergens.

Are there any foods exempt from the new labeling requirements?

Yes. Under FALCPA, raw agricultural commodities (generally fresh fruits and vegetables) are exempt as are highly refined oils derived from one of the eight major food allergens and any ingredient derived from such highly refined oil.

Can food manufacturers ask to have a product exempted from the new labeling requirements?

Yes. FALCPA provides mechanisms by which a manufacturer may request that a food ingredient covered by FALCPA may be exempt from FALCPA's labeling requirements. An ingredient may be exempt if it does not cause an allergic response that poses a risk to human health or if it does not contain allergenic protein.

How will FDA make sure food manufacturers adhere to the labeling regulations?

As a part of its routine regulatory functions, FDA inspects a variety of packaged foods to ensure that they are properly labeled.

What is cross-contact?

Cross-contact is the inadvertent introduction of an allergen into a product. It is generally the result of environmental exposure during processing or handling, which may occur when multiple foods are produced in the same facility. It may occur due to use of the same processing line, through the misuse of rework, as the result of ineffective cleaning, or from the generation of dust or aerosols containing an allergen.

Are mislabeled food products removed from the market?

Yes. A food product that contains an undeclared allergen may be subject to recall. In addition, a food product that is not properly labeled may be misbranded and subject to seizure and removed from the market place.

The number of recalls due to undeclared allergens (eight of the most common allergens only) remained steady between 1999 and 2001. In 2002, recall actions nearly doubled, rising from 68 to 116. This rise may be attributed to the increased awareness of food allergies among consumers and manufacturers and increased attention from FDA inspectors to issues related to food allergy in manufacturing plants.

How can I avoid foods to which I'm allergic?

FDA advises consumers to work with health care providers to find out what food(s) can cause an allergic reaction. In addition, consumers who are allergic to major food allergens should read the ingredient statement on food products to determine if products contain a major allergen. A "Contains _____" statement, if present on a label, can also be used to determine if the food contains a major food allergen.

But I don't understand what some of the terms mean. How will I know what they are?

FALCPA was designed to improve food labeling information so that consumers who suffer from food allergies—especially children and their caregivers—will be able to recognize the presence of an ingredient that they must avoid. For example, if a product contains the milk-derived protein casein, the product's label would have to use the term "milk" in addition to the term "casein" so that those with milk allergies would clearly understand the presence of an allergen they need to avoid.

Section 25.2

How to Read a Label for Your Food Allergy

This chapter contains text from "Food Labels Identify Allergens More Clearly," by Linda Bren, *FDA Consumer* magazine, published by the U.S. Food and Drug Administration (FDA, www.fda.gov/fdac), March-April 2006. Information under the heading "Reading Food Labels away from Home" is excerpted from "Food Allergen Labeling and Consumer Protection Act of 2004 Questions and Answers," by the U.S. Food and Drug Administration (FDA), July 18, 2006.

Food Labels Identify Allergens More Clearly

When you drink a glass of milk, are you consuming casein and lactoglobulin? How about potassium caseinate and lactalbumin?

According to food scientists, all of these substances are proteins found in milk. And until recently, food manufacturers could use technical terms such as these on food labels without further explanation, instead of listing the more common term "milk."

That changed at the beginning of 2006, when a new food labeling law, the Food Allergen Labeling and Consumer Protection Act (FALCPA), took effect.

Under FALCPA, food labels are required to state clearly whether the food contains a "major food allergen." The law identifies as a major food allergen any of eight allergenic foods: milk; eggs; fish such as bass, flounder, and cod; crustacean shellfish such as crab, lobster, and shrimp; tree nuts such as almonds, walnuts, and pecans; peanuts; wheat; and soybeans. The law also identifies as a major food allergen any ingredient that contains protein derived from any of these eight foods.

The plain language declaration requirement of FALCPA also applies to flavorings, colorings, and incidental additives that are or contain a major food allergen. "FALCPA recognizes that eight major foods or food groups account for 90 percent of all food allergies in the United States, and some allergic reactions may be severe or life-threatening," says Robert E. Brackett, PhD, director of the Food and Drug Administration's Center for Food Safety and Applied Nutrition (CFSAN).

About 2 percent of adults and 5 percent of infants and young children in the United States suffer from food allergies. About 30,000 consumers require emergency room treatment, and 150 Americans die each year because of allergic reactions to food.

There is no cure for food allergies. Avoidance of the food that causes the allergy is the only way a person can prevent a reaction. The improved label will make it easier for food allergic people and their caregivers to identify and avoid foods that contain major food allergens, says Catherine Copp, policy advisor in the CFSAN. For example, if a product contains the milk-derived protein casein, the product's label will have to use the term "milk" in addition to the term "casein" so that those with milk allergies can clearly understand the presence of the allergen they need to avoid.

"We're very excited about this change," says Anne Muñoz-Furlong, founder and CEO of The Food Allergy & Anaphylaxis Network based in Fairfax, Virginia. "People with food allergies will be able to tell right away whether a food is safe for them to eat or not."

Food allergies are on the rise in children, says Muñoz-Furlong, and the improved food labeling information will be especially helpful to children who must learn to recognize the presence of substances they need to avoid. Parents often take children with them when they shop for groceries, she says. "They want to teach children early on to start reading food labels. They have the children read the label to them and figure out if the product contains an allergy-causing food and whether it should go in the grocery cart or go back on the shelf."

"When the child is too young to read, parents will read the label to the child," adds Muñoz-Furlong. "It's almost impossible to keep the attention of a 5-year-old when you say 'ammonium caseinate,' but when you say 'milk,' the child with a milk allergy will instantly say, 'That's not good for me.'" Manufacturers must identify the presence of a major food allergen in one of two ways: In the list of ingredients, manufacturers must state the source of an allergenic ingredient in parentheses after the name of that ingredient; or after or next to the ingredient list, manufacturers must add "contains" followed by the name of the source of each allergenic ingredient in the food. For example:

- **Option 1:** Ingredients: Enriched flour (wheat flour, malted barley, niacin, reduced iron, thiamin mononitrate, riboflavin, folic acid), sugar, partially hydrogenated soybean oil, and/or cottonseed oil, high fructose corn syrup, whey (milk), eggs, vanilla, natural and artificial flavoring, salt, leavening (sodium acid pyrophosphate, monocalcium phosphate), lecithin (soy), mono- and diglycerides (emulsifier).

- **Option 2:** Contains Wheat, Milk, Eggs, and Soy

"These statements are not required if the major food allergen's common name already identifies its food source," says Copp. For example, the ingredients whole wheat flour, buttermilk, and peanut butter already state that they contain wheat, milk, and peanuts, respectively, so no further explanatory terms are required.

FALCPA applies to both domestically produced and imported packaged foods that the FDA regulates. So even if you purchase a box of candy from overseas, it should be in compliance, says Copp. Raw agricultural commodities, such as fresh fruits and vegetables, are exempt from FALCPA. So are highly refined oils made from one of the eight allergenic foods identified by the law.

FALCPA establishes two separate processes that food manufacturers can use to request an exemption for their product from the FALCPA declaration requirement—the notification and petition processes. "The notification process may be used by manufacturers who can demonstrate that their ingredient does not contain an allergenic protein; the petition process may be used by a manufacturer who can demonstrate that, although the ingredient does contain protein derived from an allergenic food, the ingredient does not cause an adverse reaction that poses a risk to human health," says Felicia Billingslea, director of the FDA's Division of Food Labeling and Standards.

The law applies only to products labeled on or after January 1, 2006, so until products labeled before that date are sold or otherwise removed from the market, consumers will continue to see some products without the plain language allergen labeling on grocery store shelves, says Copp, "particularly nonperishables such as canned goods."

Even if consumers have purchased a product in the past that does not aggravate their allergies, they should not take it for granted that it will always be nonallergenic, says Copp. "We encourage consumers to always read the ingredients list, because manufacturers may change their product formulation."

The FDA will enforce the new law. "We intend to document violations of the law when inspecting manufacturing plants," says Betty Harden, an FDA consumer safety officer in the Office of Compliance. A food product that contains an undeclared allergen may be subject to recall. In addition, a food product not properly labeled may be misbranded and subject to seizure and removal from the marketplace.

FALCPA also requires the FDA to submit a report to Congress on food allergens, particularly with respect to identifying ways to reduce or eliminate cross contact and stating the risk of cross contact on food labels. Cross contact occurs when a residue or other trace amount of an allergenic food is unintentionally incorporated into another food that is not intended to contain that allergenic food; cross contact may occur during harvesting, transportation, manufacturing, processing, or storage.

In addition, the agency is required to propose a regulation by August 2006, and to issue a final regulation by August 2008, to define the term "gluten-free" for voluntary use in food labeling. Gluten is a term that describes a group of proteins that occur naturally in certain grains, including wheat, barley, and rye. When present in certain amounts, gluten can cause a serious reaction in people with celiac disease, a chronic digestive disease that damages the small intestine and interferes with absorption of nutrients from food. About 2 million people in the United States have this disease.

"Consumers susceptible to celiac disease need accurate, complete, and informative labels on food to protect themselves," says Billingslea, "and a standardized definition of 'gluten-free' and use of the term on labels will help."

Reading Food Labels away from Home

What about food prepared in restaurants? How will I know that the food I ordered does not contain an ingredient to which I am allergic?

FALCPA only applies to packaged FDA-regulated foods. However, FDA advises consumers who are allergic to particular foods to ask questions about ingredients and preparation when eating at restaurants or any place outside the consumer's home.

How will FALCPA apply to foods purchased at bakeries, food kiosks at the mall, and carry out restaurants?

FALCPA's labeling requirements extend to retail and food-service establishments that package, label, and offer products for human consumption.

However, FALCPA's labeling requirements do not apply to foods that are placed in a wrapper or container in response to a consumer's order—such as the paper or box used to provide a sandwich ordered by a consumer.

Chapter 26

Tips on Avoiding Food Allergy Reactions

Chapter Contents

Section 26.1

A Food Diary Can Reduce Risk of Reactions

Food allergies are on the rise worldwide, as is research into possible causes and cures. But even though doctors are seeing more patients with food-related symptoms, correctly diagnosing food allergies remains tricky.

Most of us eat multiple ingredients with every bite of food we take. So stomach cramps from eating spaghetti and meatballs could be the result of tomato allergy if you used tomato sauce, egg allergy or gluten intolerance from the pasta . . . even food poisoning. Not all reactions to food are allergic reactions. In addition, food allergy symptoms can start 2 minutes or 2 hours after you eat a certain food—making it difficult to pinpoint what caused the reaction.

Food allergy tests are important diagnostic tools but aren't enough to close the case. If you test negative to a food allergen, that diagnosis sticks. But positive results are a different matter. According to Robert Wood, MD, in *Food Allergies for Dummies®*, "Up to 60 percent of all positive food skin tests turn out to be incorrect (false positive)." Why the confusion? Two possible reasons are:

- your immune system has a small amount of IgE antibodies— your defenders against invading allergens—to a food but not enough to cause an allergic reaction; or

- you are allergic to a related food or environmental allergen (like pollen). This situation is called cross reactivity.

Blood tests can be thrown off by the same scenarios. Before you take platefuls of food off your menu—and miss out on meals packed with nutrients and health benefits—use a food diary to help confirm or rule out a food allergy.

Dear Diary

Just as food journals have helped dieters around the world cut calories and fat, a food diary can help you focus in on possible food allergies. Keep a small notebook handy in your purse, briefcase, or backpack to make quick journal entries at each meal. Items to include:

- what you eat and drink;
- symptoms you think may be the result of a food allergy;
- what you were doing at the time your symptoms started.

Look out Stomach, Here It Comes

To root out the cause of food allergies, you'll need to transform yourself from casual diner to food detective. The suspect could be your breakfast cereal, steak dinner, or even that pack of breath mints. If it goes in your mouth, it should go in your food diary! Include all the ingredients, how your food is cooked (such as grilled vs. fried in peanut oil), and the amount you consume.

Hidden ingredients like flavorings, dyes, and preservatives can cause allergic reactions in some people. When food labels start to look like chemistry lists, it may be easier to just cut out and save the labels. Borrow a pocket folder from your child's school supply stash to keep labels handy and in one spot.

Most restaurants are becoming quite food allergy aware these days. When dining out, look for places that offer ingredient lists and ask the restaurant manager for labels from packaged foods used in any of the dishes you've been served. It may be easier to dine in or limit your diet to foods with few ingredients until you solve your food allergy mystery. And if you find that you haven't had symptoms since you stopped eating at your favorite Italian restaurant . . . that tells you something!

If you're eating with family or friends when symptoms strike, ask around—did anyone else eating the same food get sick? Think back to the time before you started having food issues. Had you been able to eat a suspect food without problems? How often did you eat it? Jot down notes to share with your doctor. It will help with your diagnosis.

Symptom Savvy

While you're keeping track of what goes in your mouth, add suspected food allergy symptoms that come up. Allergic reactions can range from annoying to life-threatening—and move quickly from one to the other. So take note of any possible symptoms, including:

- tingling or itching in and around the mouth;
- swelling of the tongue and throat;
- flushing of the face or neck;
- rash;
- eczema (if symptoms get worse after eating);
- hives and swelling;
- vomiting;
- abdominal cramps;
- diarrhea;
- wheezing;
- difficulty breathing;
- drop in blood pressure (feeling faint or weak);
- loss of consciousness.

Include when symptoms started and when you felt them go away, whether you were drinking alcohol when the symptoms occurred (which can increase your body's absorption of a food allergen), whether you took any medications to treat symptoms, and any other medications you were taking at the time. Get immediate medical help for severe symptoms.

Time out on the Treadmill

Exercise can also be a factor in food allergies. AANMA President Nancy Sander recently sat next to a woman on a plane who had exercise-induced anaphylaxis to tomatoes—if she exercised too soon after eating anything with tomatoes, she experienced symptoms of anaphylaxis! If you think you're having food allergy symptoms, include a note about what you were doing right before or during the time you had the reaction (like taking a walk outside or sweeping the floors).

Pinpointing Patterns

Over time (it could be days, weeks, or longer), you and your doctor may start to see patterns between what you're eating and allergy symptoms. Look for consistency: Do all milk products give you stomach cramps or do you feel ill only after drinking a glass of milk?

More than 90 percent of allergic reactions to food in the United States are due to eight foods or food groups:

- Milk

- Eggs

- Peanuts

- Tree nuts

- Fish

- Shellfish

- Soy

- Wheat

Manufacturers are now required to label allergens in these terms on food labels. You could also fall into the other 10 percent of cases ranging from avocados to yams. Your food diary can help you identify even the most unlikely of food allergy suspects.

From Diarrhea to Diagnosis

Food diaries, allergy tests, medical history . . . you and your medical care team have a range of clues to detect possible food allergies. Where do you start? In *Food Allergies for Dummies*, Dr. Wood suggests a visit to your general practitioner (GP)—family physician, internist, or pediatrician—first. Your GP will perform a physical exam and take your medical history, which is the most important step in ruling out other causes of your symptoms. If food allergies are still a possibility, your GP can refer you to a board-certified allergist experienced in diagnosing and treating food allergies. If you have asthma or allergies, you are probably already working with an allergist, so check with your allergy team on how to proceed. In either case, your food diary will help you and your medical care team identify likely food allergy culprits and start you down the road to better health.

Section 26.2

Working with a Dietitian If Your Child Has Food Allergies

"Is Your Dietitian the Right Fit?" © 2007 Kids With Food Allergies, Inc. (www.kidswithfoodallergies.org). Reprinted with permission.

As soon as your child is diagnosed with food allergies, what is the first thing you do? You think, "What will I feed my child and how will I make sure I provide foods that are nutritious but won't trigger an allergic reaction?" A dietitian may be the first person who comes to mind to answer this question. Perhaps your allergist recommended a dietitian for help in planning your child's allergen-free diet. But, can one really help? Maybe—maybe not.

Just as there are doctors who have specialties, there are dietitians who specialize in certain areas of nutrition. You would not take your child to a general practitioner to test, diagnose, and treat your child's allergies. For the same reason, you would want to find a dietitian who specializes in food allergy or pediatric nutrition.

A registered dietitian is a food and nutrition professional who has met certain academic and professional requirements as outlined by the American Dietetic Association. Registered dietitians must earn a bachelor's degree in nutrition from an accredited college or university with coursework approved by the Commission on Accreditation for Dietetics Education. They should also complete an approved practice program or internship, pass a national examination administered by the Commission on Dietetic Registration, and finish professional educational requirements in order to maintain the registration. Does this prepare a dietitian to help you with your child's allergies? Not necessarily.

After completing all of the necessary requirements for registration, many dietitians choose a field of practice they find interesting. Food allergy is not a topic regularly covered in the educational and practice training of most dietitians. Therefore, any dietitian who wants to specialize in food allergy must study on their own and work in a setting where allergy is a specialty. Many allergists are willing to have a dietitian work with them to help parents choose nutritional foods and supplements while avoiding their children's trigger foods. These dietitians learn from allergists, as well as make an effort to attend conferences and seminars specifically addressing food allergy.

Those who are experts in food allergy have studied that subject and worked in pediatric hospitals and medical practices guided by allergists who focus on nutrition and food allergy.

As a registered dietitian, it is disheartening to hear parents say, "My child's doctor referred me to a dietitian but she really didn't help us." When I was at the Kids With Food Allergies booth at a recent conference, many physicians said they did not know where to refer their patients for nutritional guidance for food allergies. This can be frustrating for physicians and parents.

When choosing a dietitian consider the following:

- Where did the dietitian train?

- How many food allergy patients has the dietitian worked with?

- Has the dietitian been involved in the diagnostic aspect of food allergy, including testing and food challenges in addition to educating patients?

- How did the dietitian gain knowledge in food allergy beyond the bachelor's degree and internship?

- What professional memberships are held (Pediatric Nutrition Practice Group, American Academy of Allergy, Asthma and Immunology, American Association of Allergy, Asthma and Immunology)?

If the dietitian has not had food allergy experience, then find one who does.

During a visit with a dietitian, your child's normal intake should be discussed along with symptoms that have occurred with the ingestion of suspected or positive test foods. The nutritional needs of your child should be compared with current intake to determine if more nutritionally dense foods or if supplements are necessary. A meal plan should be outlined, food/symptom diaries provided, lists of foods to avoid and suggestions for meals and foods to use provided. A follow-up visit should be scheduled for you to discuss progress, as well as concerns, and determine an alternate plan for suggestions that did not work.

The American Dietetic Association (www.eatright.org) has a network of registered dietitians listed by specialty and location.

Section 26.3

Avoiding Cross Contamination

Many parents of severely food-allergic children, especially those whose kids are only allergic to peanuts and/or tree nuts, choose to completely eliminate all allergenic foods from their homes. Others, especially those whose children have multiple food allergies, do not make this choice. If you choose to allow allergenic foods in your house, you run the risk that the allergenic foods will "contaminate" your home and your non-allergenic foods. There are a number of precautions you should take to avoid potential problems.

Label Foods in Your Home as "Safe" or "Not Safe"

To ensure everyone (including your children, visitors, babysitters, etc.) can easily determine which foods in your home are "safe" and which are not, it can be helpful to label the food in your pantry, refrigerator, and freezer. A convenient way to do this is to purchase a supply of red and green self-adhesive 1/2"- or 1"-diameter circle-shaped stickers from your local office supplies store. The red stickers are for the unsafe foods and the green are for the safe foods (i.e., "red" means "stop" and "green" means "go"). Apply these stickers to every food item in your house.

Avoid Pantry Mix-Ups

If you keep both "safe" and "not safe" versions of similar items in your home (for example, soy milk and cow's milk, cheese-flavored crackers, and dairy-free crackers), do not keep these products next to each other in the refrigerator or pantry. Designate particular shelves or cabinets for storing the "safe" foods.

Avoid Sippy Cup Mix-Ups

If your toddler is allergic to milk, purchase a "special" sippy cup from which he is always served his beverages (both at home and away from home), and which is never used for anyone else. Put his name on it. Once you put the lid on the average sippy cup you cannot see the contents. Having a special cup that is always used ensures that your child doesn't grab the wrong cup by mistake.

Avoid Contaminating Your Food Supply

If you keep both "safe" and "not-safe" foods in your household, you need to take steps to ensure that your non-allergenic foods do not become contaminated through casual contact:

- Hands—Teach all members of your household to wash their hands before touching the non-allergenic foods—even if they are touching it in order to serve themselves. For example, your non-allergic daughter should not stick her possibly allergen-covered hand into the box of crackers or bag of chips that are meant to be safe for her allergic sibling.

- Utensils—Do not allow allergen-covered utensils to contaminate your "safe" foods. For example, if a knife containing butter has been inserted into a jar of jam, the jam is no longer safe for a dairy-allergic individual to eat. If a knife is used to spread some butter on a piece of wheat bread toast, and the stick of butter is then touched by this now bread crumb-covered knife, the butter will be cross-contaminated with wheat (and all of the other ingredients contained in the bread).

Avoid Getting Allergenic Residue All over the House

If you allow allergenic food in your home, you need to take precautions to ensure that your entire home does not become contaminated with allergenic food residue. Teach all members of your household to always wash their hands with soap immediately after eating or touching something allergenic. In addition, consider confining all food consumption to your kitchen and dining areas.

Remember, if Dad eats dinner on the sofa and Sister walks around the house eating snacks, crumbs and other residue are likely to find their way onto your carpets, furniture, countertops, toys, and other surfaces.

Don't Forget Your Guests

When friends who have been eating allergenic foods just prior to visiting your home arrive, politely ask them (and their children!!) to wash their hands before they touch anything. If your friends have infants, you may need to take precautions to avoid allowing these infants to spit up on your carpets or furniture, especially if your food-allergic child tends to put her hands or fingers into her mouth. The food, formula, or breast milk that your friends' babies spit up is likely to be allergenic, and will therefore "contaminate" the surfaces on which it lands. Because your goal is to make your home a safe haven for your child, be sure that your friends' babies are set down on a clean blanket or other appropriate carpet or furniture protector.

Take Precautions When Cooking

Take steps to ensure that you do not contaminate your child's food with allergens during the cooking or serving process:

- If you are preparing both allergenic and non-allergenic food for the same meal (such as sandwiches with or without mayonnaise and cheese), prepare the non-allergenic meal first—before you even open the allergenic ingredients.

- Do not use the same utensils to simultaneously prepare allergenic and non-allergenic dishes.

- Place all allergen-contaminated utensils, plates, cutting boards, etc. directly into the sink or the dishwasher immediately after use. Teach all members of your household that soiled items in the sink or dishwasher are not to be used again until they have been properly washed.

- If you use your barbecue to cook both allergenic and non-allergenic foods, be sure to thoroughly clean the grill before cooking for your food-allergic child.

Wash Dishes Thoroughly

Mixing bowls, pots, pans, utensils, and so forth that have been used in the preparation of allergenic foods must be thoroughly washed in hot, sudsy water prior to being used to prepare food for your allergic child. In addition, to avoid having stray bits of dried allergenic food stick to your "clean" dishes, it is best to rinse off dirty dishes and utensils that are "contaminated" with allergenic foods prior to loading them into your dishwasher.

Part Four

Airborne, Chemical, and Other Environmental Allergy Triggers

Chapter 27

Overview of Airborne Allergens

Sneezing is not always the symptom of a cold. Sometimes, it is an allergic reaction to something in the air. Health experts estimate that 35 million Americans suffer from upper respiratory tract symptoms that are allergic reactions to airborne allergens. Pollen allergy, commonly called hay fever, is one of the most common chronic diseases in the United States. Worldwide, airborne allergens cause the most problems for people with allergies. The respiratory symptoms of asthma, which affect approximately 11 million Americans, are often provoked by airborne allergens.

Overall, allergic diseases are among the major causes of illness and disability in the United States, affecting as many as 40 to 50 million Americans.

Allergy Definition

An allergy is a specific reaction of the body's immune system to a normally harmless substance, one that does not bother most people. People who have allergies often are sensitive to more than one substance. Types of allergens that cause allergic reactions include the following:

Excerpted from "Airborne Allergens: Something in the Air," by the National Institute of Allergy and Infectious Diseases (NIAID, www.niaid.nih.gov), part of the National Institutes of Health, April 2003. Reviewed by David A. Cooke, MD, FACP, August 10, 2010.

- Pollens
- House dust mites
- Mold spores
- Food
- Latex rubber
- Insect venom
- Medicines

Why Some People Are Allergic

Scientists think that some people inherit a tendency to be allergic from one or both parents. This means they are more likely to have allergies. They probably, however, do not inherit a tendency to be allergic to any specific allergen. Children are more likely to develop allergies if one or both parents have allergies. In addition, exposure to allergens at times when the body's defenses are lowered or weakened, such as after a viral infection or during pregnancy, seems to contribute to developing allergies.

Allergic Reactions

Normally, the immune system functions as the body's defense against invading germs such as bacteria and viruses. In most allergic reactions, however, the immune system is responding to a false alarm. When an allergic person first comes into contact with an allergen, the immune system treats the allergen as an invader and gets ready to attack.

The immune system does this by generating large amounts of a type of antibody called immunoglobulin E, or IgE. Each IgE antibody is specific for one particular substance. In the case of pollen allergy, each antibody is specific for one type of pollen. For example, the immune system may produce one type of antibody to react against oak pollen and another against ragweed pollen.

The IgE molecules are special because IgE is the only type of antibody that attaches tightly to the body's mast cells, which are tissue cells, and to basophils, which are blood cells. When the allergen next encounters its specific IgE, it attaches to the antibody like a key fitting into a lock. This action signals the cell to which the IgE is attached to release (and, in some cases, to produce) powerful chemicals like histamine, which cause inflammation. These chemicals act on tissues in various parts of the body, such as the respiratory system, and cause the symptoms of allergy.

Symptoms

The signs and symptoms of airborne allergies are familiar to many:

- Sneezing, often with a runny or clogged nose
- Coughing and postnasal drip
- Itching eyes, nose, and throat
- Watering eyes
- Conjunctivitis
- Allergic shiners (dark circles under the eyes caused by increased blood flow near the sinuses)
- Allergic salute (in a child, persistent upward rubbing of the nose that causes a crease mark on the nose)

In people who are not allergic, the mucus in the nasal passages simply moves foreign particles to the throat, where they are swallowed or coughed out. But something different happens in a person who is sensitive to airborne allergens.

In sensitive people, as soon as the allergen lands on the lining inside the nose, a chain reaction occurs that leads the mast cells in these tissues to release histamine and other chemicals. The powerful chemicals contract certain cells that line some small blood vessels in the nose. This allows fluids to escape, which causes the nasal passages to swell—resulting in nasal congestion. Histamine also can cause sneezing, itching, irritation, and excess mucus production, which can result in allergic rhinitis.

Other chemicals released by mast cells, including cytokines and leukotrienes, also contribute to allergic symptoms.

Some people with allergy develop asthma, which can be a very serious condition. The symptoms of asthma include the following:

- Coughing
- Wheezing
- Shortness of breath

The shortness of breath is due to a narrowing of the airways in the lungs and to excess mucus production and inflammation. Asthma can be disabling and sometimes fatal. If wheezing and shortness of breath accompany allergy symptoms, it is a signal that the airways also have become involved.

There is no good way to tell the difference between allergy symptoms of runny nose, coughing, and sneezing and cold symptoms. Allergy symptoms, however, may last longer than cold symptoms. Anyone who has any respiratory illness that lasts longer than a week or two should consult a health care provider.

Diagnosis

People with allergy symptoms—such as the runny nose of allergic rhinitis—may at first suspect they have a cold, but the "cold" lingers on. Testing for allergies is the best way to find out if a person is allergic.

Skin Tests

Allergists (doctors who specialize in allergic diseases) use skin tests to determine whether a person has IgE antibodies in the skin that react to a specific allergen. The allergist will use weakened extracts from allergens such as dust mites, pollens, or molds commonly found in the local area. The extract of each kind of allergen is injected under a person's skin or is applied to a tiny scratch or puncture made on the arm or back.

Skin tests are one way of measuring the level of IgE antibody in a person. With a positive reaction, a small, raised, reddened area, called a wheal (hive), with a surrounding flush, called a flare, will appear at the test site. The size of the wheal can give the doctor an important diagnostic clue, but a positive reaction does not prove that a particular allergen is the cause of symptoms. Although such a reaction indicates that IgE antibody to a specific allergen is present, respiratory symptoms do not necessarily result.

Blood Tests

Skin testing is the most sensitive and least costly way to identify allergies. People with widespread skin conditions like eczema, however, should not be tested using this method.

There are other diagnostic tests that use a blood sample to detect levels of IgE antibody to a particular allergen. One such blood test is called the radioallergosorbent test (RAST), which can be performed when eczema is present or if a person has taken medicines that interfere with skin testing.

Prevention and Avoidance

Pollen and Molds

Complete avoidance of allergenic pollen or mold means moving to a place where the offending substance does not grow and where it is not present in the air. Even this extreme solution may offer only temporary relief because a person sensitive to a specific pollen or mold may develop allergies to new allergens after repeated exposure to them. For example, people allergic to ragweed may leave their ragweed-ridden communities and relocate to areas where ragweed does not grow, only to develop allergies to other weeds or even to grasses or trees in their new surroundings. Because relocating is not a reliable solution, allergy specialists do not encourage this approach.

There are other ways to reduce exposure to offending pollens.

- Remain indoors with the windows closed in the morning, for example, when the outdoor pollen levels are highest. Sunny, windy days can be especially troublesome.

- Wear a face mask designed to filter pollen out of the air and keep it from reaching nasal passages, if you must work outdoors.

- Take your vacation at the height of the expected pollinating period and choose a location where such exposure would be minimal.

- Vacationing at the seashore or on a cruise, for example, may be effective retreats for avoiding pollen allergies.

House Dust

If you have dust mite allergy, pay careful attention to dust-proofing your bedroom. The worst things to have in the bedroom are the following:

- Wall-to-wall carpet
- Blinds
- Down-filled blankets
- Feather pillows
- Stuffed animals
- Heating vents with forced hot air
- Dogs and cats
- Closets full of clothing

Carpets trap dust and make dust control impossible.

- Shag carpets are the worst type of carpet for people who are sensitive to dust mites.

- Vacuuming doesn't get rid of dust mite proteins in furniture and carpeting, but redistributes them back into the room, unless the vacuum has a special HEPA (high-efficiency particulate air) filter.

- Rugs on concrete floors encourage dust mite growth.

If possible, replace wall-to-wall carpets with washable throw rugs over hardwood, tile, or linoleum floors, and wash the rugs frequently.

Reducing the amount of dust mites in your home may mean new cleaning techniques as well as some changes in furnishings to eliminate dust collectors. Water is often the secret to effective dust removal.

- Clean washable items, including throw rugs, often, using water hotter than 130 degrees Fahrenheit. Lower temperatures will not kill dust mites.

- Clean washable items at a commercial establishment that uses high water temperature, if you cannot or do not want to set water temperature in your home at 130 degrees. (There is a danger of getting scalded if the water is more than 120 degrees.)

- Dust frequently with a damp cloth or oiled mop.

If cockroaches are a problem in your home, the U.S. Environmental Protection Agency suggests some ways to get rid of them.

- Do not leave food or garbage out.

- Store food in airtight containers.

- Clean all food crumbs or spilled liquids right away.

- Try using poison baits, boric acid (for cockroaches), or traps first, before using pesticide sprays.

If you use sprays:

- Do not spray in food preparation or storage areas.

- Do not spray in areas where children play or sleep.

- Limit the spray to the infested area.

- Follow instructions on the label carefully.

- Make sure there is plenty of fresh air when you spray.

- Keep the person with allergies or asthma out of the room while spraying.

Pets

If you or your child is allergic to furry pets, especially cats, the best way to avoid allergic reactions is to find them another home. If you are like most people who are attached to their pets, that is usually not a desirable option. There are ways, however, to help lower the levels of animal allergens in the air, which may reduce allergic reactions.

- Bathe your cat weekly and brush it more frequently (ideally, a non-allergic person should do this).
- Keep cats out of your bedroom.
- Remove carpets and soft furnishings, which collect animal allergens.
- Use a vacuum cleaner and room air cleaners with HEPA filters.
- Wear a face mask while house and cat cleaning.

Chemicals

Irritants such as chemicals can worsen airborne allergy symptoms, and you should avoid them as much as possible. For example, if you have pollen allergy, avoid unnecessary exposure to irritants such as insect sprays, tobacco smoke, air pollution, and fresh tar or paint during periods of high pollen levels.

Air Conditioners and Filters

When possible, use air conditioners inside your home or car to help prevent pollen and mold allergens from entering. Various types of air-filtering devices made with fiberglass or electrically charged plates may help reduce allergens produced in the home. You can add these to your present heating and cooling system. In addition, portable devices that can be used in individual rooms are especially helpful in reducing animal allergens.

An allergist can suggest which kind of filter is best for your home. Before buying a filtering device, rent one and use it in a closed room (the bedroom, for instance) for a month or two to see whether your allergy symptoms diminish. The airflow should be sufficient to exchange the air in the room five or six times per hour. Therefore, the size and efficiency of the filtering device should be determined in part by the size of the room.

You should be wary of exaggerated claims for appliances that cannot really clean the air. Very small air cleaners cannot remove dust and pollen. No air purifier can prevent viral or bacterial diseases such as the flu, pneumonia, or tuberculosis.

Before buying an electrostatic precipitator, you should compare the machine's ozone output with federal standards. Ozone can irritate the noses and airways of people with allergies, especially those with asthma, and can increase their allergy symptoms. Other kinds of air filters, such as HEPA filters, do not release ozone into the air. HEPA filters, however, require adequate air flow to force air through them.

Treatment with Medicines

If you cannot adequately avoid airborne allergens, your symptoms often can be controlled by medicines. You can buy medicines without a prescription that can relieve allergy symptoms. If, however, they don't give you relief or they cause unwanted side effects such as sleepiness, your health care provider can prescribe antihistamines and topical nasal steroids. You can use either medicine alone or together.

Antihistamines

As the name indicates, an antihistamine counters the effects of histamine, which is released by the mast cells in your body's tissues and contributes to your allergy symptoms. For many years, antihistamines have proven useful in relieving itching in the nose and eyes; sneezing; and in reducing nasal swelling and drainage.

Many people who take antihistamines have some distressing side effects such as drowsiness and loss of alertness and coordination. Adults may interpret such reactions in children as behavior problems.

Antihistamines that cause fewer of these side effects are available over-the-counter or by prescription. These non-sedating antihistamines are as effective as other antihistamines in preventing histamine-induced symptoms, but most do so without causing sleepiness.

Topical Nasal Steroids

You should not confuse topical nasal steroids with anabolic steroids, which athletes sometimes use to enlarge muscle mass and which can have serious side effects. The chemicals in nasal steroids are different from those in anabolic steroids.

Topical nasal steroids are anti-inflammatory medicines that stop the allergic reaction. In addition to other helpful actions, they decrease the number of mast cells in the nose and reduce mucus secretion and nasal swelling. The combination of antihistamines and nasal steroids is a very effective way to treat allergic rhinitis, especially if you have moderate or severe allergic rhinitis.

Although topical nasal steroids can have side effects, they are safe when used at recommended doses.

Cromolyn Sodium

Cromolyn sodium is a nasal spray that in some people helps prevent allergic rhinitis from starting. When used as a nasal spray, it can safely stop the release of chemicals like histamine from mast cells. It has few side effects when used as directed and significantly helps some people manage their allergies.

Decongestants

Sometimes helping the nasal passages to drain away mucus will help relieve symptoms such as congestion, swelling, excess secretions, and discomfort in the sinus areas that can be caused by nasal allergies. Your doctor may recommend using oral or nasal decongestants to reduce congestion along with an antihistamine to control allergic symptoms.

You should not, however, use over-the-counter or prescription decongestant nose drops and sprays for more than a few days. When used for longer periods, these medicines can lead to even more congestion and swelling of the nasal passages. Because of recent concern about the bad effects of decongestant sprays and drops, some have been removed from store shelves.

Immunotherapy

Immunotherapy, or a series of allergy shots, is the only available treatment that has a chance of reducing your allergy symptoms over a longer period of time. You would receive subcutaneous (under the skin) injections of increasing concentrations of the allergen(s) to which you are sensitive. These injections reduce the level of IgE antibodies in the blood and cause the body to make a protective antibody called IgG.

About 85 percent of people with allergic rhinitis will see their hay fever symptoms and need for medicines drop significantly within 12 months of starting immunotherapy. Those who benefit from allergy shots may continue it for 3 years and then consider stopping. While many are able to stop the injections with good results lasting for several years, others do get worse after the shots are stopped.

One research study shows that children treated for allergic rhinitis with immunotherapy were less likely to develop asthma. Researchers need to study this further, however. As researchers produce better allergens for immunotherapy, this technique will be become an even more effective treatment.

Chapter 28

Pollen Allergy

Chapter Contents

Section 28.1

What Is Pollen Allergy?

Excerpted from "Airborne Allergens: Something in the Air," by the National Institute of Allergy and Infectious Diseases (NIAID, www.niaid.nih.gov), part of the National Institutes of Health, April 2003. Reviewed by David A. Cooke, MD, FACP, August 10, 2010.

Each spring, summer, and fall, tiny pollen grains are released from trees, weeds, and grasses. These grains hitch rides on currents of air. Although the mission of pollen is to fertilize parts of other plants, many never reach their targets. Instead, pollen enters human noses and throats, triggering a type of seasonal allergic rhinitis called pollen allergy. Many people know this as hay fever.

Of all the things that can cause an allergy, pollen is one of the most common. Many of the foods, medicines, or animals that cause allergies can be avoided to a great extent. Even insects and household dust are escapable. But short of staying indoors, with the windows closed, when the pollen count is high—and even that may not help—there is no easy way to avoid airborne pollen.

Understanding Pollen

Plants produce tiny—too tiny to see with the naked eye—round or oval pollen grains to reproduce. In some species, the plant uses the pollen from its own flowers to fertilize itself. Other types must be cross-pollinated. Cross-pollination means that for fertilization to take place and seeds to form, pollen must be transferred from the flower of one plant to that of another of the same species. Insects do this job for certain flowering plants, while other plants rely on wind for transport.

The types of pollen that most commonly cause allergic reactions are produced by the plain-looking plants (trees, grasses, and weeds) that do not have showy flowers. These plants make small, light, dry pollen grains that are custom-made for wind transport.

Amazingly, scientists have collected samples of ragweed pollen 400 miles out at sea and 2 miles high in the air. Because airborne pollen can drift for many miles, it does little good to rid an area of an offending

312

plant. In addition, most allergenic pollen comes from plants that produce it in huge quantities. For example, a single ragweed plant can generate a million grains of pollen a day.

The type of allergens in the pollen is the main factor that determines whether the pollen is likely to cause hay fever. For example, pine tree pollen is produced in large amounts by a common tree, which would make it a good candidate for causing allergy. It is, however, a relatively rare cause of allergy because the type of allergens in pine pollen appear to make it less allergenic.

Among North American plants, weeds are the most prolific producers of allergenic pollen. Ragweed is the major culprit, but other important sources are sagebrush, redroot pigweed, lamb's quarters, Russian thistle (tumbleweed), and English plantain.

Grasses and trees, too, are important sources of allergenic pollens. Although more than 1,000 species of grass grow in North America, only a few produce highly allergenic pollen.

It is common to hear people say they are allergic to colorful or scented flowers like roses. In fact, only florists, gardeners, and others who have prolonged, close contact with flowers are likely to be sensitive to pollen from these plants. Most people have little contact with the large, heavy, waxy pollen grains of such flowering plants because this type of pollen is not carried by wind but by insects such as butterflies and bees.

Some grasses that produce pollen include the following:

- Timothy grass
- Kentucky bluegrass
- Johnson grass
- Bermuda grass
- Redtop grass
- Orchard grass
- Sweet vernal grass

Some trees that produce pollen include the following:

- Oak
- Ash
- Elm
- Hickory

- Pecan
- Box elder
- Mountain cedar

Plants and Pollen

One of the most obvious features of pollen allergy is its seasonal nature—people have symptoms only when the pollen grains to which they are allergic are in the air. Each plant has a pollinating period that is more or less the same from year to year. Exactly when a plant starts to pollinate seems to depend on the relative length of night and day—and therefore on geographical location—rather than on the weather. On the other hand, weather conditions during pollination can affect the amount of pollen produced and distributed in a specific year. Thus, in the Northern Hemisphere, the farther north you go, the later the start of the pollinating period and the later the start of the allergy season.

A pollen count, familiar to many people from local weather reports, is a measure of how much pollen is in the air. This count represents the concentration of all the pollen (or of one particular type, like ragweed) in the air in a certain area at a specific time. It is shown in grains of pollen per square meter of air collected over 24 hours. Pollen counts tend to be the highest early in the morning on warm, dry, breezy days and lowest during chilly, wet periods. Although the pollen count is an approximate measure that changes, it is useful as a general guide for when it may be wise to stay indoors and avoid contact with the pollen.

Section 28.2

Ragweed Allergy: The Most Common Type of Pollen Allergy

Come late summer, some 10 to 20 percent of Americans begin to suffer from ragweed allergy, or hay fever. Sneezing, stuffy or runny nose, itchy eyes, nose, and throat, and trouble sleeping make life miserable for these people. Some of them also must deal with asthma attacks.

All this misery can begin when ragweeds release pollen into the air, and continue almost until frost kills the plant.

What is ragweed?

Ragweeds are weeds that grow throughout the United States. They are most common in the Eastern states and the Midwest. A plant lives only one season, but that plant produces up to 1 billion pollen grains. Pollen-producing and seed-producing flowers grow on the same plant but are separate organs. After midsummer, as nights grow longer, ragweed flowers mature and release pollen. Warmth, humidity, and breezes after sunrise help the release. The pollen must then travel by air to another plant to fertilize the seed for growth the coming year.

Ragweed plants usually grow in rural areas. Near the plants, the pollen counts are highest shortly after dawn. The amount of pollen peaks in many urban areas between 10 a.m. and 3 p.m., depending on the weather. Rain and low morning temperatures (below 50 degrees Fahrenheit) slow pollen release. Ragweed pollen can travel far. It has been measured in the air 400 miles out to sea and 2 miles up in the atmosphere, but most falls out close to its source.

These annual plants are easily overgrown by turf grasses and other perennial plants that come up from established stems every year. But where the soil is disturbed by streams of water, cultivation, or chemical effects such as winter salting of roads, ragweed will grow. It is often found along roadsides and river banks, in vacant lots and

315

fields. Seeds in the soil even after many decades will grow when conditions are right.

What is ragweed allergy?

The job of immune system cells is to find foreign substances such as viruses and bacteria and get rid of them. Normally, this response protects us from dangerous diseases. People with allergies have specially sensitive immune systems that react when they contact certain harmless substances called allergens. When people who are allergic to ragweed pollen inhale its allergens from air, the common hay fever symptoms develop.

Seventeen species or types of ragweed grow in North America. Ragweed also belongs to a larger family called *Compositae*. Other members of the family that spread pollen by wind can cause symptoms. They include sage, burweed marsh elder and rabbit brush, mugworts, groundsel bush, and eupatorium. Some family members spread their pollen by insects rather than wind, and cause few allergic reactions. But sniffing these plants can cause symptoms.

Who gets ragweed allergy?

Of Americans who are allergic to pollen-producing plants, 75 percent are allergic to ragweed. People with allergies to one type of pollen tend to develop allergies to other pollens as well.

People with ragweed allergy may also get symptoms when they eat cantaloupe and banana. Chamomile tea, sunflower seeds, and honey containing pollen from *Compositae* family members occasionally cause severe reactions, including shock.

What are its symptoms?

The allergic reaction to all plants that produce pollen is commonly known as hay fever. Symptoms include eye irritation, runny nose, stuffy nose, puffy eyes, sneezing, and inflamed, itchy nose and throat. For those with severe allergies, asthma attacks, chronic sinusitis, headaches, and impaired sleep are symptoms.

How is it diagnosed?

To identify an allergy to ragweed or one of its relatives requires a careful medical history, a physical exam, and testing. The main approach to confirm a suspected allergy is the skin sensitivity test.

For this, the skin is scratched or pricked with extract of ragweed pollen. In sensitive people, the site will turn red, swollen, and itchy. Sometimes blood tests are used to see if an antibody to ragweed is present. This is sometimes necessary, but it takes longer for processing by a laboratory and it is more expensive.

What can I do about it?

There is no cure for ragweed allergy. The best control is to avoid contact with the pollen. This is difficult given the amount of ragweed pollen in the air during pollination time. There is help, though.

- Track the pollen count for your area. The news media often reports the count, especially when pollen is high. You also can call the National Allergy Bureau at 800-9-POLLEN, check it on www.aafa.org, or reach it through the American Academy of Allergy, Asthma and Immunology on the internet (www.aaaai.org). It will give you the pollen count for your region.

- Stay indoors in central air conditioning with a HEPA (high efficiency particulate air) filter attachment when the pollen count is high. This will remove pollen from the indoor air.

- Get away from the pollen where possible. People in the Eastern and Midwestern states may get some relief by going west to the Rocky Mountains and beyond. Going to sea or abroad in late summer can greatly reduce exposure. But check the area abroad you plan to visit. It may have a ragweed season as well.

You might even consider moving to get away from ragweed. Although this often helps people feel better for a short time, it is common for them to develop allergies to plants in the new location within a few years. A well thought out treatment plan is a better way to live with your allergies.

- Take antihistamine medications. These work well to control hay fever symptoms, whatever the cause. The drowsiness caused by older products is less of a problem with antihistamines now on the market. Anti-inflammatory nose sprays or drops also help and have few side effects. Similar agents can reduce eye symptoms, but other remedies are needed for the less common, pollen-induced asthma.

- If medication does not give enough relief, consider immunotherapy ("allergy shots"). This approach reduces the allergic response to specific allergens. For it to work, the allergens must be carefully identified. The allergens are injected over several months or years. If diagnosis and treatment are well directed, you may see major improvements in symptoms.

Section 28.3

Ragweed Therapy Offers Allergy Sufferers Longer Relief

"Experimental Ragweed Therapy Offers Allergy Sufferers Longer Relief with Fewer Shots," by the National Institute of Allergy and Infectious Diseases (NIAID, www.niaid.nih.gov), part of the National Institutes of Health, October 4, 2006.

Americans accustomed to the seasonal misery of sneezing, runny noses, and itchy, watery eyes caused by ragweed pollen might one day benefit from an experimental allergy treatment that not only requires fewer injections than standard immunotherapy, but leads to a marked reduction in symptoms that persists for at least a year after therapy has stopped, according to a study in the October 5 [2006] issue of the *New England Journal of Medicine (NEJM)*. The research was sponsored by the Immune Tolerance Network, which is funded by the National Institute of Allergy and Infectious Diseases (NIAID) and the National Institute of Diabetes and Digestive and Kidney Diseases (NIDDK), both components of the National Institutes of Health (NIH), and the Juvenile Diabetes Research Foundation International.

"As many as 40 million Americans suffer from seasonal allergies caused by airborne pollens produced by grasses, trees, and weeds," says NIH Director Elias A. Zerhouni, MD. "Finding new therapies for allergy sufferers is certainly an important research goal."

"This innovative research holds great promise for helping people with allergies," says NIAID Director Anthony S. Fauci, MD. "A short course of immunotherapy that reduces allergic symptoms over an extended period of time will significantly improve the quality of life for many people."

Ragweed is one of the most common pollens in the United States and is prevalent in the Northeast, Midwest, and the South. In Baltimore, where the *NEJM* study was conducted, the ragweed pollen season lasts from mid-August to October.

Physicians treat people suffering from mild and moderate ragweed allergies with antihistamines or nasal corticosteroids. However, when people with allergies do not respond to these treatments or experience severe symptoms, the next therapeutic option is a course of subcutaneous injections of the allergen, which is called allergen immunotherapy. Although this standard immunotherapy is often effective, it has two major drawbacks. First, it can cause systemic allergic reactions, such as anaphylaxis, a hypersensitivity reaction that can lead to severe and sometimes life-threatening physical symptoms. Second, to provide long-lasting relief, standard immunotherapy may require frequent injections over a 3- to 5-year period. The large number of injections over such an extended period of time often results in many people not completing the treatment.

In the study detailed in *NEJM*, lead investigator Peter Creticos, MD, medical director of the Johns Hopkins Asthma and Allergy Center in Baltimore, and his research team found that an investigational therapy based on the major ragweed allergen, Amb a 1, coupled to a unique short, synthetic sequence of DNA that stimulates the immune system, reduced allergy symptoms in adults for at least one year when given just once a week over a 6-week period. The therapeutic agent was provided by Dynavax Technologies Corp., based in Berkeley, CA.

"For almost 100 years, we've been using the tedious process of giving allergy sufferers one to two shots a week for up to 4 to 5 years to ensure its success," Dr. Creticos says. "This study is an important immunotherapy advance in that we've shown you can induce long-lasting relief from allergic rhinitis with just a few weeks of injections."

The study initially involved 25 adult volunteers, ages 23 to 60, with a history of seasonal allergic rhinitis, positive skin test reactions to ragweed pollen, and an immediate reaction when nasally challenged with ragweed. Prior to the start of the 2001 fall ragweed season, the study participants received six injections, each a week apart, of either the investigational therapy in increasingly higher doses or a placebo. They received no other injections throughout the course of the study. Fourteen volunteers received the study drug; 11 were given the placebo. The therapy was well-tolerated and caused only limited local reactions, which required neither medication nor change in treatment dose. No clinically significant, therapy-related adverse events occurred.

Throughout the 2001 and 2002 ragweed seasons, the volunteers were monitored for allergy-related symptoms, including the number of sneezes and the degree of postnasal drip, allergy medication use, and quality-of-life scores. Compared with the placebo recipients, the group that received the therapy experienced dramatically better outcomes that continued throughout the 2002 ragweed season even though therapy ended 1 year earlier.

Clearly, the regimen of only six injections showed therapeutic promise when compared with the current therapy, the study authors note. However, because the results are based on a small number of volunteers and the long-term safety of the therapy is unknown, they say additional clinical trials with longer-term follow-up to adequately assess the therapy's safety and effectiveness are necessary.

How the experimental therapy relieves ragweed allergy symptoms is not fully understood at this time. When exposed to ragweed pollen, people who are allergic to ragweed experience an increase in IgE (immunoglobulin E) antibodies; immunotherapy blocks this increase in IgE. Researchers believe the experimental therapy tempers the release of immune regulatory proteins called cytokines, which blocks increases in the level of IgE antibodies.

"Using ragweed as a model allergen system with a predictable seasonal pattern of symptoms and pollen counts, it is possible to correlate pollen levels with symptoms and measure treatment effects on symptoms. This enables us to better understand immune response to allergens and serves as an approach to similar therapies to manage other allergic reactions for which there are currently no treatments, such as food allergies," says Marshall Plaut, MD, chief of the Allergic Mechanisms Section of NIAID's Division of Allergy, Immunology, and Transplantation.

References

PS Creticos et al. Immunotherapy with a ragweed-TLR9 agonist vaccine for allergic rhinitis. The *New England Journal of Medicine* DOI: 10.1056/NEJMoa052196 (2006).

Section 28.4

Understanding Pollen Counts

A sure sign of spring (or summer or fall) in many regions of the United States is news media reports of pollen counts. These counts are of interest to some 35 million Americans who get hay fever because they are allergic to pollen.

People also look for counts of mold or fungus spores. These are another major cause of seasonal allergic reactions. Pollen and mold counts are important in helping many people with allergies plan their day.

What is the pollen count?

The pollen count tells us how many grains of plant pollen were in a certain amount of air (often 1 cubic meter) during a set period of time (usually 24 hours). Pollen is a very fine powder released by trees, weeds, and grasses. It is carried to another plant of the same kind, to fertilize the forerunner of new seeds. This is called pollination.

The pollen of some plants is carried from plant to plant by bees and other insects. These plants usually have brightly colored flowers and sweet scents to attract insects. They seldom cause allergic reactions. Other plants rely on the wind to carry pollen from plant to plant. These plants have small, drab flowers and little scent. These are the plants that cause most allergic reactions, or hay fever.

When conditions are right, a plant starts to pollinate. Weather affects how much pollen is carried in the air each year, but it has less effect on when pollination occurs. As a rule, weeds pollinate in late summer and fall. The weed that causes 75 percent of all hay fever is ragweed which has numerous species. One ragweed plant is estimated to produce up to 1 billion pollen grains. Other weeds that cause allergic reactions are cocklebur, lamb's quarters, plantain, pigweed, tumbleweed, or Russian thistle and sagebrush.

- Trees pollinate in late winter and spring. Ash, beech, birch, cedar, cottonwood, box, elder, elm, hickory, maple, and oak pollen can trigger allergies.

- Grasses pollinate in late spring and summer. Those that cause allergic reactions include Kentucky bluegrass, timothy, Johnson, Bermuda, redtop, orchard, rye, and sweet vernal grasses.

Much pollen is released early in the morning, shortly after dawn. This results in high counts near the source plants. Pollen travels best on warm, dry, breezy days and peaks in urban areas midday. Pollen counts are lowest during chilly, wet periods.

What is the mold count?

Mold and mildew are fungi. They differ from plants or animals in how they reproduce and grow. The "seeds," called spores, are spread by the wind. Allergic reactions to mold are most common from July to late summer.

Although there are many types of molds, only a few dozen cause allergic reactions. *Alternaria, Cladosporium (Hormodendrum), Aspergillus, Penicillium, Helminthosporium, Epicoccum, Fusarium, Mucor, Rhizopus,* and *Aureobasidium (Pullularia)* are the major culprits. Some common spores can be identified when viewed under a microscope. Some form recognizable growth patterns, or colonies.

Many molds grow on rotting logs and fallen leaves, in compost piles, and on grasses and grains. Unlike pollens, molds do not die with the first killing frost. Most outdoor molds become dormant during the winter. In the spring they grow on vegetation killed by the cold.

Mold counts are likely to change quickly, depending on the weather. Certain spore types reach peak levels in dry, breezy weather. Some need high humidity, fog, or dew to release spores. This group is abundant at night and during rainy periods.

What are the symptoms for hay fever?

Pollen allergies cause sneezing, runny or stuffy nose, coughing, postnasal drip, itchy nose and throat, dark circles under the eyes, and swollen, watery, and itchy eyes. For people with severe allergies, asthma attacks can occur.

Mold spores can contact the lining of the nose and cause hay fever symptoms. They also can reach the lungs, to cause asthma or another serious illness called allergic bronchopulmonary aspergillosis.

How are pollen and mold measured?

To collect a sample of particulates in the air, a plastic rod or similar device is covered with a greasy substance. The device spins in the air at a controlled speed for a set amount of time—usually over a 24-hour period. At the end of that time, a trained analyst studies the surface under a microscope. Pollen and mold that have collected on the surface are identified by size and shape as well as other characteristics. A formula is then used to calculate that day's particle count.

The counts reported are always for a past time period and may not describe what is currently in the air. Some counts reflect poorly collected samples and poor analytical skills. Some monitoring services give "total pollen" counts. They may not break out the particular pollen or mold that causes your allergies. This means that allergy symptoms may not relate closely to the published count. But knowing the count can help you decide when to stay indoors.

How can I prevent a reaction to pollen or mold?

Allergies cannot be cured. But the symptoms of the allergy can be reduced by avoiding contact with the allergen.

- Limit outdoor activity during pollination periods when the pollen or mold count is high. This will lessen the amount you inhale. The National Allergy Bureau (NAB) tracks pollen counts for different regions of the country. Contact the NAB through the American Academy of Allergy, Asthma and Immunology website. Pollen.com is also a reliable source of "pollen forecasts" in your zip code area, maintained by Surveillance Data Inc., a national monitor of medical and environmental statistics.

- Use central air conditioning set on "recirculate" which exclude much of the pollen and mold from the air in your home.

- Vacationing away from an area with a high concentration of the plants that cause your allergies may clear up symptoms.

However, if you move to such an area, within a few years you are prone to develop allergies to plants and other offenders in the new location.

Chapter 29

Household Allergens: Animal Dander, Cockroach, Dust Mite, and Mold Allergy

Chapter Contents

Section 29.1

Dust Mite Allergy

"Dust Mites," reprinted with permission from the Asthma and Allergy
Foundation of America, © 2005. All rights reserved. Reviewed by
David A. Cooke, MD, FACP, June 28, 2010.

If you have allergies or asthma, a tiny creature living in your home
could be making big problems for you. Although you can't see them, if
you have allergies or asthma you may be feeling their effects only too
well. They are dust mites, and they live in many homes throughout
the world.

Dust mites may be the most common cause of year-round allergy
and asthma. About 20 million Americans have dust mite allergy. Dust
mites are well adapted to most areas of the world—they are found on
every continent except Antarctica. It may not be possible to rid your
home entirely of these creatures, but there are ways in which you can
lessen your allergic reactions to them.

What is a dust mite?

Too small to be seen with the naked eye, a dust mite measures only
about one quarter to one third of a millimeter. Under a microscope,
they can be seen as whitish bugs. Having eight rather than six legs,
mites are technically not insects but arthropods, like spiders.

Mites are primitive creatures that have no developed respiratory system and no eyes. They spend their lives moving about, eating, reproduc-
ing, and eliminating waste products. A mite's life cycle consists of several
stages, from egg to adult. A female may lay as many as 100 eggs in her
lifetime. Depending on the species, it takes anywhere from 2 to 5 weeks for
an adult mite to develop from an egg. Adults may live for 2 to 4 months.

Dust mites thrive in temperatures of 68 to 77 degrees Fahrenheit
and relative humidity levels of 70 percent to 80 percent. There are at
least 13 species of mites, all of which are well adapted to the environment inside your home. They feed chiefly on the tiny flakes of human
skin that people normally shed each day. These flakes work their way
deep into the inner layers of furniture, carpets, bedding, and even

stuffed toys. These are the places where mites thrive. An average adult person may shed up to 1.5 grams of skin in a day—this is enough to feed 1 million dust mites!

What is dust mite allergy?

Household dust is not a single substance but rather a mixture of many materials. Dust may contain tiny fibers shed from different kinds of fabric, as well as tiny particles of feathers, dander from pet dogs or cats, bacteria, food, plant and insect parts, and mold and fungus spores. It also contains many microscopic mites and their waste products.

These waste products, not the mites themselves, are what cause allergic reactions. Dust mite waste contains a protein that is an allergen—a substance that provokes an allergic immune reaction—for many people. Throughout its life a single dust mite may produce as much as 200 times its body weight in waste.

Most dust mites die when exposed to low humidity levels or extreme temperatures. But they leave their waste behind, which continues to cause allergic reactions. In a warm, humid house, dust mites can easily survive year round.

What can I do?

Unless you live in Antarctica or in an extremely dry climate, there is probably no practical way to completely rid your home of dust mites. But you can take action to lessen their effects.

Having dust mites doesn't mean that your house isn't clean. In most areas of the world, these creatures are in every house, no matter how immaculate. But it is true that keeping your home as free of dust as possible can lessen dust mite allergy.

Studies show that more dust mites live in the bedroom than anywhere else in the home. So to attack the problem of dust mite allergy, the bedroom is the best place to start.

Unfortunately, vacuuming is not enough to remove mites and mite waste. Up to 95 percent of mites may remain after vacuuming, because they live deep inside the stuffing of sofas, chairs, mattresses, pillows, and carpeting.

The first and most important step to reduce dust mites is to cover mattresses and pillows in zippered dust-proof covers. These covers are made of a material with pores too small to let dust mites and their waste product through and are called allergen-impermeable. Plastic or vinyl covers are the least expensive but some people find them uncomfortable.

Other fabric allergen impermeable covers can be purchased from allergy supply companies as well as many regular bedding stores.

The next most important step is to wash the sheets and blankets weekly in hot water. Temperatures of at least 130 degrees Fahrenheit are needed to kill dust mites.

Other desirable, but not as critical, steps are to rid the bedroom of all types of materials that mites love. Avoid having wall-to-wall carpeting, blinds, wool blankets, upholstered furniture, and down-filled covers and pillows in the bedroom. Keep pets out of this room as well. Windows should have roll-type shades for the windows instead of curtains; if you do have curtains, be sure to wash them often.

It is ideal for someone without dust mite allergy to do the cleaning of the bedroom. If this is not possible, wear a filtering mask when dusting or vacuuming. Many drug stores carry these items. Because dusting and vacuuming stir up dust, try to do these chores at a time of day when you can stay out of the bedroom for a while afterward.

Special filters for vacuum cleaners can help to keep mites and mite waste from circulating back into the air. These filters can be bought from an allergy supply company or in some specialty vacuum stores.

Other rooms in your house can be treated similarly to the bedroom. Avoid having wall-to-wall carpeting, if possible. If you do use carpeting, the type with a short, tight pile is less hospitable to mites than the loose-pile or shag type. Better still are washable throw rugs over regularly damp-mopped wood, linoleum, or tiled floors.

Wash rugs in hot water whenever possible. Cold water leaves up to 10 percent of mites behind. Dry cleaning kills all mites and is also good for removing dust from fabrics.

Reduce the humidity in your home to less than 50 percent by using a dehumidifier and/or air conditioner. If you have taken as many of these actions as practically possible and are still having allergic reactions to house dust mites, allergy shots may help. A dust mite extract can be formulated to boost your immune system's response specifically to dust mite allergen. Shots for this purpose have been shown to be very effective.

Dust mites are probably impossible to avoid completely. Still, they don't have to make your life miserable. There are many ways you can change the environment inside your home to reduce the numbers of these unwanted "guests."

Your doctor is an important resource in helping you to keep dust mite allergies under control. Talk to him or her about measures you can take, sources of more information and of allergy products, and whether immunizing shots may be right for you. Together you can prevail against the effects of house dust mites.

Section 29.2

Cockroach Allergy

What is cockroach allergy?

When most people think of allergy "triggers," they often focus on plant pollens, dust, animals, and stinging insects. In fact, cockroaches also can trigger allergies and asthma.

Cockroach allergy was first reported in 1943, when skin rashes appeared immediately after the insects crawled over patients' skin. Skin tests first confirmed patients had cockroach allergy in 1959.

In the 1970s, studies made it clear that patients with cockroach allergies develop acute asthma attacks. The attacks occur after inhaling cockroach allergens and last for hours. Asthma has steadily increased over the past 30 years. It is the most common chronic disease of childhood. Now we know that the frequent hospital admissions of inner-city children with asthma often is directly related to their contact with cockroach allergens—the substances that cause allergies. From 23 percent to 60 percent of urban residents with asthma are sensitive to the cockroach allergen.

The increase in asthma is not fully understood. Experts think one reason for the increase among children is that they play indoors more than in past years and thus have increased contact with the allergen. This is especially true in the inner cities where they stay inside because of safety concerns.

What causes the allergic reaction?

The job of immune system cells is to find foreign substances such as viruses and bacteria and get rid of them. Normally, this response protects us from dangerous diseases. People with allergies have supersensitive immune systems that react when they inhale, swallow, or touch certain harmless substances such as pollen or cockroaches. These substances are the allergens.

Cockroach allergen is believed to derive from feces, saliva, and the bodies of these insects. Cockroaches live all over the world, from tropical areas to the coldest spots on earth. Studies show that 78 percent to 98 percent of urban homes have cockroaches. Each home has from 900 to 330,000 of the insects.

Private homes also harbor them, especially if the homes are well insulated. When one roach is seen in the basement or kitchen, it is safe to assume that at least 800 roaches are hidden under the kitchen sink, in closets, and the like. They are carried in with groceries, furniture, and luggage used on trips. Once they are in the home, they are hard to get rid of.

The amount of roach allergen in house dust or air can be measured. In dwellings where the amount is high, exposure is high and the rate of hospitalization for asthma goes up. Allergen particles are large and settle rapidly on surfaces. They become airborne when the air is stirred by people moving around or by children at play.

Who develops cockroach allergy?

People with chronic severe bronchial asthma are most likely to have cockroach allergy. Also likely to have it are people with a chronic stuffy nose, skin rash, constant sinus infection, repeat ear infection, and asthma.

Cockroach allergy is a problem among people who live in inner cities or in the South and are of low socioeconomic status. In one study of inner-city children, 37 percent were allergic to cockroaches, 35 percent to dust mites, and 23 percent to cats. Those who were allergic to cockroaches and were exposed to the insects were hospitalized for asthma 3.3 times more often than other children. This was true even when compared with those who were allergic to dust mites or cats.

Cockroach allergy is more common among poor African Americans. Experts believe that this is not because of racial differences; rather, it is because of the disproportionate number of African Americans living in the inner cities.

What are its symptoms?

Symptoms vary. They may be a mildly itchy skin, scratchy throat, or itchy eyes and nose. Or the allergy symptoms can become stronger, including severe, persistent asthma in some people. Asthma symptoms often are a problem all year, not just in some seasons. This can make it hard to determine that a cockroach allergy is the cause of the asthma.

How is cockroach allergy diagnosed?

The National Heart, Lung, and Blood Institute recommends that all patients with persistent asthma be tested for allergic response to cockroach as well as to the other chief allergens, dust mites, cats, dogs, and mold.

Diagnosis can be made only by skin tests. The doctor scratches or pricks the skin with cockroach extract. Redness, an itchy rash, or swelling at the site suggests you are allergic to the insect.

Cockroaches should be suspected, though, when allergy symptoms—stuffy nose, inflamed eyes or ears, skin rash, or bronchial asthma—persist year round.

How can I manage cockroach allergy?

If you have cockroach allergy, avoid contact with roaches and their droppings.

- The first step is to rid your home of the roaches. Because they resist many control measures, it is best to call in pest control experts.

- For ongoing control, use poison baits, boric acid, and traps.

- Don't use chemical agents. They can irritate allergies and asthma.

- Do not leave food and garbage uncovered.

- To manage nasal and sinus symptoms, use antihistamines, decongestants, and anti-inflammatory medications. Your doctor will also prescribe anti-inflammatory medications and bronchodilators if you have asthma.

- If you keep having serious allergic symptoms, see an allergist about "allergy injections" with the cockroach extract. They can reduce symptoms over time.

Section 29.3

Animal Dander Allergy

"Allergies to Pets," © 2010 Humane Society of the United States.
Reprinted with permission. For additional information,
visit www.humanesociety.org.

The benefits of having a pet usually outweigh the drawbacks of pet allergies for many people. You'd be surprised to know how many people, with non-life-threatening allergies, live with pets despite having allergies to them!

It's Not You, It's Me

Any and all cats and dogs may cause reactions for people who are allergic to animals. Cats tend to cause more reactions than dogs for allergic people, although some people are more sensitive to dogs than cats. Contrary to popular belief, there are no "non-allergenic" breeds of dogs or cats; even hairless breeds may cause symptoms.

Dogs with soft, constantly-growing hair—like Poodles or the Bichon Frise—may be less irritating to some individuals, although this may be because they are bathed and groomed more frequently. One dog or cat may be more irritating to an individual allergy sufferer than another animal of the same species.

What to Do

If someone in your household has been diagnosed with a pet allergy by an allergist, carefully consider whether you can live with the symptoms before you bring a new pet home. Except in the case of children, who sometimes outgrow allergies, few people with allergies become accustomed to pets to which they are allergic. Too many allergic owners obtain pets without thinking through the challenges of living with allergies.

If your or a family member's allergies are simply miserable, but not life-threatening, take these five steps to reduce the symptoms:

1. Create an "allergy free" zone in your home—preferably the allergic person's bedroom—and strictly prohibit the pet's

access to it. Use a high-efficiency HEPA [high efficiency particulate air] air cleaner, and consider using impermeable covers for the mattress and pillows.

2. Use HEPA air cleaners throughout the rest of the home, and avoid dust-and-dander-catching furnishings such as cloth curtains and blinds and carpeted floors. Clean frequently and thoroughly to remove dust and dander, washing articles such as couch covers and pillows, curtains, and pet beds.

3. Bathing your pet on a weekly basis can reduce the level of allergy-causing dander (shed old skin cells). Cats can get used to being bathed, but it's critical to only use products labeled for them; kittens may need a shampoo safe for kittens. Check with your veterinarian's staff or a good book on pet care for directions about safe bathing, It's a good idea to use a shampoo recommended by your veterinarian or other animal care professional.

4. Don't be quick to blame the family pet for allergies. Ask your allergist to specifically test for allergies to pet dander. Many allergy sufferers are sensitive to more than one allergen. Reduce the overall allergen level in your environment by concentrating on all of the causes, not just the pet allergy.

5. Try treatments. Additional treatments for allergies to pets are include immunotherapy (allergy shots), steroidal and antihistamine nose sprays, and antihistamine pills. It is important to find an allergist who understands your commitment to living with your pet. A combination of approaches—medical control of symptoms, good housecleaning methods, and immunotherapy—is most likely to succeed in allowing an allergic person to live with pets.

Section 29.4

Mold Allergy

If you have an allergy that never ends when seasons change, you may be allergic to the spores of molds or other fungi. Molds live everywhere, and disturbing a mold source can disperse the spores into the air.

What is mold allergy?

Mold and mildew are fungi. They differ from plants or animals in how they reproduce and grow. The "seeds," called spores, are spread by the wind outdoors and by air indoors. Some spores are released in dry, windy weather. Others are released with the fog or dew when humidity is high.

Inhaling the spores causes allergic reactions in some people. Allergic symptoms from fungus spores are most common from July to late summer. But with fungi growing in so many places, allergic reactions can occur year round.

Although there are many types of molds, only a few dozen cause allergic reactions. *Alternaria, Cladosporium (Hormodendrum), Aspergillus, Penicillium, Helminthosporium, Epicoccum, Fusarium, Mucor, Rhizopus,* and *Aureobasidium (Pullularia)* are the major culprits. Some common spores can be identified when viewed under a microscope. Some form recognizable growth or colonies.

Many molds grow on rotting logs and fallen leaves, in compost piles, and on grasses and grains. Unlike pollens, molds do not die with the first killing frost. Most outdoor molds become dormant during the winter. In the spring they grow on plants killed by the cold.

Indoors, fungi grow in damp areas, particularly in the bathroom, kitchen, or basement.

Who gets the allergy?

It is common for people to get mold allergy if they or other family members are allergic to substances such as pollen or animal dander.

People may become allergic to only mold or fungi, or they may also have problems with dust mites, pollens, and other spores. If you are allergic to only fungi, it is unlikely that you would be bothered by all fungi. The different types of fungi spores have only limited similarities.

People in some occupations have more exposure to mold and are at greater risk of developing allergies. Farmers, dairymen, loggers, bakers, mill workers, carpenters, greenhouse employees, wine makers, and furniture repairers are at increased risk.

There is only weak evidence that allergic symptoms are caused by food fungi (e.g., mushrooms, dried fruit, foods containing yeast, vinegar, or soy sauce). It is more likely that reactions to food fungi are caused by the food's direct effect on blood vessels. For example, histamine may be present because of the fermentation of red wines.

Fungi on house plants can cause an allergic reaction, but this is only likely to happen if the soil is disturbed.

Fungi can even grow in the human body. If not properly treated, intense inflammation can recur often. It can permanently damage airway walls. This is not common, though.

What are the symptoms?

The symptoms of mold allergy are very similar to the symptoms of other allergies, such as sneezing, itching, nasal discharge, congestion, and dry, scaling skin. Some people with mold allergies may have allergy symptoms the entire summer because of outdoor molds or year-round if symptoms are due to indoor molds.

Mold spores can deposit on the lining of the nose and cause hay fever symptoms. They also can reach the lungs, to cause asthma or another serious illness called allergic bronchopulmonary aspergillosis.

Sometimes the reaction is immediate, and sometimes the reaction is delayed. Symptoms often worsen in a damp or moldy room such as a basement; this may suggest mold allergy.

How is mold allergy diagnosed?

To diagnose an allergy to mold or fungi, the doctor will take a complete medical history. If mold allergy is suspected, the doctor often will do skin tests. Extracts of different types of fungi will be used to scratch or prick the skin. If there is no reaction, allergy is not suggested. In some people with allergy, irritation alone can cause a reaction. Therefore the doctor uses the patient's medical history, the skin testing results, and the physical examination combined to diagnose mold allergy.

How is mold allergy treated?

As with most allergies, patients should:

- Avoid contact with the spores. Wear a dust mask when cutting grass, digging around plants, picking up leaves, and disturbing other plant materials. Reduce the humidity indoors to prevent fungi from growing. These measures will reduce symptoms.

- Take medications for nasal or other allergic symptoms. Antihistamines and decongestants are available over the counter—without a prescription. Because these antihistamines can cause drowsiness, they are best taken at bedtime. If drowsiness continues to be a problem, talk to your doctor about taking non-sedating antihistamines, which require a prescription. For moderate and severe allergy symptoms, your doctor may prescribe corticosteroid nasal sprays.

- If these medications are inadequate, talk to your doctor or allergist about taking allergy shots (immunotherapy). This works for some carefully selected patients.

How can I prevent a reaction to mold?

Allergies cannot be cured. But the symptoms of the allergy can be reduced by avoiding contact with the spores. Several measures will help:

- Stay indoors during periods when the published mold count is high. This will lessen the amount you inhale. Mold spores are "counted" by collecting a sample of particulates in the air then identifying and counting the mold spores in the sample. The amount of airborne spores are likely to change quickly, depending on the weather. The counts reported are always for a past time period and may not reflect what is currently in the air. The mold that causes your allergic reaction may not be counted separately. This means that allergy symptoms may not relate closely to the published count. But knowing the count can help you decide when to stay indoors.

- Use central air conditioning with a HEPA (high efficiency particulate air) filter attachment. It will help trap spores before they reach you. Air conditioning with a HEPA filter attached works better than electrostatic air-cleaning devices and much better than freestanding air cleaners. Devices that treat air with heat, ions, or ozone are not recommended. No air cleaners will help if excess moisture remains. If indoor humidity is above 50 percent, risks of fungus growth rise steeply. Hygrometers can be used to measure humidity accurately. The goal is to keep humidity below 45 percent, and preferably about 35 percent. If humidifiers are necessary, scrub the fluid reservoirs at least twice a week to prevent mold growth. Air conditioners and dehumidifiers can also be a source of mold and should be cleaned.

- To prevent mold and mildew build up inside the home, especially in bathrooms, basements, and laundry areas, be aggressive about reducing dampness:

  - Put an exhaust fan or open a window in the bathroom.

  - Quickly repair any plumbing leaks.

  - Remove bathroom carpeting where moisture is a concern.

  - Scour sinks and tubs at least monthly. Fungi thrive on soap and other films that coat tiles and grout. For problem areas, use ordinary laundry bleach (1 ounce diluted in a quart of water). Fungicides (chemicals that kill fungus) are less important than a good scrubbing. Fungicides may be added to paint, primer, or wallpaper paste to slow fungus growth on treated areas. But this will have little effect if excess moisture remains.

  - Clean garbage pails frequently.

  - Clean refrigerator door gaskets and drip pans.

  - Repair basement plumbing leaks, blocked drains, poorly vented clothes dryers, and water seepage through walls.

  - Use an electric dehumidifier to remove moisture from the basement. Be sure to drain the dehumidifier regularly and clean the condensation coils and collection bucket.

  - Raise the temperature in the basement to help lower humidity levels. Small space heaters or a low-wattage light bulb may be useful in damp closets. Be careful where they are placed, though, to avoid creating a fire hazard.

  - Polyurethane and rubber foams seem especially prone to fungus invasion. If bedding is made with these foams, it should be covered in plastic.

  - Throw away or recycle old books, newspapers, clothing, or bedding.

- Promote ground water drainage away from a house. Remove leaves and dead vegetation near the foundation and in the rain gutters. Completely shaded homes dry out slowly, and dense bushes and other plants around the foundation often promote dampness. In the winter, condensation on cold walls encourages mold growth, but even thick insulation can be invaded if vapor barriers in exterior walls are not effective.

Chapter 30

Air Quality, Allergies, and Your Health

"It's a code red day for ozone."

"Particle pollution levels are forecast to be unhealthy for sensitive groups."

"Local air quality is very unhealthy today."

You may hear these alerts on radio or TV or read them in the newspaper. But what do they mean if you:

- are active outdoors?

- have children who play outdoors?

- are an older adult?

- have heart or lung disease?

This text will help you understand how to find out about air quality in your area and protect your health.

Why is air quality important?

Local air quality affects how you live and breathe. Like the weather, it can change from day to day or even hour to hour. The U.S. Environmental Protection Agency (EPA) and your local air quality agency have been working to make information about outdoor air quality as easy to find and understand as weather forecasts. A key tool in this effort

---

Excerpted from "Air Quality Index: A Guide to Air Quality and Your Health," by the Environmental Protection Agency (EPA, www.epa.gov), August 2009.

is the Air Quality Index, or AQI. EPA and local officials use the AQI to provide simple information about your local air quality, how unhealthy air may affect you, and how you can protect your health.

What is the AQI?

The AQI is an index for reporting daily air quality. It tells you how clean or unhealthy your air is, and what associated health effects might be a concern. The AQI focuses on health effects you may experience within a few hours or days after breathing unhealthy air. The AQI is calculated for four major air pollutants regulated by the Clean Air Act: Ground level ozone, particle pollution, carbon monoxide, and sulfur dioxide. For each of these pollutants, EPA has established national air quality standards to protect public health.

EPA is currently reviewing the national air quality standard for nitrogen dioxide. If the standard is revised, the AQI will be revised as well.

How does the AQI work?

Think of the AQI as a yardstick that runs from 0 to 500. The higher the AQI value, the greater the level of air pollution and the greater the health concern. For example, an AQI value of 50 represents good air quality with little or no potential to affect public health, while an AQI value over 300 represents air quality so hazardous that everyone may experience serious effects.

An AQI value of 100 generally corresponds to the national air quality standard for the pollutant, which is the level EPA has set to protect public health. AQI values at or below 100 are generally thought of as satisfactory. When AQI values are above 100, air quality is considered to be unhealthy—at first for certain sensitive groups of people, then for everyone as AQI values increase.

What do the AQI values mean?

The purpose of the AQI is to help you understand what local air quality means to your health. To make it easier to understand, the AQI is divided into six levels of health concern, as indicated in Table 30.1.

Each category corresponds to a different level of health concern:

- **Good:** The AQI value for your community is between 0 and 50. Air quality is satisfactory and poses little or no health risk.

- **Moderate:** The AQI is between 51 and 100. Air quality is acceptable; however, pollution in this range may pose a moderate health concern for a very small number of individuals. People who are unusually sensitive to ozone or particle pollution may experience respiratory symptoms.

- **Unhealthy for sensitive groups:** When AQI values are between 101 and 150, members of sensitive groups may experience health effects, but the general public is unlikely to be affected.

  - **Ozone:** People with lung disease, children, older adults, and people who are active outdoors are considered sensitive and therefore at greater risk.

  - **Particle pollution:** People with heart or lung disease, older adults, and children are considered sensitive and therefore at greater risk.

- **Unhealthy:** Everyone may begin to experience health effects when AQI values are between 151 and 200. Members of sensitive groups may experience more serious health effects.

- **Very unhealthy:** AQI values between 201 and 300 trigger a health alert, meaning everyone may experience more serious health effects.

- **Hazardous:** AQI values over 300 trigger health warnings of emergency conditions. The entire population is even more likely to be affected by serious health effects.

Table 30.1. Air Quality Index Values and What They Mean

Air Quality Index (AQI) Values	Levels of Health Concern	Colors
When the AQI is in this range:	air quality conditions are:	as symbolized by this color.
0 to 50	Good	Green
51 to 100	Moderate	Yellow
101 to 150	Unhealthy for sensitive groups	Orange
151 to 200	Unhealthy	Red
201 to 300	Very Unhealthy	Purple
301 to 500	Hazardous	Maroon

How is a community's AQI calculated and reported?

Each day, monitors record concentrations of the major pollutants at more than a thousand locations across the country.

These raw measurements are converted into a separate AQI value for each pollutant (ground-level ozone, particle pollution, carbon monoxide, and sulfur dioxide) using standard formulas developed by EPA. The highest of these AQI values is reported as the AQI value for that day.

In large cities (more than 350,000 people), state and local agencies are required to report the AQI to the public daily. Many smaller communities also report the AQI as a public health service.

When the AQI is above 100, agencies must also report which groups, such as children or people with asthma or heart disease, may be sensitive to that pollutant. If two or more pollutants have AQI values above 100 on a given day, agencies must report all the groups that are sensitive to those pollutants. For example, if a community's AQI is 130 for ozone and 101 for particle pollution, the AQI value for that day would be announced as 130 for ozone. The announcements would note that particle pollution levels were also high and would alert groups sensitive to ozone or particle pollution about how to protect their health.

Many cities also provide forecasts for the next day's AQI. These forecasts help local residents protect their health by alerting them to plan their strenuous outdoor activities for a time when air quality is better.

The AQI is a national index, so the values and colors used
to show local air quality and the levels of health concern are the same everywhere in the United States.

Where can I find the AQI?

Checking local air quality is as easy as checking the weather. You can find the latest AQI values on the internet, in your local media, and on many state and local telephone hotlines. You can also sign up to receive AQI forecasts by e-mail.

Here's the type of report you might hear: "Tomorrow will be a code red air quality day for Center City. The cold winter air, morning traffic, and wood smoke are expected to cause particle pollution to rise to unhealthy levels. People with heart or lung disease, older adults, and children should avoid prolonged or heavy physical activities."

What are typical AQI values in most communities?

In many U.S. communities, AQI values are usually below 100, with higher values occurring just a few times a year. Larger cities typically have more air pollution than smaller cities, so their AQI values may exceed 100 more often. AQI values higher than 200 are infrequent, and AQI values above 300 are extremely rare—they generally occur only during events such as forest fires. You can compare the air quality of U.S. cities and find out about quality trends in your area by visiting "Air Compare" at www.epa.gov/aircompare.

AQI values can vary from one season to another. In winter, carbon monoxide may be high in some areas because cold weather makes it difficult for car emission control systems to operate effectively. Ozone is often higher in warmer months, because heat and sunlight increase ozone formation. Particle pollution can be elevated any time of the year.

AQI values also can vary depending on the time of day. Ozone levels often peak in the afternoon to early evening. Carbon monoxide may be a problem during morning or evening rush hours. And particle pollution can be high any time of day, and is often elevated near busy roadways, especially during morning or evening rush hours.

How can I avoid being exposed to unhealthy air?

You can take simple steps to reduce your exposure to unhealthy air. First, you need to find out whether AQI levels are a concern in your area. You can do this, by visiting the AIRNow website, signing up for EnviroFlash, or checking your local media. If the AQI for ozone, particle pollution, carbon monoxide, or sulfur dioxide is a concern in your area, you can learn what steps to take to protect your health. Two important terms you will need to understand are:

- **Prolonged exertion:** This means any outdoor activity that you'll be doing intermittently for several hours and that makes you breathe slightly harder than normal. A good example of this is working in the yard for part of a day. When air quality is unhealthy, you can protect your health by reducing how much time you spend on this type of activity.

- **Heavy exertion:** This means intense outdoor activities that cause you to breathe hard. When air quality is unhealthy, you can protect your health by reducing how much time you spend on this type of activity, or by substituting a less intense activity—for example, go for a walk instead of a jog. Be sure to reduce your activity level if you experience any unusual coughing, chest discomfort, wheezing, breathing difficulty, or unusual fatigue.

What is ozone?

Ozone is a gas found in the air we breathe. Ozone can be good or bad, depending where it occurs:

- Good ozone is present naturally in the Earth's upper atmosphere—approximately 6 to 30 miles above the Earth's surface. This natural ozone shields us from the sun's harmful ultraviolet rays.

- Bad ozone forms near the ground when pollutants (emitted by sources such as cars, power plants, industrial boilers, refineries, and chemical plants) react chemically in sunlight. Ozone pollution is more likely to form during warmer months. This is when the weather conditions normally needed to form ground-level ozone—lots of sun—occur.

Who is most at risk?

Several groups of people are particularly sensitive to ozone, especially when they are active outdoors. This is because ozone levels are higher outdoors, and physical activity causes faster and deeper breathing, drawing more ozone into the body.

- People with lung diseases, such as asthma, chronic bronchitis, and emphysema, can be particularly sensitive to ozone. They will generally experience more serious health effects at lower levels. Ozone can aggravate their diseases, leading to increased medication use, doctor and emergency room visits, and hospital admissions.

- Children are at higher risk from ozone exposure because they often play outdoors in warmer weather when ozone levels are higher, they are more likely to have asthma (which may be aggravated by ozone exposure), and their lungs are still developing.

- Older adults may be more affected by ozone exposure, possibly because they are more likely to have pre-existing lung disease.

- Active people of all ages who exercise or work vigorously outdoors are at increased risk.

- Some healthy people are more sensitive to ozone. They may experience health effects at lower ozone levels than the average person even though they have none of the risk factors listed above. There may be a genetic basis for this increased sensitivity.

In general, as concentrations of ground-level ozone increase, more people begin to experience more serious health effects. When levels are very high, everyone should be concerned about ozone exposure.

What are the health effects?

Ozone affects the lungs and respiratory system in many ways. It can do the following:

- It can irritate the respiratory system, causing coughing, throat soreness, airway irritation, chest tightness, or chest pain when taking a deep breath.

- It can reduce lung function, making it more difficult to breathe as deeply and vigorously as you normally would, especially when exercising. Breathing may start to feel uncomfortable, and you may notice that you are taking more rapid and shallow breaths than normal.

- It can inflame and damage the cells that line the lungs. Within a few days, the damaged cells are replaced and the old cells are shed—much like the way your skin peels after sunburn. Studies suggest that if this type of inflammation happens repeatedly, lung tissue may become permanently scarred and lung function may be permanently reduced.

- It can make the lungs more susceptible to infection. Ozone reduces the lung's defenses by damaging the cells that move particles and bacteria out of the airways and by reducing the number and effectiveness of white blood cells in the lungs.

- It can aggravate asthma. When ozone levels are unhealthy, more people with asthma have symptoms that require a doctor's attention or the use of medication. Ozone makes people more sensitive to allergens—the most common triggers for asthma attacks. Also, asthmatics may be more severely affected by reduced lung function and airway inflammation. People with asthma should ask their doctor for an asthma action plan and follow it carefully when ozone levels are unhealthy.

- It can aggravate other chronic lung diseases such as emphysema and bronchitis. As concentrations of ground-level ozone increase, more people with lung disease visit doctors or emergency rooms and are admitted to the hospital.

- It can cause permanent lung damage. Repeated short-term ozone damage to children's developing lungs may lead to reduced lung function in adulthood. In adults, ozone exposure may accelerate the natural decline in lung function that occurs with age.

What is particle pollution?

Particle pollution (also known as "particulate matter") consists of a mixture of solids and liquid droplets. Some particles are emitted directly; others form when pollutants emitted by various sources react in the atmosphere. Particle pollution levels can be very unhealthy and even hazardous during events such as forest fires. Particle levels can be elevated indoors, especially when outdoor particle levels are high.

Particles come in a wide range of sizes. Those less than 10 micrometers in diameter (smaller than the width of a single human hair) are so small that they can get into the lungs, where they can cause serious health problems.

- Fine particles: The smallest particles (those 2.5 micrometers or less in diameter) are called "fine" particles. These particles are so small they can be detected only with an electron microscope. Major sources of fine particles include motor vehicles, power plants, residential wood burning, forest fires, agricultural burning, some industrial processes, and other combustion processes.

- Coarse particles: Particles between 2.5 and 10 micrometers in diameter are referred to as "coarse." Sources of coarse particles include crushing or grinding operations, and dust stirred up by vehicles traveling on roads.

What are the health effects and who is most at risk?

Particles smaller than 10 micrometers in diameter can cause or aggravate a number of health problems and have been linked with illnesses and deaths from heart or lung disease. These effects have been associated with both short-term exposures (usually over 24 hours, but possibly as short as one hour) and long-term exposures (years).

Sensitive groups for particle pollution include people with heart or lung disease (including heart failure and coronary artery disease, or asthma and chronic obstructive pulmonary disease), older adults (who may have undiagnosed heart or lung disease), and children. The risk of heart attacks, and thus the risk from particle pollution, may begin as early as the mid-40s for men and mid-50s for women.

- When exposed to particle pollution, people with heart or lung diseases and older adults are more likely to visit emergency rooms, be admitted to hospitals, or in some cases, even die.

- Exposure to particle pollution may cause people with heart disease to experience chest pain, palpitations, shortness of breath, and fatigue. Particle pollution has also been associated with cardiac arrhythmias and heart attacks.

- When exposed to high levels of particle pollution, people with existing lung disease may not be able to breathe as deeply or vigorously as they normally would. They may experience symptoms such as coughing and shortness of breath. Healthy people also may experience these effects, although they are unlikely to experience more serious effects.

- Particle pollution also can increase susceptibility to respiratory infections and can aggravate existing respiratory diseases, such as asthma and chronic bronchitis, causing more use of medication and more doctor visits.

What is carbon monoxide?

Carbon monoxide is an odorless, colorless gas. It forms when the carbon in fuels does not completely burn. Vehicle exhaust contributes roughly 75 percent of all carbon monoxide emissions nationwide, and up to 95 percent in cities. Other sources include fuel combustion in industrial processes and natural sources such as wildfires. Carbon monoxide levels typically are highest during cold weather, because cold temperatures make combustion less complete and cause inversions that trap pollutants close to the ground.

What are the health effects and who is most at risk?

Carbon monoxide enters the bloodstream through the lungs and binds to hemoglobin, the substance in blood that carries oxygen to cells. It reduces the amount of oxygen reaching the body's organs and tissues.

- People with cardiovascular disease, such as coronary artery disease, are most at risk. They may experience chest pain and other cardiovascular symptoms if they are exposed to carbon monoxide, particularly while exercising.

- People with marginal or compromised cardiovascular and respiratory systems (for example, individuals with congestive heart failure, cerebrovascular disease, anemia, or chronic obstructive lung disease), and possibly young infants and fetuses, also may be at greater risk from carbon monoxide pollution.

- In healthy individuals, exposure to higher levels of carbon monoxide can affect mental alertness and vision.

What is sulfur dioxide?

Sulfur dioxide, a colorless, reactive gas, is produced when sulfur-containing fuels such as coal and oil are burned. Generally, the highest levels of sulfur dioxide are found near large industrial complexes. Major sources include power plants, refineries, and industrial boilers.

What are the health effects and who is most at risk?

Sulfur dioxide is an irritant gas that is removed by the nasal passages. Moderate activity levels that trigger mouth breathing, such as a brisk walk, are needed for sulfur dioxide to cause health effects in most people.

- People with asthma who are physically active outdoors are most likely to experience the health effects of sulfur dioxide. The main effect, even with very brief exposure (minutes), is a narrowing of the airways (called bronchoconstriction). This may be accompanied by wheezing, chest tightness, and shortness of breath, which may require use of medication that opens the airways. Symptoms increase as sulfur dioxide levels or breathing rate increases. When exposure to sulfur dioxide ceases, lung function typically returns to normal within an hour, even without medication.

- At very high levels, sulfur dioxide may cause wheezing, chest tightness, and shortness of breath even in healthy people who do not have asthma.

- Long-term exposure to sulfur dioxide may cause respiratory symptoms and illness, and aggravate asthma. People with asthma are the most susceptible to sulfur dioxide. However, people with other chronic lung diseases or cardiovascular disease, as well as children and older adults, may also be susceptible to these effects.

Where can I get more information?

For information and resources about air quality, visit the AIRNow website at www.airnow.gov. There you can do the following:

- Access maps and information on air quality in your area. Find out how to protect your health and how to reduce air pollution.

- Sign up for EnviroFlash (www.environflash.info), a free service that will alert you via e-mail when air quality in your area is forecast to be a concern.

- Access brochures, movies, games, and other air quality educational resources for adults and kids.

- Visit Air Compare (www.epa.gov/aircompare), where you can compare the air quality of U.S. cities and find out about air quality trends in your area.

- Access cameras that provide real-time pictures of visibility at many locations across the United States.

- Access training and tools. If you are a health care provider, teacher, or weathercaster, you can use these resources to help adults and children understand how air pollution affects their health and how they can protect their health.

Chapter 31

Tobacco Smoke

Most people know about the dangers of cigarette smoking, thanks in large part to increased efforts to educate the public. Smoking is estimated to be the single largest cause of preventable deaths in the United States. What many people are less aware of though, is that tobacco can pose risks to your health even if you are not the one doing the smoking.

Environmental tobacco smoke, or ETS, refers to the smoke that is released in the air when a smoker exhales, combined with the smoke released from a burning cigarette, cigar, or pipe. In 1993, the U.S. Environmental Protection Agency issued a report that outlined the dangers of ETS or "passive smoking." It found that ETS causes about 3,000 deaths from lung cancer each year in the United States. It also stated that passive smoking is an important cause of respiratory illness.

Children who live with a smoker are especially at risk for health problems. Their growing lungs are at increased risk for illnesses such as bronchitis, pneumonia, tracheitis (inflammation of the upper airway), and asthma. And infants exposed to ETS are more likely to develop otitis media (middle ear infection).

What's in tobacco smoke?

Secondhand smoke is the combination of the smoke given off by a burning cigarette, pipe, or cigar and the smoke exhaled as a person smokes. The tobacco is treated with chemicals so that it will keep burning even when it is not being smoked.

Secondhand smoke contains up to 4,000 chemicals, including trace amounts of poisons like formaldehyde, arsenic, DDT [dichlorodiphenyltrichloroethane], and cyanide. More than 40 of the substances in ETS are known to cause cancer. Many more cause irritation of the lungs and airways. Secondhand smoke has been classified by the U.S. Environmental Protection Agency as a Group A carcinogen (cancer causing agent). Group A carcinogens are the most harmful.

How is ETS linked to allergies and asthma in children?

Children are at special risk of lung damage and illness from inhaled smoke. Studies have shown a clear link between ETS and asthma in young people. Passive smoking worsens asthma in teens and may cause up to 26,000 new cases of asthma each year. It is also linked to hundreds of thousands of infections of the lower respiratory tract (the lungs and lower airways) in infants under 18 months. These infections in turn lead to thousands of hospitalizations of children each year. The incidence of sudden infant death syndrome quadruples if either mother or both parents are smokers.

Children exposed to ETS are more likely to have reduced lung function and symptoms of respiratory irritation, such as coughing, wheezing, and excess phlegm (fluid in the lungs and airways). Children with allergies and nasal congestion who are also exposed to tobacco smoke are up to six times more likely than others to have persistent middle ear infections requiring the surgical insertion of tubes.

Smoke and minors: Exposure to ETS is responsible for increased frequency of asthma episodes in adolescents. There is also evidence which suggests that adolescents exposed to ETS may have decreased pulmonary function tests, higher cholesterol levels, and may increase their risks of heart disease as adults.

Surveys show a disturbing trend of smoking among young people. The most recent data shows that more than a third of high school students (grades 9–12) report that they currently smoke. The rate is highest among high school seniors. In addition, about one tenth of high school students report that they use smokeless (chewing) tobacco.

Tobacco advertising that seems to be aimed at young people is troubling. Many communities and local governments are increasing their efforts to control such marketing practices and the topic has received a good deal of attention in the media in recent years. In some states, parental smoking is an important issue in deciding questions of custody in divorce cases.

How to reduce secondhand smoke exposure?

As a parent, you can limit your children's exposure to secondhand smoke. As in most things, the first and most important steps begin at home—by quitting smoking yourself, if you are a smoker. You can also set down a policy of having a smoke-free home by asking guests not to light up in your house.

Quitting is seldom easy, but it is possible. Smoking-cessation programs, counseling, and methods such as nicotine gum or patches have helped many people give up tobacco for good. Your doctor should be able to steer you toward resources to help you on the road to kicking the habit and addiction. Until you quit, do not smoke within the airspace of your child, not in your home or in your car.

Choose childcare carefully so that your children will not suffer from the harmful effects of ETS.

Remember: Children exposed to secondhand smoke are at risk of illness. Protecting them from exposure is good preventive medicine. Your child's health depends on it.

Chapter 32

Sensitivity to Fragrances and Chemicals

Chapter Contents

Section 32.1

Fragrance Sensitivity

Excerpted from "Accommodation and Compliance Series: Employees
with Fragrance Sensitivity," by the Job Accommodation Network
(JAN, www.jan.wvu.edu), September 5, 2008.

What is fragrance sensitivity?

Fragrance sensitivity may be an actual allergy or a simple irritation. It can be difficult to diagnose which is occurring. In addition, fragrances are composed of many different chemicals. This can make it difficult to identify if the sensitivity is to one particular chemical or to a combination of chemicals.

Typical reactions to fragrances include breathing problems, asthma, and contact dermatitis (an itchy and inflamed skin rash). Once a person has developed fragrance irritation it is likely that the sensitivity will grow over time and with repeated exposure. Certain chemicals may be sensitizers at high levels of exposure and can result in sensitivity to the chemical at much lower levels after initial exposure.

What are the symptoms of fragrance sensitivity?

Fragrances can enter the body through inhalation, ingestion, or absorption. The first indicator of a fragrance irritation or allergy is usually a skin rash after the use of a perfume, cream, or lotion. Reactions can also take other forms, including: hives; nausea; dizziness; headache; itchy skin, eyes, and nose; runny nose; wheezing; coughing; eczema; difficulty breathing; sore throat; asthma attacks or asthma-like symptoms; and strange tastes in the mouth. The severity of symptoms varies from one individual to another. Symptoms can show up over a wide time range from a few minutes to 7 to 10 days.

How is fragrance sensitivity prevented and treated?

The best way to prevent fragrance sensitivity is to avoid the offending substance. Discussing the fragrance sensitivity with people at work and at home will help to limit exposure to other people's fragrances.

Careful examination of product labels is also important. A product labeled "unscented" does not mean it is fragrance free, merely that it has no perceptible scent. A fragrance may have been added to the product to mask scent. While such a trace amount of fragrance is unlikely to cause irritation, it may trigger allergic reactions in people with fragrance allergies.

Fragrances added to products to mask scent do not have to be labeled as ingredients. A label that is marked "perfume free" or "fragrance free" is more likely to contain no fragrances. Sensitive people may wish to consult a dermatologist for recommendations on fragrance-free skin products or an allergist for recommendations on avoiding a variety of scented products.

Is fragrance sensitivity a disability under the Americans with Disabilities Act (ADA)?

The ADA does not contain a list of medical conditions that constitute disabilities. Instead, the ADA has a general definition of disability that each person must meet. Therefore, some people with fragrance sensitivity will have a disability under the ADA and some will not.

A person has a disability if he/she has a physical or mental impairment that substantially limits one or more major life activities, a record of such an impairment, or is regarded as having such an impairment.

Is an employer required to implement a fragrance policy as an accommodation?

The implementation of a fragrance policy is an option to consider when addressing possible accommodations. An employer could choose to make a request that employees voluntarily refrain from wearing fragrances or the employer could go as far as creating a policy that requires employees to refrain. An employer has the right to decide how far is reasonable when implementing accommodations. Employers who have concerns about the legalities of implementing a fragrance policy as an accommodation should consult an appropriate legal professional.

Section 32.2

Sensitivity to Multiple Chemicals

Excerpted from "Employees with Multiple Chemical Sensitivity (MCS) and Environmental Illness (EI)," by the Job Accommodation Network (JAN, www.jan.wvu.edu), March 23, 2010.

What is MCS/EI?

Defining MCS/EI has been a difficult task for the environmental health community. MCS/EI is generally an inability to tolerate an environmental chemical or class of foreign chemicals. It develops from exposure to substances in the environment and may result in intolerance to even very low level exposure to chemicals. Symptoms can occur in more than one organ system in the body, such as the nervous system, the lungs, and the vascular system (heart problems).

Exposures can come through the air, from food and water, or through the skin.

What are the symptoms of MCS/EI?

MCS/EI causes different symptoms in different people. Symptoms may include: headaches, dizziness, fatigue, nausea, breathing difficulties, tightening of the throat, difficulty concentrating, memory loss, learning disorders, eczema, arthritis-like sensations, and muscle pain. A person who experiences limitations due to MCS/EI may have any of the above mentioned symptoms when exposed to such irritants as fragrances, cleaning agents, smoke, pesticides, molds, office machines, car exhaust, paint, new carpeting, solvents, and poor indoor air quality among other irritants.

Is MCS/EI considered a disability under the Americans with Disabilities Act (ADA)?

The ADA does not contain a list of medical conditions that constitute disabilities. Instead, the ADA has a general definition of disability that each person must meet. Therefore, some people will have a disability under the ADA and some will not.

A person has a disability if he/she has a physical or mental impairment that substantially limits one or more major life activities, a record of such an impairment, or is regarded as having such an impairment. Questions to consider:

- What limitations is the employee experiencing?

- How do these limitations affect the employee and the employee's job performance?

- What specific job tasks are problematic as a result of these limitations?

- What accommodations are available to reduce or eliminate these problems? Are all possible resources being used to determine possible accommodations?

- Has the employee been consulted regarding possible accommodations?

- Once accommodations are in place, would it be useful to meet with the employee to evaluate the effectiveness of the accommodations and to determine whether additional accommodations are needed?

- Do supervisory personnel and employees need training?

What are some accommodation ideas?

Ventilation and indoor air quality issues:

- Provide an office or workspace that has working windows.

- Make certain the ventilation system is not distributing pollutants throughout the work-site from locations within or outside of the building.

- Use HEPA [high-efficiency particulate air] filters in the ventilation system if possible and have ducts maintained.

- Have an air quality test performed by an industrial hygiene professional to assess poor air quality, dust, mold or mildew accumulation, VOC [volatile organic compound] concentration, etc.

- Work with specialists in the industrial hygiene field by contacting resources like the American Industrial Hygiene Association for a member referral.

- Use air purification systems throughout the building or in personal workstations. Work with specialists in the air filtration field by contacting resources like The National Air Filtration Association for a member referral.

- Maintain a work environment that is free of pollutants such as fragrances, toxic cleaning agents, pesticides, exhaust fumes, tobacco smoke, etc.

- Provide adequate exhaust systems to remove fumes from copiers and similar office machines.

Construction, remodeling, and cleaning issues:

- Provide prenotification of events such as remodeling, painting, pesticide applications, floor waxing, and carpet shampooing by way of signs, memos, e-mail, or an employee register. A voluntary registry can be created for people to be notified on a regular basis.

- Allow for alternative work arrangements for those people who may be sensitive to the chemical agents used in the above activities such as offering the use of another office, work on another floor of the building, work outside, or work from home.

- Use non-toxic building materials, furnishings, and supplies.

- Use non-toxic carpeting or alternative floor covering such as tile or cotton throw rugs. Products can be used to reduce the outgassing of newly laid carpeting.

- If industrial products are being used such as solvents, primers, stains, paints, lubricants, etc., consider any alternative products that could possibly be used that may not illicit an MCS/EI reaction.

- If possible, have cleaning, maintenance, and remodeling activities performed when the building is not occupied to reduce employee exposure to these activities.

- Discontinue the use of toxic pesticides and opt for an alternative pest management policy. Contact resources like the National Pesticide Telecommunications Network or the National Coalition Against the Misuse of Pesticides to find out more about alternative pest management practices.

- Discontinue the use of synthetic lawn care products.

Chapter 33

Sick Building Syndrome

The term "sick building syndrome" (SBS) is used to describe situations in which building occupants experience acute health and comfort effects that appear to be linked to time spent in a building, but no specific illness or cause can be identified. The complaints may be localized in a particular room or zone, or may be widespread throughout the building. In contrast, the term "building related illness" (BRI) is used when symptoms of diagnosable illness are identified and can be attributed directly to airborne building contaminants.

A 1984 World Health Organization Committee report suggested that up to 30 percent of new and remodeled buildings worldwide may be the subject of excessive complaints related to indoor air quality (IAQ). Often this condition is temporary, but some buildings have long-term problems. Frequently, problems result when a building is operated or maintained in a manner that is inconsistent with its original design or prescribed operating procedures. Sometimes indoor air problems are a result of poor building design or occupant activities.

Indicators of SBS include: Building occupants complain of symptoms associated with acute discomfort, e.g., headache; eye, nose, or throat irritation; dry cough; dry or itchy skin; dizziness and nausea; difficulty in concentrating; fatigue; and sensitivity to odors. The cause of the symptoms is not known. Most of the complainants report relief soon after leaving the building.

Excerpted from "Indoor Air Facts No. 4 Sick Building Syndrome," by the Environmental Protection Agency (EPA, www.epa.gov), February 20, 2008.

Indicators of BRI include: Building occupants complain of symptoms such as cough; chest tightness; fever, chills; and muscle aches. The symptoms can be clinically defined and have clearly identifiable causes. Complainants may require prolonged recovery times after leaving the building.

It is important to note that complaints may result from other causes. These may include an illness contracted outside the building, acute sensitivity (e.g., allergies), job related stress or dissatisfaction, and other psychosocial factors. Nevertheless, studies show that symptoms may be caused or exacerbated by indoor air quality problems.

Causes of Sick Building Syndrome

The following have been cited causes of or contributing factors to sick building syndrome:

Inadequate ventilation: In the early and mid 1900s, building ventilation standards called for approximately 15 cubic feet per minute (cfm) of outside air for each building occupant, primarily to dilute and remove body odors. As a result of the 1973 oil embargo, however, national energy conservation measures called for a reduction in the amount of outdoor air provided for ventilation to 5 cfm per occupant. In many cases these reduced outdoor air ventilation rates were found to be inadequate to maintain the health and comfort of building occupants. Inadequate ventilation, which may also occur if heating, ventilating, and air conditioning (HVAC) systems do not effectively distribute air to people in the building, is thought to be an important factor in SBS. In an effort to achieve acceptable IAQ while minimizing energy consumption, the American Society of Heating, Refrigerating and Air-Conditioning Engineers (ASHRAE) recently revised its ventilation standard to provide a minimum of 15 cfm of outdoor air per person (20 cfm/person in office spaces). Up to 60 cfm/person may be required in some spaces (such as smoking lounges) depending on the activities that normally occur in that space.

Chemical contaminants from indoor sources: Most indoor air pollution comes from sources inside the building. For example, adhesives, carpeting, upholstery, manufactured wood products, copy machines, pesticides, and cleaning agents may emit volatile organic compounds (VOCs), including formaldehyde. Environmental tobacco smoke contributes high levels of VOCs, other toxic compounds, and respirable particulate matter. Research shows that some VOCs can cause chronic and acute health effects at high concentrations, and some are known carcinogens. Low to moderate levels of multiple VOCs may also produce acute reactions. Combustion products such as carbon monoxide, nitrogen dioxide, as well as respirable particles, can come from unvented kerosene and gas space heaters, woodstoves, fireplaces and gas stoves.

Chemical contaminants from outdoor sources: The outdoor air that enters a building can be a source of indoor air pollution. For example, pollutants from motor vehicle exhausts; plumbing vents, and building exhausts (e.g., bathrooms and kitchens) can enter the building through poorly located air intake vents, windows, and other openings. In addition, combustion products can enter a building from a nearby garage.

Biological contaminants: Bacteria, molds, pollen, and viruses are types of biological contaminants. These contaminants may breed in stagnant water that has accumulated in ducts, humidifiers and drain pans, or where water has collected on ceiling tiles, carpeting, or insulation. Sometimes insects or bird droppings can be a source of biological contaminants. Physical symptoms related to biological contamination include cough, chest tightness, fever, chills, muscle aches, and allergic responses such as mucous membrane irritation and upper respiratory congestion. One indoor bacterium, *Legionella*, has caused both Legionnaire's Disease and Pontiac Fever.

These elements may act in combination, and may supplement other complaints such as inadequate temperature, humidity, or lighting. Even after a building investigation, however, the specific causes of the complaints may remain unknown.

Building Investigation Procedures

The goal of a building investigation is to identify and solve indoor air quality complaints in a way that prevents them from recurring and which avoids the creation of other problems. To achieve this goal, it is necessary for the investigator(s) to discover whether a complaint is actually related to indoor air quality, identify the cause of the complaint, and determine the most appropriate corrective actions.

An indoor air quality investigation procedure is best characterized as a cycle of information gathering, hypothesis formation, and hypothesis testing. It generally begins with a walkthrough inspection of the problem area to provide information about the four basic factors that influence indoor air quality:

- The occupants
- The HVAC system
- Possible pollutant pathways
- Possible contaminant sources

Preparation for a walkthrough should include documenting easily obtainable information about the history of the building and of the complaints; identifying known HVAC zones and complaint areas; notifying occupants of the upcoming investigation; and, identifying key individuals needed for information and access. The walkthrough itself entails visual inspection of critical building areas and consultation with occupants and staff.

The initial walkthrough should allow the investigator to develop some possible explanations for the complaint. At this point, the investigator may have sufficient information to formulate a hypothesis, test the hypothesis, and see if the problem is solved. If it is, steps should be taken to ensure that it does not recur. However, if insufficient information is obtained from the walk through to construct a hypothesis, or if initial tests fail to reveal the problem, the investigator should move on to collect additional information to allow formulation of additional hypotheses. The process of formulating hypotheses, testing them, and evaluating them continues until the problem is solved.

Although air sampling for contaminants might seem to be the logical response to occupant complaints, it seldom provides information about possible causes. While certain basic measurements, e.g., temperature, relative humidity, CO_2, and air movement, can provide a useful "snapshot" of current building conditions, sampling for specific pollutant concentrations is often not required to solve the problem and can even be misleading. Contaminant concentration levels rarely exceed existing standards and guidelines even when occupants continue to report health complaints. Air sampling should not be undertaken until considerable information on the factors listed above has been collected, and any sampling strategy should be based on a comprehensive understanding of how the building operates and the nature of the complaints.

Solutions to Sick Building Syndrome

Solutions to sick building syndrome usually include combinations of the following.

Pollutant source removal or modification is an effective approach to resolving an IAQ problem when sources are known and control is feasible. Examples include routine maintenance of HVAC systems, e.g., periodic cleaning or replacement of filters; replacement of water-stained ceiling tile and carpeting; institution of smoking restrictions; venting contaminant source emissions to the outdoors; storage and use of paints, adhesives, solvents, and pesticides in well ventilated areas, and use of these pollutant sources during periods of non-occupancy; and allowing time for building materials in new or remodeled areas to off-gas pollutants before occupancy. Several of these options may be exercised at one time.

Increasing ventilation rates and air distribution often can be a cost effective means of reducing indoor pollutant levels. HVAC systems should be designed, at a minimum, to meet ventilation standards in local building codes; however, many systems are not operated or maintained to ensure that these design ventilation rates are provided. In many buildings, IAQ can be improved by operating the HVAC system to at least its design standard. When there are strong pollutant sources, local exhaust ventilation may be appropriate to exhaust contaminated air directly from the building. Local exhaust ventilation is particularly recommended to remove pollutants that accumulate in specific areas such as rest rooms, copy rooms, and printing facilities.

Air cleaning can be a useful adjunct to source control and ventilation but has certain limitations. Particle control devices such as the typical furnace filter are inexpensive but do not effectively capture small particles; high performance air filters capture the smaller, respirable particles but are relatively expensive to install and operate. Mechanical filters do not remove gaseous pollutants. Some specific gaseous pollutants may be removed by adsorbent beds, but these devices can be expensive and require frequent replacement of the adsorbent material. In sum, air cleaners can be useful, but have limited application.

Education and communication are important elements in both remedial and preventive indoor air quality management programs. When building occupants, management, and maintenance personnel fully communicate and understand the causes and consequences of IAQ problems, they can work more effectively together to prevent problems from occurring, or to solve them if they do.

Chapter 34

Insect Sting Allergy

Most people are not allergic to insect stings. Recognizing the difference between an allergic reaction and a normal reaction will reduce anxiety and prevent unnecessary medical expense.

More than 500,000 people enter hospital emergency rooms every year suffering from insect stings. A severe allergic reaction known as anaphylaxis occurs in 0.5 percent to 5 percent of the U.S. population as a result of insect stings. At least 40 deaths per year result from insect sting anaphylaxis.

The majority of insect stings in the United States come from wasps, yellow jackets, hornets, and bees. The red or black imported fire ant now infests more than 260 million acres in the southern United States, where it has become a significant health hazard and may be the number one agent of insect stings.

What is a normal reaction to an insect sting, and how is it treated?

The severity of an insect sting reaction varies from person to person. A normal reaction will result in pain, swelling, and redness confined to the sting site. Simply disinfect the area (washing with soap and water will do) and apply ice to reduce the swelling.

A large local reaction will result in swelling that extends beyond the sting site. For example, a sting on the forearm could result in the entire arm swelling. Although alarming in appearance, this condition is often treated the same as a normal reaction. An unusually painful or very large local reaction may need medical attention. Because this condition may persist for 2 to 3 days, antihistamines and corticosteroids are sometimes prescribed to lessen the discomfort.

Fire ants, yellow jackets, hornets, and wasps can sting repeatedly. Honeybees have barbed stingers that are left behind in their victim's skin. These stingers are best removed by a scraping action, rather than a pulling motion, to avoid squeezing more venom into the skin.

Almost all people stung by fire ants develop an itchy, localized hive or lump at the sting site, which usually subsides within 30 to 60 minutes. This is followed by a small blister within 4 hours. This usually appears to become filled with pus-like material by 8 to 24 hours. However, what is seen is really dead tissue, and the blister has little chance of being infected unless it is opened. When healed, these lesions may leave scars.

Treatment for fire ant stings is aimed at preventing secondary bacterial infection, which may occur if the pustule is scratched or broken. Clean the blisters with soap and water to prevent secondary infection. Do not break the blister. Topical corticosteroid ointments and oral antihistamines may relieve the itching associated with these reactions.

What are symptoms of insect sting allergy?

The most serious reaction to an insect sting is an allergic one. This condition requires immediate medical attention. Symptoms of an allergic reaction may include one or more of the following:

- Hives, itching, and swelling in areas other than the sting site
- Abdominal cramping, vomiting, intense nausea, or diarrhea
- Tightness in the chest and difficulty in breathing
- Hoarse voice or swelling of the tongue or throat or difficulty swallowing

An even more severe allergic reaction, or anaphylaxis, can occur within minutes after the sting and may be life-threatening. Symptoms may include:

- dizziness or a sharp drop in blood pressure;
- unconsciousness or cardiac arrest.

People who have experienced an allergic reaction to an insect sting have a 60 percent chance of a similar or worse reaction if stung again.

How are allergic reactions to insect stings treated?

Insect sting allergy is treated in a two-step approach:

1. The first step is the emergency treatment of the symptoms of a serious reaction when they occur.

2. The second step is preventive treatment of the underlying allergy with venom immunotherapy.

Life-threatening allergic reactions can progress very rapidly and require immediate medical attention. Emergency treatment usually includes administration of certain drugs, such as epinephrine, antihistamines, and in some cases, corticosteroids, intravenous fluids, oxygen, and other treatments. Once stabilized, these patients sometimes require close observation in the hospital overnight.

Injectable epinephrine (EpiPen® or Twinject®) for self-administration is often prescribed as emergency rescue medication for treating an allergic reaction. People who have had previous allergic reactions and rely on epinephrine must remember to carry it with them at all times. Also, because one dose may not be enough to reverse the reaction, immediate medical attention following an insect sting is recommended.

What is venom immunotherapy?

The long-term treatment of insect sting allergy is called venom immunotherapy, a highly effective program administered by an allergist-immunologist, which can prevent future allergic reactions to insect stings.

Venom immunotherapy involves administering gradually increasing doses of venom to decrease a patient's sensitivity to the venom. This can reduce the risk of a future allergic reaction to that of the general population. In a matter of weeks to months, people who previously lived under the constant threat of severe reactions to insect stings can return to leading normal lives.

If you think you might be allergic to insect stings, ask your doctor to send a consult to an allergist-immunologist, a physician who is a specialist in the diagnosis and treatment of allergic diseases. Based on your past history and certain tests, the allergist will determine if you are a candidate for skin testing and immunotherapy.

How can I avoid insect stings?

Knowing how to avoid stings from fire ants, bees, wasps, hornets, and yellow jackets leads to a more enjoyable summer for everyone. Stinging insects are most active during the late spring, summer, and early fall. Insect repellents do not work against stinging insects.

Yellow jackets will nest in the ground and in walls. Hornets and wasps will nest in bushes, trees, and on buildings. Use extreme caution when working or playing in these areas. Avoid open garbage cans and exposed food at picnics, which attract yellow jackets. Also, try to reduce the amount of exposed skin when outdoors.

Effective methods for insecticide treatment of fire ant mounds use attractant baits. These baits often contain soybean oil, corn grits combined with chemical agents. The bait is picked up by the worker ants and taken deeper into the mound to the queen. It can take weeks for these insecticides to work.

Allergists-immunologists recommend the following additional precautions to avoid insect stings:

- Avoid wearing sandals or walking barefoot in the grass.

- Honeybees and bumblebees forage on white clover, a weed that grows in lawns throughout the country.

- Never swat at a flying insect. If need be, gently brush it aside or patiently wait for it to leave.

- Do not drink from open beverage cans. Stinging insects will crawl inside a can attracted by the sweet beverage.

- When eating outdoors, try to keep food covered at all times.

- Garbage cans stored outside should be covered with tight-fitting lids.

- Avoid sweet-smelling perfumes, hair sprays, colognes, and deodorants.

- Avoid wearing bright-colored clothing.

- Yard work and gardening should be done with caution. Wearing shoes and socks and using work gloves will prevent stings on hands and feet and provide time to get away from an unexpected mound.

- Keep window and door screens in good repair. Drive with car windows closed.

- Keep prescribed medications handy at all times and follow the attached instructions if you are stung. These medications are for immediate emergency use while en route to a hospital emergency room for observation and further treatment.

If you have had an allergic reaction to an insect sting, it's important that you see an allergist-immunologist.

Chapter 35

Allergies to Medicines and Medical Products

Chapter Contents

Section 35.1

Medications and Drug Allergic Reactions

"Drug Allergies," © 2010 A.D.A.M., Inc. Reprinted with permission.

Drug allergies are a group of symptoms caused by an allergic reaction to a drug (medication).

Causes

Adverse reactions to drugs are common, and almost any drug can cause an adverse reaction. Reactions range from irritating or mild side effects such as nausea and vomiting to life-threatening anaphylaxis.

A true drug allergy results from a series of chemical steps within the body that produce the allergic reaction to a medication. One time (often the first time you take the drug), your immune system launches an incorrect response that is not noticeable. The next time you take the drug, an immune response occurs, and your body produces antibodies and histamine.

Most drug allergies cause minor skin rashes and hives. Serum sickness is a delayed type of drug allergy that occurs a week or more after exposure to a medication or vaccine.

Penicillin and related antibiotics are the most common cause of drug allergies. Other common allergy-causing drugs include:

- sulfa drugs;
- anticonvulsants;
- insulin preparations (particularly animal sources of insulin);
- iodinated (containing iodine) x-ray contrast dyes (these can cause allergy-like anaphylactoid reactions).

Most side effects of drugs are not due to an allergic reaction. For example, aspirin can cause nonallergic hives or trigger asthma. Some drug reactions are considered "idiosyncratic." This means the reaction is an unusual effect of the medication, not due to a predictable chemical effect of the drug. Many people confuse an uncomfortable, but not serious, side effect of a medicine (such as nausea) with a true drug allergy, which can be life threatening.

Symptoms

- Anaphylaxis, or severe allergic reaction
- Hives (a less common type of rash)
- Itching of the skin or eyes (common)
- Skin rash (common)
- Swelling of the lips, tongue, or face
- Wheezing

Symptoms of anaphylaxis include:

- abdominal pain or cramping;
- confusion;
- diarrhea;
- difficulty breathing with wheeze or hoarse voice;
- dizziness;
- fainting, lightheadedness;
- hives over different parts of the body;
- nausea, vomiting;
- rapid pulse;
- sensation of feeling the heart beat (palpitations).

Exams and Tests

An examination of the skin and face may show hives, rash, or angioedema (swelling of the lips, face, or tongue). Decreased blood pressure, wheezing, and other signs may indicate an anaphylactic reaction.

Skin testing may confirm allergy to penicillin-type medications. Testing may be ineffective (or in some cases, dangerous) for other medications. A history of allergic-type reaction after use of a medication is often considered proof enough of drug allergy—no further testing is required. The same applies to other substances that are not considered drugs but are used in hospitals, such as x-ray contrast dyes.

Treatment

The treatment goal is to relieve symptoms and prevent a severe reaction. Treatment may include:

- antihistamines to relieve mild symptoms such as rash, hives, and itching;

- bronchodilators such as albuterol to reduce asthma-like symptoms (moderate wheezing or cough);

- corticosteroids applied to the skin, given by mouth, or given intravenously (directly into a vein);

- epinephrine by injection to treat anaphylaxis.

The offending medication and similar drugs should be avoided. Make sure all your health care providers—including dentists and hospital personnel—know about any drug allergies that you or your children have.

Identifying jewelry or cards (such as Medic-Alert or others) may be recommended. Occasionally, a penicillin (or other drug) allergy responds to desensitization, where increasing doses of a medicine are given to improve a person's tolerance of the drug. This should only be done by an allergist.

Outlook (Prognosis)

Most drug allergies respond readily to treatment. A few cases cause severe asthma, anaphylaxis, or death.

Possible Complications

- Anaphylaxis (life-threatening)

- Asthma

- Death

When to Contact a Medical Professional

Call your health care provider if you are taking a medication and seem to be having a reaction to it.

Go to the emergency room or call the local emergency number (such as 911) if you have difficulty breathing or develop other symptoms of severe asthma or anaphylaxis. These are emergency conditions.

Prevention

There is generally no way to prevent development of a drug allergy.

If you have a known drug allergy, avoiding the medication is the best way to prevent an allergic reaction. You may also be told to avoid similar medicines. For example, if you are allergic to penicillin, you should also avoid amoxicillin or ampicillin.

In some cases, a doctor may approve use of a drug that causes an allergy if you are pretreated with corticosteroids (such as prednisone) and antihistamines (such as diphenhydramine). Do not try this without a doctor's supervision. Pretreatment with corticosteroids and antihistamines has been shown to prevent anaphylaxis in people needing to get iodinated x-ray contrast dye.

Section 35.2

Latex in Medical Products

From "Latex Allergy: A Prevention Guide," by the National Institute for Occupational Safety and Health (NIOSH, www.cdc.gov/niosh), part of the Centers for Disease Control and Prevention, 1998. Reviewed by David A. Cooke, MD, FACP, August 10, 2010.

Latex gloves have proved effective in preventing transmission of many infectious diseases to health care workers. But for some workers, exposures to latex may result in allergic reactions. Reports of such reactions have increased in recent years—especially among health care workers.

What is latex?

The term "latex" refers to natural rubber latex, the product manufactured from a milky fluid derived from the rubber tree, *Hevea brasiliensis*. Several types of synthetic rubber are also referred to as latex, but these do not release the proteins that cause allergic reactions.

What is latex allergy?

Latex allergy is a reaction to certain proteins in latex rubber. The amount of latex exposure needed to produce sensitization or an allergic reaction is unknown. Increasing the exposure to latex proteins increases the risk of developing allergic symptoms. In sensitized persons, symptoms usually begin within minutes of exposure; but they can occur hours later and can be quite varied. Mild reactions to latex involve skin redness, rash, hives, or itching. More severe reactions may involve respiratory symptoms such as runny nose, sneezing, itchy eyes, scratchy throat, and asthma (difficult breathing, coughing spells, and wheezing). Rarely, shock may occur; however, a life-threatening reaction is seldom the first sign of latex allergy.

Who is at risk of developing latex allergy?

Health care workers are at risk of developing latex allergy because they use latex gloves frequently. Workers with less glove use (such as housekeepers, hairdressers, and workers in industries that manufacture latex products) are also at risk.

Is skin contact the only type of latex exposure?

No. Latex proteins become fastened to the lubricant powder used in some gloves. When workers change gloves, the protein/powder particles become airborne and can be inhaled.

How is latex allergy treated?

Detecting symptoms early, reducing exposure to latex, and obtaining medical advice are important to prevent long-term health effects. Once a worker becomes allergic to latex, special precautions are needed to prevent exposures. Certain medications may reduce the allergy symptoms, but complete latex avoidance, though quite difficult, is the most effective approach.

Are there other types of reactions to latex besides latex allergy?

Yes. The most common reaction to latex products is irritant contact dermatitis—the development of dry, itchy, irritated areas on the skin, usually the hands. This reaction is caused by irritation from wearing gloves and by exposure to the powders added to them. Irritant contact dermatitis is not a true allergy. Allergic contact dermatitis (sometimes called chemical sensitivity dermatitis) results from the chemicals added to latex during harvesting, processing, or manufacturing. These chemicals can cause a skin rash similar to that of poison ivy. Neither irritant contact dermatitis nor chemical sensitivity dermatitis is a true allergy.

How can I protect myself from latex allergy?

Take the following steps to protect yourself from latex exposure and allergy in the workplace:

- Use nonlatex gloves for activities that are not likely to involve contact with infectious materials (food preparation, routine housekeeping, general maintenance, etc.).

- Appropriate barrier protection is necessary when handling infectious materials. If you choose latex gloves, use powder-free gloves with reduced protein content. Such gloves reduce exposures to latex protein and thus reduce the risk of latex allergy. So-called hypoallergenic latex gloves do not reduce the risk of latex allergy. However, they may reduce reactions to chemical additives in the latex (allergic contact dermatitis).

- Use appropriate work practices to reduce the chance of reactions to latex.

  - When wearing latex gloves, do not use oil-based hand creams or lotions (which can cause glove deterioration).

  - After removing latex gloves, wash hands with a mild soap and dry thoroughly.

  - Practice good housekeeping. Frequently clean areas and equipment contaminated with latex-containing dust.

- Take advantage of all latex allergy education and training provided by your employer and become familiar with procedures for preventing latex allergy.

- Learn to recognize the symptoms of latex allergy, including skin rash; hives; flushing; itching; nasal, eye, or sinus symptoms; asthma; and (rarely) shock.

What if I think I have latex allergy?

If you develop symptoms of latex allergy, avoid direct contact with latex gloves and other latex-containing products until you can see a physician experienced in treating latex allergy.

If you have latex allergy, consult your physician regarding the following precautions:

- Avoid contact with latex gloves and products.

- Avoid areas where you might inhale the powder from latex gloves worn by other workers.

- Tell your employer and health care providers (physicians, nurses, dentists, etc.) that you have latex allergy.

- Wear a medical alert bracelet.

Part Five

Diagnosing and
Treating Allergies

Chapter 36

When You Should See an Allergist

Asthma and other allergic diseases are two of the most common health problems. Approximately 50 million Americans have asthma, hay fever, or other allergy-related conditions.

Some allergy problems—such as a mild case of hay fever—may not need any treatment. Sometimes allergies can be controlled with the occasional use of an over-the-counter medication. However, sometimes allergies can interfere with day-to-day activities or decrease the quality of life. Allergies can even be life threatening.

The Allergist Treats Asthma and Allergies

An allergist is a physician who specializes in the diagnosis and treatment of asthma and other allergic diseases. The allergist is specially trained to identify the factors that trigger asthma or allergies. Allergists help people treat or prevent their allergy problems. After earning a medical degree, the allergist completes a 3-year residency-training program in either internal medicine or pediatrics. Next the allergist completes 2 or 3 more years of study in the field of allergy and immunology. You can be certain that your doctor has met these requirements if he or she is certified by the American Board of Allergy and Immunology.

What Is an Allergy?

One of the marvels of the human body is that it can defend itself against harmful invaders such as viruses or bacteria. But sometimes the defenses are too aggressive and harmless substances such as dust, molds, or pollen are mistakenly identified as dangerous. The immune system then rallies its defenses, which include several chemicals, to attack and destroy the supposed enemy. In the process, some unpleasant and, in extreme cases, life-threatening symptoms may be experienced in the allergy-prone individual.

The Cause of Allergic Reactions

There are hundreds of ordinary substances that can trigger allergic reactions. Among the most common are plant pollens, molds, household dust (dust mites), cockroaches, pets, industrial chemicals, foods, medicines, feathers, and insect stings. These triggers are called allergens.

Who Develops Asthma or Allergies?

Asthma and allergies can affect anyone, regardless of age, gender, race, or socioeconomic factors. While it's true that asthma and allergies are more common in children, they can occur for the first time at any age. Sometimes allergy symptoms start in childhood, disappear for many years, and then start up again during adult life.

Although the exact genetic factors are not yet understood, there is a hereditary tendency to asthma and allergies. In susceptible people, factors such as hormones, stress, smoke, perfume, or other environmental irritants also may play a role.

Types of Allergy Problems

An allergic reaction may occur anywhere in the body but usually appears in the nose, eyes, lungs, lining of the stomach, sinuses, throat, and skin. These are places where special immune system cells are stationed to fight off invaders that are inhaled, swallowed, or come in contact with the skin.

Allergic Rhinitis (Hay Fever)

Allergic rhinitis is a general term used to describe the allergic reactions that take place in the nose. Symptoms may include sneezing, congestion, runny nose, and itching of the nose, the eyes and/or the roof of the mouth. When this problem is triggered by pollens or outdoor molds, during the spring, summer, or fall, the condition is often called hay fever. When the problem is year-round, it might be caused by exposure to house dust mites, household pets, indoor molds, or allergens at school or in the workplace.

Asthma

Asthma symptoms occur when airway muscle spasms block the flow of air to the lungs and/or the linings of the bronchial tubes become inflamed. Excess mucus may clog the airways. An asthma attack is characterized by labored or restricted breathing, a tight feeling in the chest, coughing, and/or wheezing. Sometimes a chronic cough is the only symptom. Asthma trouble can cause only mild discomfort or it can cause life-threatening attacks in which breathing stops altogether.

Contact Dermatitis/Skin Allergies

Contact dermatitis, eczema, and hives are skin conditions that can be caused by allergens and other irritants. Often the reaction may take hours or days to develop, as in the case of poison ivy. The most common allergic causes of rashes are medicines, insect stings, foods, animals, and chemicals used at home or work. Allergies may be aggravated by emotional stress.

Anaphylaxis

Anaphylaxis is a rare, potentially fatal allergic reaction that affects many parts of the body at the same time. The trigger may be an insect sting, a food (such as peanuts) or a medication. Symptoms may include:

- vomiting or diarrhea;
- a dangerous drop in blood pressure;
- redness of the skin and/or hives;
- difficulty breathing;
- swelling of the throat and/or tongue;
- loss of consciousness.

Frequently these symptoms start without warning and get worse rapidly. At the first sign of an anaphylactic reaction, the affected person must go immediately to the closest Emergency Room or call 911.

When to See an Allergist

Often, the symptoms of asthma or allergies develop gradually over time.

Allergy sufferers may become used to frequent symptoms such as sneezing, nasal congestion, or wheezing. With the help of an allergist, these symptoms usually can be prevented or controlled with major improvement in quality of life.

Effectively controlling asthma and allergies requires planning, skill and patience. The allergist, with his or her specialized training, can develop a treatment plan for your individual condition. The goal will be to enable you to lead a life that is as normal and symptom-free as possible.

A visit to the allergist might include:

- Allergy testing: The allergist will usually perform tests to determine what allergens are involved.

- Prevention education: The most effective approach to treating asthma or allergies is to avoid the factors that trigger the condition in the first place. Even when it is not possible to completely avoid allergens, an allergist can help you decrease exposure to allergens.

- Medication prescriptions: A number of new and effective medications are available to treat both asthma and allergies.

- Immunotherapy (allergy shots): In this treatment, patients are given injections every week or two of some or all of the allergens that cause their allergy problems. Gradually the injections get stronger and stronger. In most cases, the allergy problems get less and less over time.

You should see an allergist if:

- your allergies are causing symptoms such as chronic sinus infections, nasal congestion, or difficulty breathing;

- you experience hay fever or other allergy symptoms several months out of the year;

- antihistamines and over-the-counter medications do not control your allergy symptoms or create unacceptable side effects, such as drowsiness;

- your asthma or allergies are interfering with your ability to carry on day-to-day activities;

- your asthma or allergies decrease the quality of your life; or
- you are experiencing warning signs of serious asthma such as:
  - you sometimes have to struggle to catch your breath;
  - you often wheeze or cough, especially at night or after exercise;
  - you are frequently short of breath or feel tightness in your chest;
  - you have previously been diagnosed with asthma, and you have frequent asthma attacks even though you are taking asthma medication.

Chapter 37

Health Insurance Issues for People with Allergies and Asthma

Most Americans have insurance for asthma treatment and medical supplies. But many insurance plans have payment limits and other rules. Even if your insurance covers a treatment, getting the insurer to pay can sometimes be difficult. This text will help you get the most from your plan and pay the least from your own pocket.[1]

I don't have health insurance. How can I get it?

You may be eligible for a government program such as Medicaid at little or no cost. Call your state's local social services office for details. If you are not eligible for a government program, Blue Cross plans in most states have a yearly "open enrollment" period. You can't be turned down for this coverage if you pay the premium. Some states have "high-risk pool" programs in which you are assigned to one of several plans. This also requires you to pay a premium, but the state may help fund it.

Did you have coverage within the last 18 months through your own or your spouse's private employer? If so, and the employer has at least 50 workers, you can buy what's called COBRA Continuation coverage. You pay the plan's full premium plus a 2 percent fee. COBRA coverage is a better value than an individual or high-risk plan. Contact your former employer for details.[2]

When I choose a health plan, what issues should I consider?

No specific plan is best for everyone. The three most important issues are the health services covered, the choice of providers, and the plan's cost to you. These issues are discussed in the next few answers.

You also should consider whether the plan will cover just you ("self only") or—if you have a family—them as well (a "family" plan). Finally, a plan offered through a "group" such as your employer usually will be a better value than an "individual" plan.

What should I know about coverage of asthma-related services?

Each plan has different rules for the services it covers. Most plans pay for doctor and hospital treatment for asthma if the provider is approved by the plan. But many plans limit coverage of asthma medications and medical equipment. And only a few plans—mainly "Health Maintenance Organizations"—cover preventive care.

In addition to rules specifically for asthma, plans may have rules applying to several medical conditions. Two frequent rules are preexisting condition limits and chronic condition limits.

What are preexisting and chronic condition limits?

A preexisting condition limit means that if you already have a medical condition when you sign up for a plan, the plan will limit its payments for that condition for a certain time. Some "individual" and "small group" plans have this rule, and it can be a major problem for people with asthma. Government plans usually don't have this limit and, if you change plans that are employer-sponsored, the rule generally can't be used if the employer has at least 50 workers.

A chronic condition limit means that if a medical condition is not expected to show improvement within a certain time, then services for it won't be covered. In rare cases, this can apply to asthma.[3]

What choice of providers do plans give me, and why is that important?

Almost every plan has a list of "approved" providers the plan will pay best, while some plans pay nothing to a "non-approved" provider. Most or all of a plan's "approved" providers are listed in its "Provider Directory." You can get a copy by asking the plan.

Because you must pay more to use a non-approved provider, the larger the plan's approved list, the better. But provider choice isn't just about saving money. Some providers specialize in treating asthma, some are located near you, and so on. Usually, managed care plans have the fewest approved providers.

What are the types of managed-care plans and how do they limit my choice of provider?

There are three types of managed care plans: preferred provider organizations, health maintenance organizations, and "point of service" plans. A preferred provider organization (PPO) allows the patient to choose any provider, but pays approved ("preferred") providers a higher amount than non-approved providers. The plan might cover all of a PPO doctor's charge but only 80 percent of a non-PPO doctor's bill.

A health maintenance organization (HMO) pays nothing for non-emergency care if from a provider lacking a contract with the HMO. So an HMO patient has a strong financial reason to use only HMO providers. An HMO also requires you to choose a "primary care" doctor. He or she must approve referrals to "specialist" providers such as pulmonology doctors and respiratory therapists.

The third managed-care plan, called "point of service" (POS), is a cross between an HMO and a PPO. Like an HMO, it requires you to choose a primary-care doctor. Like a PPO, if you want to see a non-HMO provider, the plan will pay some amount for that care, but less than if you used an HMO provider.

Compared to traditional insurance, managed care plans are cheaper or offer more benefits. But they always have fewer choices of providers.

What out-of-pocket costs should I consider in choosing a plan?

You may have to pay four types of costs. These are:

- premiums (periodic fees charged regardless of how many services you use);

- deductible (yearly total amounts you must pay for one or more services before the plan will begin paying);

- copayments (small amounts you pay each time you get a service);

- uncovered out-of-pocket costs (your spending for services the plan doesn't cover, in contrast to premiums, deductibles, and copayments).

Most plans have a "catastrophic," "stop-loss" or "hold harmless" feature that limits the total yearly amount you must pay. But that cap doesn't apply to the premium. The higher the total premium, the lower the other three types of costs.

Many people prefer to pay a higher premium to reduce their other costs. That protects them from large unexpected bills. It's especially good if you're likely to get many treatments for a major medical condition.

How can I get the best mix of covered services, provider choice, and costs?

What is best depends on your situation. Because you or a family member has asthma, it's good to have a plan with broad coverage for that condition. But you may not be able to afford a high-cost plan.

If you've long been treated by a doctor who's not contracted with any plans, you'll need to get a non-managed care plan to keep that doctor. But if you just moved to a new city, being able to see a particular provider is not as important. Your doctor's staff or a community group such as a senior citizen association can advise you what plan is best.

What is "assignment of benefits" and how can it help me?

Assignment of benefits ("assignment" for short) means your provider agrees to send a claim to your plan and accept the plan's "allowed" payment as full payment.

You don't have to pay out-of-pocket for the entire bill when you're treated. You also may save money and you don't have to mail a claim. And if the claim is denied, your provider usually can file an appeal on your behalf.

All providers contracting with managed care plans, and all Medicare and Medicaid "participating" providers must accept assignment for those plans. But some providers whose services are in high demand don't accept assignment because they can pick and choose the patients they treat. Assignment is always good financially, but it doesn't concern the quality of your care.

Should I get coverage under more than one plan?

It's not good to pay the full premium of more than one plan. The plans usually will duplicate each other but you won't be paid double. Yet sometimes having two plans makes sense.

If you have a plan such as Medicare that has major limits, you can buy a supplemental plan such as "Medigap." If both spouses in a family have family plans, each plan may cover limits in the other.

There are three "dual coverage" rules on which plan pays first. Some plans (e.g., Medigap) always pay after another plan (e.g., Medicare). Read the plan's rules to determine which plan pays first.

If you and your spouse both have family plans, your plan will always pay first for your own care. Your spouse's plan will pay first for your spouse's care. After the first ("primary") plan has paid, if there's any unpaid balance, the other ("secondary") plan should be billed.

When there are two family plans and a child is treated, the "birthday rule" usually applies. The plan of the parent with the birthday earliest in the year will pay first. If the mother's birthday is January 2, and the father's is June 7, the mother's plan would pay first for the child's care. But plans in a few states use different rules.

What can I do if a plan refuses to enroll me, denies a claim, or causes other problems?

Different plans have different "appeal" rules. It's important to know these rules because if you don't follow them, your problem won't be solved. In some plans, you must appeal in as little as 30 days.

You're entitled to a pamphlet summarizing your plan's rules. This "insurance policy" booklet is called an Outline of Coverage, Summary Benefits Plan Description, Medicare Handbook, or similar name. You should read this. If you don't have it, you can get a copy from your plan.

Government plans such as Medicare and Medicaid give you many rights. They usually allow you to appeal several times if you disagree with a decision.

Private plans are run by insurers such as Blue Cross. Their rules are less detailed than government plans. You become eligible for a private plan if you or your spouse's employer offers it or if you pay individual premiums.

Some private plans are allowed to turn down your enrollment even if you can pay the premium. Private plans may be either "true insurance" overseen by your state government or "self-insured" plans. Self-insured plans give you fewer appeal rights. In general, plans sold to individuals and to small companies are insured plans. Those sold to large employers are self-insured. If your plan booklet does not say which type it is, contact the plan or your state's insurance commission in your state capitol.

If a claim is denied, the Explanation of Benefits notice you get must give a reason why. Some reasons are easier to overturn than others. If the plan says your care wasn't "medically necessary," that's a poor explanation and often can be reversed.

If your care went beyond what the plan covers, such as medications costing more than the plan's $500 yearly limit, it's unlikely the plan will reverse its decision. But it may do that if you convince the plan it would save by avoiding bigger costs. For example, asthma medication may keep you from going to the hospital. The plan doesn't have to make exceptions. When it does, that's called an "extra-contractual" benefit.[4]

Can I see a specialist?

HMOs and POS plans require all non-emergency services from specialty providers to be preapproved by the plan and your primary-care doctor. This also applies if you are already being treated by a specialist and you switch to a new HMO.

What if I have a medical emergency while traveling?

If you think your life could be endangered or the functioning of an organ such as your lungs permanently damaged, seek the nearest medical treatment. In most cases, your plan will pay for this care. If your condition is less serious and you are enrolled in a managed-care plan, you must call the plan's "preauthorization" number on your insurance card and follow the plan's direction in order for the care to be paid.[5]

Can I get my plan to pay for a second opinion?

Most plans cover second opinions for major procedures such as surgeries. For details, call your plan before getting the second opinion. If your question is about nonsurgical treatment such as prescribing one medicine rather than another, most plans won't pay for a second opinion. So ask your doctor why the specific treatment is recommended.

When I have a problem, how can I get help?

If you have a question about your plan, call the plan's customer service department, using the phone number on your enrollment card or plan brochure. Your employer's benefits office, your local labor union, or a consumer advocacy group can help.

Your doctor or hospital office also may help, especially for a denied claim when the provider accepted assignment. And you can contact your state's Insurance Commission in your state capital.[6]

If you follow all the rules and still have a problem, you can hire a lawyer. The lawyer can sue the plan for "breach of contract." But that is expensive and you aren't likely to win. This is why some people think the laws should be changed to give patients more rights.

Health insurance is valuable, but many problems can occur. It is important to be well informed so you can get the kind of insurance you want and pay less for it.

Health Reference Series Medical Advisor's Notes and Updates

1. In 2010, the Federal Affordable Care Act (commonly referred to as "The Health Care Reform Bill") was passed by Congress and signed into law by President Obama. This will expand insurance coverage and patient protections significantly, with individual elements phasing in between 2010 and 2014. As a result, rules will be changing significantly year to year, but the net effect should be progressively fewer insurance restrictions for people with allergy or asthma problems.

2. The Affordable Care Act created additional options for people who have difficulty getting health insurance. Pre-Existing Condition Insurance Plans have been created for people who have been uninsured for at least 6 months because of a preexisting condition. In some states, this is administered by the state, while in others it is a Federal government program. You may be eligible for coverage under these programs, which took effect in 2010.

Additionally, the Affordable Care Act also requires insurers to allow children up to age 26 to receive care under their parents' plan, unless the children have access to other insurance plans.

The Affordable Care Act requires that all Americans carry some form of health insurance starting in 2014. Many larger employers already provide insurance to their employees. Small employers will be able to purchase insurance plans for their employees through state-run insurance exchanges. State Medicaid programs will be expanded to cover many people who do not currently qualify. Medicare will continue to provide coverage for older adults and disabled people. People who cannot receive insurance through their employers or government programs also will be able to purchase insurance directly through the insurance exchanges.

3. The Affordable Care Act bars insurers from applying preexisting conditions limits to children under 19 on their parents' health care plans, effective September 23, 2010. Under the same law, health insurers will no longer be able to exclude individuals for preexisting conditions starting 2014.

The Affordable Care Act also eliminates lifetime dollar limits on coverage starting 2010, and annual dollar limits will be phased out completely by 2014.

4. The Affordable Care Act creates new appeal rights for patients and an external review process for denied coverage and claims, starting September 23, 2010.

5. The Federal Affordable Care Act of 2010 bars insurers from charging higher copays or coinsurance for emergency care received outside the insurer's network.

6. Following the passage of the Affordable Care Act, a new website, http://www.healthcare.gov, was created to provide information on the provisions of the health care reform law. You can find information on rule changes and new patient protections on this site.

Chapter 38

Allergy Tests

Chapter Contents

Section 38.1

Tests to Diagnose Allergies

"Allergy Testing," © 2010 A.D.A.M., Inc. Reprinted with permission.

Allergy tests are any of several tests used to determine the substances to which a person is allergic.

How the Test Is Performed

There are many methods of allergy testing. Among the more common are:

- skin tests;
- elimination-type tests
- blood tests (including the radioallergosorbent, or RAST, test).

Skin Tests

Skin tests are the most common. Specific methods vary.

One of the most common methods is the prick test. This test involves placing a small amount of suspected allergy-causing substances on the skin, usually the forearm, upper arm, or the back. Then, the skin is pricked so the allergen goes under the skin's surface. The health care provider closely watches the skin for signs of a reaction, usually swelling and redness of the site. Results are usually seen within 15–20 minutes. Several allergens can be tested at the same time.

A similar method involves injecting a small amount of allergen into the skin and watching for a reaction at the site. This is called an intradermal skin test. It is more likely to be used when testing is being done to find out if you are allergic to something specific, such as bee venom or penicillin.

Patch testing is a method to diagnose allergic reactions on the skin. Possible allergens are taped to the skin for 48 hours. The health care provider will look at the area in 24 hours, and then again 48 hours later.

Skin tests are most useful for diagnosing:

- food allergy;

- mold, pollen, animal, and other allergies that cause allergic rhinitis and asthma;

- penicillin allergy;*

- venom allergy;

- allergic contact dermatitis.

Elimination Tests

An elimination diet can be used to check for food allergies. An elimination diet is one in which foods that may be causing symptoms are removed from the diet for several weeks and then slowly re-introduced one at a time while the person is watched for signs of an allergic reaction.

Another method is the double-blind test. This method involves giving foods and harmless substances in a disguised form. The person being tested and the provider are both unaware of whether the substance tested in that session is the harmless substance or the suspected food. A third party knows the identity of the substances and identifies them with some sort of code. This test requires several sessions if more than one substance is under investigation.

While the double-blind strategy is useful and practical for mild allergic reactions, it must be done carefully in individuals with suspected severe reactions to foods. Blood tests may be a safer first approach.

Blood Tests

Blood tests can be done to measure the amount of immunoglobulin (Ig) E antibodies to a specific allergen in the blood. This test may be used when skin testing is not helpful or cannot be done.

Other blood tests include:

- absolute eosinophil count;

- total IgE level;

- serum immunoglobulin electrophoresis.

Provocation

Provocation (challenge) testing involves exposing a person to a suspected allergen under controlled circumstances. This may be done in the diet or by breathing in the suspected allergen. This type of test may provoke severe allergic reactions. Challenge testing should only be done by a doctor.

How to Prepare for the Test

Before any allergy testing, the health care provider will ask for a very detailed medical history. This may include questions about such things as illnesses, emotional and social conditions, work, entertainment, lifestyle, foods, and eating habits.

If skin testing will be performed, you should **not** take antihistamines before the test. This may lead to a false-negative result, falsely reassuring you that a substance is unlikely to cause a severe allergic reaction. Your doctor will tell you which medicines to avoid and when to stop taking them before the test.

How the Test Will Feel

Skin tests may cause very mild discomfort when the skin is pricked. Itching may occur if you have a positive reaction to the allergen.

Why the Test Is Performed

Allergy tests are done to determine the specific substances that cause an allergic reaction in a person.

Your doctor may order allergy tests if you have:

- allergic rhinitis and asthma symptoms that are not easily controlled with medications;
- angioedema and hives;
- food allergies;
- contact dermatitis;
- penicillin allergy.*

Note: Allergies to penicillin and closely related medications are the only drug allergies that can be tested using skin tests. Skin tests for allergies to other drugs can be dangerous.

The prick skin test may also be used to diagnose food allergies. Intradermal tests are not used to test for food allergies because of high false-positive results and the danger of causing a severe allergic reaction.

Normal Results

In a nonallergic person, allergy tests should be negative (no response to the allergen).

What Abnormal Results Mean

A positive result means you reacted to a specific substance. Often, but not always, a positive result means the symptoms that you are having are due to exposure to the substance in question. In general, a stronger response means you are more sensitive to the substance.

People can have a positive response with allergy skin testing, but not have any problems with the specific substance in everyday life.

The skin tests are generally reliable. However, if the dose of allergen is excessive, a positive reaction will occur even in persons who are not allergic.

Risks

Risks related to skin and food allergy tests may include:

- allergic reaction;
- life-threatening anaphylactic reaction.

Considerations

The accuracy of allergy testing varies quite a bit. Even the same test performed at different times on a person may give different results. A person may react to a substance during testing, but never react during normal exposure. Rarely, a person may also have a negative allergy test and still be allergic to the substance.

Section 38.2

Elimination Diet and Food Challenge Test

What is a controlled food challenge?

In a controlled environment such as an intensive care hospital unit, the doctor (usually a board-certified allergist) may conduct a food challenge test to determine if a food allergy exists or to confirm a suspected food allergy.

Samples of the suspected offending food may be mixed with another food or may be disguised as an ingredient in another food. These food preparation techniques are used to prevent undue influence on the outcome of the test (if the person recognizes the food by sight or taste). Another method is to have you take a capsule containing the allergen.

You eat the food or take the capsule under strict supervision. After eating the food or taking the capsule, you will be monitored to see if a reaction occurs.

The ideal way to perform the food challenge test is as a "double-blind, placebo-controlled test." With this method, neither the allergist nor the patient is aware of which capsule, or food, contains the suspected allergen. In order for the test to be effective, you must also take capsules or eat food that does not contain the allergen. This will help the allergist make sure the reaction, if any, being observed is due to the allergen and not some other factor.

Someone with a history of severe reactions cannot participate in a food challenge test. In addition, multiple food allergies are difficult to evaluate with this test.

Since this test takes a lot of time to perform, it is costly and done infrequently. This type of testing is generally used when the doctor needs to confirm or eliminate specific food allergens.

Section 38.3

Unproven Diagnostic Tests

Some methods of allergy testing are considered controversial, since no definitive studies have shown that they are effective in diagnosing food allergies. Here, we discuss some of the more common tests that have not been scientifically proven to give accurate results. None of these tests is recommended for the diagnosis of food allergies, and those that involve the ingestion or injection of allergens may increase the risk of a reaction. Please keep in mind that these are not necessarily the only tests that may be questionable. If you have concerns or questions about any diagnostic method, please contact the American Academy of Allergy, Asthma, and Immunology (AAAAI).

Applied Kinesiology and NAET Testing

Kinesiological testing exposes you to a suspect food (either by having you hold it or by bringing it close to your body) and then measures changes in your muscle strength. Similarly, the NAET (short for Nambudripad's Allergy Elimination Test) is based on the concept that a food can weaken your body by blocking your energy field. Your muscles are tested to determine whether or not you show signs of weakness after exposure to a particular food. Acupuncture or acupressure is then used to "cure" your allergy. There is no scientific evidence to support these tests or the theories behind them.

Body Chemical Analysis

This type of test analyzes a sample of your hair, body fluids, or tissue to diagnose a mineral deficiency or confirm the presence of toxic substances. Either of these supposedly leads to food allergies or other diseases. Again, there is no scientific evidence to support these claims.

Cytotoxic Testing

In this test, the white blood cells are extracted from a sample of your blood. Then, samples of the white blood cells are applied to slides that contain dried extracts of suspect foods. A technician views the slides under a microscope and analyzes them for changes that supposedly indicate whether you are allergic to any of those foods. AAAAI has concluded that there is no scientific basis for this test.

ELISA/ACT (Enzyme-Linked Immunosorbent Assay/ Activated Cell Test)

A sample of your blood is drawn and cultures of the white blood cells are analyzed for their reactions to up to 300 food allergens or other substances. Studies have shown that this test is not effective in diagnosing food or other allergies. Other questionable diagnostic methods that involve white blood cell analysis are the ALCAT [antigen leukocyte cellular antibody test] and NuTron tests.

Electrodermal Diagnosis

This test uses a galvanometer (an instrument that detects and measures electric currents) to gauge your body's resistance when you come in contact with a suspect food. Increased resistance to the electric current is supposed to indicate that you are allergic to the food being tested.

IgG Testing

This test checks your blood for the presence of food-specific immunoglobulin G (IgG) antibodies. Unlike IgE antibodies, which occur in abnormally large quantities in people with allergies, IgG antibodies are found in both allergic and non-allergic people. Experts believe that the production of IgG antibodies is a normal response to eating food and that this test is not helpful in diagnosing a food allergy.

Provocation and Neutralization

These tests involve injecting a solution containing a suspect food under your skin or administering it sublingually (as drops under your tongue). Increasing amounts are given in an effort to provoke a reaction. When symptoms appear, you are given increasingly weaker doses of the solution until your symptoms disappear. The last and weakest dose, which supposedly eliminates your symptoms, is called the "neutralizing dose." This solution may then be provided as a treatment for your food allergy. Provocation tests are not only ineffective, but increase the risk of an allergic reaction. There is no scientific proof that neutralization can prevent or control a reaction.

Pulse Testing

This test is based on the notion that, if you are allergic to a particular food, your pulse (the rate of your heartbeat) will go up after you eat that food. There is no scientific evidence to support this claim.

Chapter 39

Lung Function Tests

Lung function tests measure the size of your lungs, how much air you can breathe in and out, how fast you can breathe air out, and how well your lungs deliver oxygen to your blood. These tests also are called pulmonary function tests.

Lung function tests are used to look for the cause of breathing problems (like shortness of breath). These tests are used to check for conditions such as asthma, lung tissue scarring, sarcoidosis, and COPD (chronic obstructive pulmonary disease).

Lung function tests also are used to see how well treatments for breathing problems, such as asthma medicines, are working. The tests may be used to check on whether a condition, such lung tissue scarring, is getting worse.

Overview

Lung function tests measure the following:

- How much air you can take into your lungs (This amount is compared to that of other people your age, height, and sex. This allows your doctor to see whether you're in the normal range.)

- How much air you can blow out of your lungs and how fast you can do it

---

"Lung Function Tests," by the National Heart, Lung, and Blood Institute (NHLBI, www.nhlbi.nih.gov), part of the National Institutes of Health, February 2008.

- How well your lungs deliver oxygen to your blood
- How strong your breathing muscles are

Breathing Tests

The breathing tests most often used are the following:

- Spirometry: This test measures how much air you can breathe in and out. It also measures how fast you can blow air out.
- Peak flow meter: This meter is a small, handheld device that's sometimes used by people who have asthma. The meter helps track their breathing.
- Lung volume measurement: This test, in addition to spirometry, measures how much air you have left in your lungs after you breathe out completely.
- Lung diffusing capacity: This test measures how well oxygen passes from your lungs to your bloodstream.

These tests may not show what's causing breathing problems. Other tests, such as a cardiopulmonary exercise test, also may be done. This test measures how well your lungs and heart work while you exercise on a treadmill or bicycle.

Tests to Measure Oxygen Level

Pulse oximetry and arterial blood gas are two tests used to measure the oxygen level in the blood. They're also called blood oxygen tests.

Pulse oximetry measures blood oxygen levels using a special light. During an arterial blood gas test, your doctor inserts a small needle into an artery, usually in your wrist, and takes a sample of blood. The oxygen level of the blood sample is then checked.

Outlook

Lung function tests usually are painless and rarely cause side effects. You may feel some discomfort during the arterial blood gas test when the needle is inserted into the artery.

Types of Lung Function Tests

Breathing Tests

Spirometry: Spirometry measures how much air you breathe in and out and how fast you blow it out. This is measured in two ways:

peak expiratory flow rate (PEFR) and forced expiratory volume in 1 second (FEV1). PEFR refers to the amount of air you can blow air out as quickly as possible. FEV1 refers to the amount of air you can blow out in 1 second.

During the test, a technician will ask you to take a deep breath in and then blow as hard as you can into a tube connected to a small machine. Your doctor may have you inhale a medicine that helps open your airways. He or she will want to see whether the medicine changes or improves the test results.

Spirometry is done to look for diseases and conditions that affect how much air you can breathe in, such as sarcoidosis or lung tissue scarring. It's also done to look for diseases that affect how fast you can breathe air out, like asthma and COPD (chronic obstructive pulmonary disease).

Peak flow meter: A peak flow meter is a small, handheld device that you blow into. It shows how well air moves out of your lungs. People who have asthma sometimes use this device. It helps them (and their doctors) check their breathing. A peak flow meter can be used at home or in a doctor's office.

Lung volume measurement: This test measures the size of your lungs and how much air you can breathe in and out. During the test, you sit inside a glass booth and breathe into a tube that's hooked to a computer.

Sometimes you breathe in nitrogen or helium gas and then blow it out. The gas you breathe out is then measured to test how much air your lungs can hold.

The test can help diagnose lung tissue scarring or a stiff and/or weak chest wall.

Lung diffusion capacity: This test measures how well oxygen passes from your lungs to your bloodstream. During this test, you breathe in a gas through a tube. You hold your breath for a brief moment and then blow the gas out.

Abnormal test results may suggest loss of lung tissue, emphysema (a type of COPD), very bad scarring, or problems with blood flow through the body's arteries.

Tests to Measure Oxygen Level

Pulse oximetry and arterial blood gas tests show how much oxygen is in your blood. During pulse oximetry, a small light is placed over your fingertip, earlobe, or toe to measure the oxygen. This test is painless and no needles are used.

During an arterial blood gas test, your doctor inserts a small needle into an artery, usually in your wrist. He or she takes a sample of blood. The oxygen level of the blood is checked in a lab.

Testing in Infants and Young Children

Spirometry and other measures of lung function usually can be done in children older than 6 years, if they can follow directions well. Spirometry may be tried in children as young as 5 years. However, technicians who have special training with young children may need to do the testing.

Instead of spirometry, a growing number of medical centers measure respiratory system resistance. This is another way to test lung function in young children.

The child wears nose clips and has his or her cheeks supported with an adult's hands. The child breathes in and out quietly on a mouthpiece, while the technician measures changes in pressure at the mouth. During these lung function tests, parents can help comfort their children and encourage them to cooperate.

Very young children (younger than 2 years) may need an infant lung function test. This requires special equipment and medical staff. This type of test is only available at a few centers. The doctor gives the child medicine to help him or her sleep through the test.

A technician places a mask over your child's nose and mouth and a vest around your child's chest. The mask and vest are attached to a lung function machine. The machine gently pushes air into your child's lungs through the mask. As your child exhales, the vest slightly squeezes his or her chest. This helps push more air out of the lungs. The exhaled air is then measured.

In children younger than 5 years, the doctor likely will use signs and symptoms, medical history, and a physical exam to diagnose lung problems.

Pulse oximetry and arterial blood gas tests may be used for children of all ages.

Other Names for Lung Function Tests

- Lung diffusion testing; also called diffusing capacity and diffusing capacity of the lung for carbon monoxide, or DLCO

- Pulmonary function tests, or PFTs

Arterial blood gas tests also are called blood gas analyses, or ABGs.

Who Needs Lung Function Tests?

People who have breathing problems, such as shortness of breath, may need lung function tests. These tests help find the cause of breathing problems. They're used to check for conditions such as asthma, lung tissue scarring, sarcoidosis, and COPD (chronic obstructive pulmonary disease).

Lung function tests also are used to see how well treatments for breathing problems, such as asthma medicines, are working.

Diagnosing Lung Conditions

Your doctor will diagnose a lung condition based on your medical history, a physical exam, and test results.

Medical history: Your doctor will ask you questions, such as the following:

- Do you ever feel like you can't get enough air?

- Does your chest feel tight sometimes?

- Do you have periods of coughing or wheezing (a whistling sound when you breathe)?

- Do you ever have chest pain?

- Can you walk or run as fast as other people your age?

Your doctor also will ask if you or anyone in your family has ever experienced the following:

- Had asthma and/or allergies

- Had heart disease

- Smoked

- Traveled to places where you may have been exposed to tuberculosis

- Had a job that exposed you to dust, fumes, or particles (like asbestos)

Physical exam: Your doctor will measure your heart rate, breathing rate, and blood pressure. He or she also will listen to your heart and lungs with a stethoscope and feel your abdomen and limbs.

Your doctor will look for signs of heart or lung disease, or another disease that could cause your symptoms.

Lung and heart tests: Based on your medical history and physical exam, your doctor will decide what tests you need. A chest x-ray usually is the first test done to find the cause of breathing problems. This test takes pictures of the organs and structures inside your chest.

Your doctor may do lung function tests to find out even more about how well your lungs work.

Your doctor also may do tests to check your heart, such as an EKG (electrocardiogram) or a stress test. An EKG detects and records your heart's electrical activity. A stress test shows how well your heart works during physical activity.

What to Expect before Lung Function Tests

If you take breathing medicines, your doctor may ask you to stop them for a short time before spirometry, a lung volume measurement test, or a lung diffusion capacity test.

No special preparation is needed before pulse oximetry and arterial blood gas tests. If you're being treated with oxygen, your doctor may ask you to stop using it for a short time before the tests. This is done to check your blood oxygen level without the added oxygen.

What to Expect during Lung Function Tests

Breathing Tests

Spirometry tests may be done in your doctor's office or in a special lung function lab. Your doctor may ask you to use a peak flow meter in the office and suggest that you also do the test at home. The lung volume measurement and lung diffusion capacity tests are done in a special lab or clinic.

For the lung volume measurement and lung diffusion capacity tests, you sit in a chair next to a machine that measures your breathing. For spirometry, you sit or stand next to the machine.

Before the tests, a technician places soft clips on your nose. This allows you to breathe only through a tube that's attached to the testing machine. The technician will tell you how to breathe into the tube. For example, you may be asked to breathe normally, slowly, or rapidly.

The deep breathing done in some of the tests may make you feel short of breath, dizzy, or lightheaded, or it may make you cough.

Spirometry: In this test, you take a deep breath and then exhale as fast and as hard as you can into the tube. With spirometry, your doctor may give you a medicine that helps open your airways. Your doctor will want to see whether it changes or improves the test results.

Peak flow meter: In this test, you take a deep breath and then exhale as fast and as hard as you can into a small, handheld device that's connected to a mouthpiece.

Lung volume measurement: For this test, you sit in a clear glass booth and breathe through the tube attached to the testing machine. The changes in pressure inside the booth are measured to show how much air you can breathe into your lungs.

Sometimes you breathe in nitrogen or helium gas and then breathe it out. The gas that you exhale is then measured.

Lung diffusion capacity: During this test, you breathe in gas through the tube, hold your breath for 10 seconds, and then rapidly blow it out. The gas contains a small amount of carbon monoxide, which won't harm you.

Tests to Measure Oxygen Level

Pulse oximetry is done in a doctor's office or hospital. Arterial blood gas tests are done in a lab or hospital.

Pulse oximetry: During this test, a small light is placed over your fingertip, earlobe, or toe using a clip or flexible tape. It's then attached to a cable that leads to a small machine called an oximeter. The oximeter shows the amount of oxygen in your blood. This test is painless and no needles are used.

Arterial blood gas: During this test, your doctor or technician inserts a small needle into an artery, usually in your wrist, and takes a sample of blood. You may feel some discomfort when the needle is inserted. The oxygen level of the blood sample is then checked in a lab.

After the needle is removed, you may feel mild pressure or throbbing at the needle site. Applying pressure to the area for 5 to 10 minutes should stop the bleeding. You will be given a small bandage to place on the area.

What to Expect after Lung Function Tests

You can return to your normal activities and restart your medicines after lung function tests. Talk to your doctor about when you'll get the test results.

What Do Lung Function Tests Show?

Breathing Tests

Spirometry: Spirometry can show whether you have the following:

- Blockage (obstruction) in your airways—This may be a sign of asthma, COPD (chronic obstructive pulmonary disease), or another obstructive lung condition.

- Smaller than normal lungs (restriction)—This may be a sign of heart failure, damage or scarring of the lung tissues, or another restrictive lung condition.

Peak flow meter: A peak flow meter shows the fastest rate at which you can blow air out of your lungs. People who have asthma use this device to help track their breathing.

Lung volume measurement: This test shows the size of your lungs. Abnormal test results may show that you have lung tissue scarring or a stiff chest wall.

Lung diffusion capacity: This test can show a problem with oxygen moving from your lungs into your bloodstream. This may be a sign of loss of lung tissue, emphysema (a type of COPD), or problems with blood flow through the body's arteries.

Tests to Measure Oxygen Level

Pulse oximetry and arterial blood gas tests measure the oxygen level in your blood. These tests show how well your lungs are taking in oxygen and moving it into the bloodstream. A low level of oxygen in the blood may be a sign of a lung or heart condition.

What Are the Risks of Lung Function Tests?

Breathing Tests

Spirometry, peak flow meter, lung volume measurement, and lung diffusion capacity tests usually are safe. These tests rarely cause problems.

Tests to Measure Oxygen Level

Pulse oximetry has no risks. Side effects from arterial blood gas tests are rare.

Chapter 40

Allergy Medications

Chapter Contents

Section 40.1

Types of Allergy Medicines

"Types of Allergy Medication," © 2010 A.D.A.M., Inc.
Reprinted with permission.

If you are still having symptoms despite your efforts to avoid allergens, you might explore medication options. Regardless of which medications you select, read the product labels and know the side effects. The following list includes the most common allergy treatments (both over-the-counter and prescription) and the specific allergic conditions they treat. Particularly when treating children for allergies, it is wise to consult with your health care provider. Some of the medications are not as effective in children, and some of the medications can affect behavior and sleep, as well as cause more serious side effects.

Antihistamines: As the name implies, antihistamines counter the effects of histamine released during an allergic reaction. They are widely used to treat many allergy-related conditions. They are often combined with decongestants and are available in a variety of over-the-counter formulas (such as Advil Allergy Sinus, Alavert Allergy & Sinus, Benadryl, Chlor-Trimeton, Claritin, Contac, Dimetapp, Robitussin Cough & Allergy, Triaminic Cold and Allergy, and Tylenol Allergy) and by prescription (such as Allegra, Clarinex, and Zyrtec). You should always ask your pharmacist if your antihistamine also contains a decongestant, especially any you give to children. Some antihistamines may cause drowsiness and slowed reaction time. Others do not. Antihistamine nasal sprays are also available to treat allergic rhinitis (such as Astelin). Antihistamine eye drops may also be used for quick relief of itchy eyes associated with allergies (such as Patanol).

Leukotriene blockers: Leukotrienes are another substance released in the body that trigger allergic symptoms such as a stuffy or runny nose, sneezing, itchy eyes, postnasal drip, or wheezing. Montelukast sodium (Singulair) is a prescription medicine that can prevent symptoms by blocking leukotrienes. It is used in adults and in children as young as 2 years. It is also used to treat asthma.

Decongestants: People who experience nasal congestion (stuffy nose) due to allergies or sinusitis sometimes consider oral or nasal spray decongestants for relief. Decongestants are also included in eye drops to decrease redness caused by conjunctivitis. They work by constricting blood vessels and reducing swelling. Be careful when using some nasal spray decongestants. If you use them for a prolonged period (longer than 3–4 days), you may experience a "rebound" effect, where nasal congestion symptoms return. Concerns have been raised about oral decongestants and their side effects (especially for children) and potential for misuse. They are now available behind the counter. Ask your pharmacist; you should ask your child's pediatrician about decongestant use in children.

Corticosteroids: These anti-inflammatory agents are used to treat the itching and swelling associated with a variety of allergic disorders. The most commonly used forms are corticosteroid nasal sprays for allergic rhinitis and sinusitis (such as Flonase, Nasalide, Nasacort, Nasonex, Rhinocort), over-the-counter topical corticosteroid creams for hives, dermatitis, and insect sting reactions, and inhaled corticosteroids for asthma. Oral or injected corticosteroids are used less frequently for more severe cases of asthma, dermatitis, or other allergic reactions.

Cromolyn sodium/Nedocromil sodium: These are another type of anti-inflammatory medication. Cromolyn sodium nasal spray can be used to treat and sometimes prevent allergic rhinitis. It works by preventing the release of histamine from mast cells. Cromolyn nasal spray is available over the counter and is gentle and effective. It generally takes a few days to start working. Eye drop versions are available for itchy, bloodshot eyes. Inhaled nedocromil sodium is used to treat inflammation due to asthma, which can be exacerbated by allergies. It is more often used in children.

Epinephrine: Epinephrine (adrenalin) is used for emergency treatment in cases of anaphylaxis due to insect sting, food, or drug allergies. It is most commonly administered with a device called an injectable epinephrine kit (such as EpiPen or Twinject). Epinephrine constricts the small blood vessels in the skin and mucous membranes, which increases blood pressure and heart rate back to normal levels. Epinephrine also is an antihistamine.

Section 40.2

Allergy Medicines for Children

"Allergy Medicines," © 2009 Children's Hospitals and Clinics of Minnesota (www.childrensmn.org). Reprinted with permission.

You and your child should know the name of each medicine your child is taking. Each person's allergies are different and medicines that help one person may not help another. Always use the medicines in the amount and method prescribed by your child's doctor. Always make sure you have enough medicines on hand.

Anti-Inflammatory Nose Sprays

Brand Name (Generic Name)

- Beconase®; Beconase AQ®; Vancenase®; Vancenase AQ®; Vancenase AQ® double strength (beclomethasone)
- Flonase® (fluticasone)
- Nasacort®; Nasacort AQ (triamcinolone)
- NasalCrom® (cromolyn)
- Nasarel® (flunisolide)
- Nasonex® (mometasone furoate monohydrate)
- Rhinocort® (budesonide)

Things to Know

- Decreases swelling and inflammation in the nose
- Takes days or weeks to work
- Must be used daily to prevent inflammation

Side Effects

- Stinging or irritation to the nose

Antihistamines

For best results use a long-acting preparation (such as a 12-hour type) to control allergy symptoms. Generic products work as well as brand names.

Brand Name (Generic Name)

- Dimetane® or other brands (brompheniramine)
- Chlor-Trimeton® or other brands (chlorpheniramine)
- Tavist® (clemastine)
- Periactin® (cyproheptadine)
- Benadryl® or other brands (diphenhydramine)
- Atarax® (hydroxyzine)

Things to Know

- Usually starts working in 15–30 minutes
- May take with or without food

Side Effects

- The most common side effect is drowsiness; take it at bedtime.
- It may thicken mucus; drink plenty of fluids.
- In young children antihistamines may cause stimulation or hyperactivity.
- Call the doctor if your child is too sleepy or has blurred vision or dilated pupils.

Non-Sedating Antihistamines

Brand Name (Generic Name)

- Allegra® (fexofenadine)
- Clarinex® (desloratadine)
- Claritin® (loratadine)
- Zyrtec® (cetirizine)

Things to Know

- Take only as directed by your doctor.

- Do not take other antihistamines while on one of these medicines.

- Do not take erythromycin while taking these medicines without asking your doctor or pharmacist.

Side Effects

- It may thicken mucus; drink plenty of fluids.

- May cause nausea (upset stomach) or vomiting (throwing up). Call your child's doctor if this becomes a problem.

Nasal Decongestants

These medicines are often combined with an antihistamine. Decongestants do not treat allergies but may help relieve a runny or stuffed-up nose. If you do not have this symptom, you do not need a decongestant. Use generic products when available.

Brand Name (Generic Name)

- Afrin® (oxymetazoline)

- Neo-Synephrine® (phenylephrine)

- Privine® (naphazoline)

- Sudafed®; PediaCare® (pseudoephedrine)

- Various combinations (phenylephrine)

Things to Know

- Usually begins working in 10 to 15 minutes

- Stop using nose sprays after 3 days.

- Stop using oral medicines when symptoms are gone.

Side Effects

- Increased activity, hard to fall asleep, rapid heartbeat, shakiness, dizziness

Cough Medicines

When choosing an over-the-counter medicine, check with your doctor or pharmacist. Cough suppressants or expectorants like Robitussin® (guaifenesin) or Robitussin® DM (dextromethorphan) have not been shown to relieve allergy symptoms. Many times they are in allergy medicines, but are not needed.

Section 40.3

Rhinitis Medications

"Medications for the Treatment of Rhinitis,"
Copyright © 2009 American College of Allergy, Asthma and
Immunology (www.acaai.org). Reprinted with permission.

When allergy symptoms are not well controlled with avoidance measures, allergy medications can help to reduce nasal congestion, runny nose, sneezing, and itching. They are available in many forms, including oral tablets, liquid medication, nasal sprays, and eye drops. Some medications may cause side effects, so it is best to consult your allergist if there's a problem.

Intranasal corticosteroids: Intranasal corticosteroids are the single most effective drug class for treatment of allergic rhinitis. They can significantly reduce nasal congestion as well as sneezing, itching, and runny nose. These drugs are frequently prescribed, and are of particular value when rhinitis symptoms are more severe. They are most effective when taken daily, as directed by your health care provider, but may have some benefit when taken as needed.

These medications are safe when used under physician supervision. They are designed to avoid the side effects that may occur from steroids when they are taken by mouth or injection. However, care must be taken not to spray them against the center portion of the nose (the nasal septum). The most common side effects are local irritation and nasal bleeding. Some older preparations have been shown to have some effect on children's growth, but data about some newer nasal steroids have not shown an effect on growth.

419

Antihistamines: Antihistamines are inexpensive and commonly used to treat allergic rhinitis. These medications counter the effects of histamine, the irritating chemical released within your body when an allergic reaction takes place. Although other chemicals are involved, histamine is primarily responsible for causing the symptoms.

Antihistamines do not cure, but help relieve nasal allergy symptoms such as:

- sneezing, itchy, and runny nose;
- eye itching, burning, tearing, and redness;
- itchy skin, hives, and eczema;
- certain other allergic conditions.

There are dozens of different antihistamines and wide variations in how patients respond to them. Some are available over-the-counter and others require a prescription.

Generally, the newer (second generation) products work well and produce only minor side effects. Some people find that an antihistamine becomes less effective as the allergy season worsens or their allergies change over time. If an antihistamine loses its "strength," notify your physician, who may then recommend an antihistamine of a different class or strength. Persons with excessive nasal dryness or thick nasal mucus should avoid taking antihistamines without consulting a physician. Contact your physician for advice if an antihistamine causes drowsiness or other side effects.

Proper use: Short-acting antihistamines can be taken every 4 to 6 hours, while timed-release antihistamines are taken every 12 to 24 hours. The short-acting antihistamines are often most helpful taken 30 minutes before an anticipated allergic exposure (such as a picnic during ragweed season). Timed-release antihistamines are better suited to chronic (long-term) use for those who need daily medications.

Proper use of these drugs is just as important as their selection. The most effective way to use them is before symptoms develop. A dose taken early can eliminate the need for many later doses to reduce established symptoms. Many times a patient will say that he "took one, and it didn't work." If he or she had taken the antihistamine regularly for 3 to 4 days, and built up blood levels, it might have been effective.

Side effects: Older (first generation) antihistamines may cause drowsiness and/or performance impairment, which can lead to accidents and personal injury. Even when these medications are taken only at bedtime, they can still cause considerable impairment the following day. Impairment can occur even in people who do not feel drowsy. For this reason, it is important that you do not drive a car or work with dangerous machinery when you take a potentially sedating antihistamine. Some of the newer antihistamines do not cause drowsiness.

Another frequently encountered side effect is excessive dryness of the mouth, nose, and eyes. Less common side effects include restlessness, nervousness, overexcitability, insomnia, dizziness, headaches, euphoria, fainting, visual disturbances, decreased appetite, nausea, vomiting, abdominal distress, constipation, diarrhea, increased or decreased urination, urinary retention, high or low blood pressure, nightmares (especially in children), sore throat, unusual bleeding or bruising, chest tightness, or palpitations. Men with prostate enlargement may encounter urinary problems while on antihistamines. Consult your allergist should these reactions occur.

Alcohol and tranquilizers increase the sedation side effects of antihistamines.

Important precautions:

- Never take anyone else's medication.
- Do not use more than one antihistamine at a time, unless prescribed.
- Keep these medications out of the reach of children.
- Know the effect of the medication on you before working with heavy machinery, driving or doing other performance-intensive tasks; some products can slow your reaction time.
- Follow your physician's instructions.

Some antihistamines appear to be safe, but there have not been enough studies to determine absolute safety of antihistamines in pregnancy. Again, consult your allergist or obstetrician if antihistamines must be taken.

While antihistamines have been taken safely by millions of people in the last 50 years, don't take antihistamines before telling your allergist if you are allergic to or intolerant of any medicine; are pregnant or intend to become pregnant while using this medication; are breastfeeding; have glaucoma or enlarged prostate; or have any medical illness.

Decongestants: Decongestants help relieve the stuffiness and pressure caused by swollen nasal tissue. They do not contain antihistamines, so they do not cause antihistaminic side effects. They do not relieve the other symptoms of allergic rhinitis, such as runny nose, postnasal drip, and sneezing. Decongestants are available as prescription and non-prescription medications and are often seen in combination with antihistamines or other medications. It is not uncommon for patients using decongestants to experience insomnia if taking the medication in the afternoon or evening. If this occurs, a dose reduction may be needed.

At times, men with prostate enlargement may encounter urinary problems while on decongestants. Patients using medications for the management of emotional or behavioral problems should discuss this with their physicians before using decongestants. Pregnant patients should also check with their physician before starting decongestants.

Non-prescription decongestant nasal sprays work within minutes and last for hours, but should not be used for more than a few days at a time without a physician's order. Prolonged use can cause rhinitis medicamentosa, or rebound swelling of the nasal tissue. Stopping the use of the decongestant nasal spray will cure rhinitis medicamentosa, providing that there is no underlying disorder.

Oral decongestants are found in many over-the-counter and prescription medications, and may be the treatment of choice for nasal congestion. They don't cause rhinitis medicamentosa but need to be avoided by some patients with high blood pressure. If you have high blood pressure, you should check with your physician before using them.

Non-prescription saline nasal sprays will help counteract symptoms of dry nasal passages or thick nasal mucus. Unlike decongestant nose sprays, a saline nose spray can be used as often as needed. Sometimes, your physician may recommend washing (douching) of the nasal passage. There are many over the counter preparations for saline rinses, including neti pots and saline rinse bottles.

Nasal cromolyn is a medication that blocks the body's release of allergy-causing substances. It does not work in all patients. The full dosage is four times daily, and improvement may take several weeks to occur. Nasal cromolyn can help prevent allergic nasal reactions if taken prior to an allergen exposure.

Nasal ipratropium bromide spray (Atrovent) can help reduce nasal drainage from allergic rhinitis or some forms of non-allergic rhinitis.

Montelukast is a tablet medication approved for treatment of allergic rhinitis, as well as asthma. It works against substances called leukotrienes that can cause symptoms of allergic rhinitis.

Antibiotics are for the treatment of bacterial infections. They do not affect the course of uncomplicated common colds and are of no benefit for non-infectious rhinitis, including allergic rhinitis.

Immunotherapy—Allergen immunotherapy, known as "allergy shots," may be recommended for persons who don't respond well to treatment with medications, experience side effects from medications, who have allergen exposure that is unavoidable, or desire a more permanent solution to their allergic problem. Immunotherapy can be very effective in controlling allergic symptoms. Immunotherapy does not help the symptoms produced by non-allergic rhinitis.

Allergy injections are usually given at variable intervals over a period of 3 to 5 years. An immunotherapy treatment program consists of injections of a diluted allergy extract, administered frequently in increasing doses until a maintenance dose is reached. Then, the injection schedule is changed so that the same dose is given with longer intervals between injections. Immunotherapy helps the body build resistance to the effects of the allergen, reduces the intensity of symptoms caused by allergen exposure, and sometimes can actually make skin test reactions disappear. As resistance develops, symptoms should improve, but the improvement from immunotherapy will take several months to occur.

Nasal surgery is of no benefit in allergic rhinitis, but it may help if patients have nasal polyps or chronic sinusitis not responsive to prolonged antibiotics and nasal steroid sprays.

Eye allergy preparations are used when the eyes are affected by the same allergens that trigger rhinitis, causing redness, watery eyes, and itching. Over-the-counter (OTC) eye drops and oral medications are commonly used for short-term relief of some eye allergy symptoms. However, they may not relieve all symptoms, and prolonged use of some OTC eye drops may actually cause your condition to become worse.

Prescription eye drops and oral medications also are used to treat eye allergies. Prescription eye drops provide both short- and long-term targeted relief of eye allergy symptoms, and they can be used to manage eye allergy symptoms.

Check with your physician or pharmacist if you are unsure about a specific drug or formula.

Medications for the Treatment of Rhinitis (Brand Names)

Non-Prescription Antihistamines

Newer antihistamines now available without a prescription are "second generation" antihistamines and generally do not cause drowsiness, slowed reaction time, and dry mouth in most people.

- Claritin, or generic loratadine
- Alavert and other generic products (consult with your physician)
- Zyrtec, or generic cetirizine

Older non-prescription antihistamines (some combined with decongestants/analgesics) are "first generation" antihistamines and generally cause drowsiness, slowed reaction time, and dry mouth in most people. Following are some examples:

- Actifed
- Alka Seltzer Plus
- Allerest
- Benadryl
- Chlor-Trimeton
- Comtrex
- Contac

- Dimetapp
- Drixoral
- PediaCare Sudafed
- Tavist
- Triaminic
- Tylenol Sinus or Allergy
- Vicks

Many brand name and generic formulas are available without prescription. If you are in doubt as to whether or not a product contains an antihistamine, consult your physician or pharmacist.

Prescription Antihistamines

The following medications are second generation antihistamines that do not generally cause the side effects of first generation antihistamines, such as drowsiness, slowed reaction time, and dry mouth.

- Allegra, or generic fexofenadine
- Clarinex
- Xyzal

The following contain first generation antihistamines (some combined with other medications) that can cause drowsiness, slowed reaction time, and dry mouth.

- Atarax, or generic hydroxyzine
- Dallergy
- Periactin
- Temaril
- Trinalin
- Vistaril

Non-Prescription Oral Decongestants

- Chlor-Trimeton Decongestant
- Dimetapp Decongestant
- Drixoral Nasal Decongestant
- Efidac/24
- PediaCare Infants' Decongestant Drops
- Sudafed 12 Hour
- Triaminic Decongestant Formula
- Prescription Oral Decongestants
- AlleRx
- Respaire
- Guaifed

Non-Prescription Decongestant Nasal Sprays

Prolonged use may cause rebound congestion.
- Afrin (and related products)
- Dristan 12 Hour Nasal Spray
- Nasacon
- Neo-Synephrine 12 Hour
- Nostrilla 12 Hour Decongestant
- Otrivin (and related products)
- Vicks Sinex 12 Hour

Non-Prescription Anti-Allergy Nasal Spray

- NasalCrom (cromolyn)

Non-Prescription Saline Nasal Sprays

- Afrin Saline Mist
- Ayr
- Breathe Right
- NaSal Moisturizer AF
- Ocean
- Salinex

Prescription Antihistamine Nasal Spray

- Astelin
- Astepro
- Patanase

Prescription Atropine-Like Nasal Spray

- Atrovent

Prescription Nasal Corticosteroid Sprays

These do not contain antihistamines or decongestants.

- Beconase
- Flonase, or generic fluticasone
- Nasacort
- Nasalide, Nasarel, or generic flunisolide
- Nasonex
- Omnaris
- Rhinocort
- Rhinocort Aqua
- Vancenase
- Veramyst

Prescription Oral Leukotriene Pathway Inhibitors

- Accolate
- Singulair

Prescription Eye Drops

Antihistamines/mast stabilizer dual-action therapies:

- Elestat
- Optivar
- Pataday
- Patanol

Antihistamine:

- Livostin

Mast cell stabilizers:

- Alamast
- Alocril

Non-Prescription Eye Drops

Antihistamine/mast cell stabilizer dual action therapies:

- Alaway
- Refresh
- Visine
- Zaditor

There are many ways of treating allergies, and each person's treatment must be individualized based on the frequency, severity, and duration of symptoms and on the degree of allergic sensitivity. If you have more questions, your allergist will be happy to answer them.

Section 40.4

Medications for Sinusitis

"Sinus Infection Treatment Guide," © 2010 Oregon Alliance Working for Antibiotic Resistance Education (AWARE), Oregon Department of Human Services. Reprinted with permission.

What You Need to Know

What is sinusitis?

Sinusitis is inflammation of the sinuses. Most cases of sinusitis are caused by viruses. Other causes include:

- allergies;
- exposure to smoke, dust, or other irritants in the home, school, or workplace;
- bacterial infection.

Do antibiotics help sinusitis?

Antibiotics only help sinusitis when it is caused by a bacterial infection. Because sinusitis is usually caused by a virus, antibiotics won't help most cases of sinusitis.

Taking antibiotics won't prevent a stuffy nose from turning into a bacterial sinus infection. In fact, taking unnecessary antibiotics puts your family at risk for developing resistant infections later.

What about yellow or green mucus?

The color of mucus does not reliably predict whether or not you have a bacterial sinus infection or need antibiotics. It's normal for mucus to change color from clear to yellow, green, or white when your body's immune system is fighting a virus.

Sinus Treatment Guide for Parents

Antibiotics are rarely needed unless your child has one or more of the following:

- Pain or pressure on one side of the face
- Swelling around the eye area
- Symptoms have lasted 10 or more days

Medical attention is recommended for:

- high fever (104 degrees Fahrenheit or above);
- fever that lasts more than 24 hours;
- symptoms that are severe or have lasted more than 10 days.

Otherwise—If your child does not have a fever, and has only mild symptoms that have lasted less than 10 days, treat as a virus:

- Get lots of rest.
- Avoid cigarette smoke.
- Encourage sinus drainage by:
  - offering plenty of fluids;
  - breathing steam from a shower or bath;
  - using non-medicated saline nose drops or spray several times a day;
  - elevating the head of the child's bed;
  - using warm facial packs for three to four times a day for 5–10 minutes.

Acetaminophen (Tylenol or generic equivalent) may be taken for fever or pain. Ibuprofen (Advil, Motrin, or generic equivalent) may be given if your child is over 6 months. Ibuprofen should not be given if the child is dehydrated or vomiting continuously. Over-the-counter decongestants should not be given to children under the age of 3 years.

Aspirin should never be used in children with fever due to the risk of stomach upset, intestinal bleeding, and Reye syndrome.

Adult Sinus Treatment Guide

Cough and runny nose by themselves are unlikely to be caused by a bacterial sinus infection unless those symptoms have been present for more than 10 days. Antibiotics are rarely required unless the following symptoms are present:

- Pain or pressure on one side of the face
- Toothache in the upper jaw in the absence of dental problems
- Worsening of symptoms after initial improvement

Medical attention is recommended for:

- typical symptoms of bacterial infection (see above) that are severe or have lasted more than 10 days;
- persistent fever.

Otherwise—If symptoms are mild or have lasted less than 10 days:

- get lots of rest;
- avoid cigarette smoke;
- help your sinuses drain by:
  - drinking plenty of fluids (try to avoid caffeine and alcohol);
  - breathing steam from a shower or bath;
  - using non-medicated saline nose drops or spray several times a day;
  - elevating the head of your bed;
  - using warm facial packs for three to four times a day for 5–10 minutes.
- Acetaminophen (Tylenol or generic equivalent) or ibuprofen (Advil, Motrin, or generic equivalent) may be taken for fever or pain.

Over-the-counter decongestants like Sudafed or Benadryl may also be helpful.

Section 40.5

Decongestants

Excerpted from "Itching for Allergy Relief?" by the U.S. Food and
Drug Administration (FDA, www.fda.gov), April 29, 2009.

Pollen grains from trees, grasses, and weeds can float through the air in
spring, summer, or fall. But on their way to fertilize plants and tree flowers,
pollen particles often end up in our noses, eyes, ears, and mouths. The result
can be sneezing spells, watery eyes, congestion, and an itchy throat.

The collection of symptoms that affect the nose when you breathe in
something you are allergic to is called allergic rhinitis; when the symptoms affect the eyes, it's called allergic conjunctivitis. Allergic rhinitis
caused by plant pollen is commonly called hay fever—although it's not a
reaction to hay and it doesn't cause fever.

Pollen allergy affects about one out of 10 Americans, according to the
National Institute of Allergy and Infectious Diseases (NIAID). For some,
symptoms can be controlled by using over-the-counter (OTC) medicine
occasionally. Others have reactions that may more seriously disrupt
the quality of their lives. Allergies can trigger or worsen asthma and
lead to other health problems such as sinus infection (sinusitis) and ear
infections in children.

"You can distinguish allergy symptoms from a cold because a cold
tends to be short-lived, results in thicker nasal secretions, and is usually associated with sore throat, hoarseness, malaise, and fever," says
Badrul Chowdhury, MD, PhD, an allergist and immunologist in the
Food and Drug Administration (FDA).

Many people with allergic rhinitis notice a seasonal pattern with
their symptoms, but others may need a health care professional's help
to find out for sure if pollen is the source of their misery. If symptoms
crop up year-round, dust mites, pet dander, or another indoor allergy
trigger (allergen) could be the culprit. This year-round condition is
known as perennial allergic rhinitis.

When to Get Treatment

Chowdhury suggests seeing a health care professional if you experience allergies for the first time, your symptoms interfere with your

ability to function, you don't find relief from OTC drugs, or you experience allergy symptoms over a long period.

You may need an allergy test, the most common of which is a skin test that shows how you react to different allergens, including specific pollen allergens like ragweed and grass pollen.

Avoid Pollen

Once you know you have seasonal allergies, try to avoid pollen as much as possible, says Chowdhury. Pay attention to pollen counts and try to stay indoors when pollen levels are highest. Pollen counts measure how much pollen is in the air (pollen level) and are expressed in grains of pollen per square meter of air collected during a 24-hour period.

- In the late summer and early fall, during ragweed pollen season, pollen levels are highest in the morning.

- In the spring and summer, during the grass pollen season, pollen levels are highest in the evening.

- Some molds, another allergy trigger, may also be seasonal. For example, leaf mold is more common in the fall.

- Sunny, windy days can be especially troublesome for pollen allergy sufferers.

It may also help to:

- keep windows closed in your house and car and run the air conditioner;

- avoid mowing grass and doing other yard work, if possible;

- wear a face mask designed to filter pollen out of the air and keep it from reaching nasal passages, if you must work outdoors.

Decongestants

FDA regulates many medications that offer allergy relief. Decongestants, available both by prescription and OTC, come in oral and nasal spray forms. They are sometimes recommended in combination with antihistamines, which used alone do not have an effect on nasal congestion. Allegra D is an example of a drug that contains both an antihistamine (fexofenadine) and a decongestant (pseudoephedrine).

Drugs that contain pseudoephedrine are available without a prescription but are kept behind the pharmacy counter as a safeguard

431

because of their use in making methamphetamine—a powerful, highly addictive stimulant often produced illegally in home laboratories. You will need to ask your pharmacist and show identification to purchase drugs that contain pseudoephedrine.

Using nose sprays and drops more than a few days may give you a "rebound" effect—your nasal congestion will get worse. These drugs are more useful for short-term use to relieve nasal congestion.

Section 40.6

Saline Nasal Sprays and Irrigation

"Saline Nasal Sprays and Irrigation," February 2008, reprinted with permission of the University of Michigan Health System. © 2008 Regents of the University of Michigan. All rights reserved.

This information is not a tool for self-diagnosis or a substitute for medical treatment. You should speak to your health-care provider or make an appointment to be seen if you have questions or concerns about this information or your medical condition.

How do saline nasal sprays work?

Saline nasal sprays provide moisture to the nasal passages, especially during the winter when the environment is cold and dry outside, hot and dry inside. When your nasal passages are dry, mild nasal crusting may occur, and bacterial infections can develop under these crusts. Saline sprays clean the nasal passages of crusts and mucus and also help the natural cleaning system of your nasal passages.

Where can I purchase saline nasal sprays?

Saline sprays are available over the counter at most drug stores. Some national brands include Saline, Ocean Spray, and Ayr. Many pharmacies and stores carry their own brands. Preservative-free saline sprays are also available at most pharmacies, including Meijer, Walgreens, and Rite Aid.

Are there any side effects?

Nasal sprays may sting slightly. You may experience irritation caused by the preservative in the saline spray. If this happens, use "Simply Saline," a preservative-free saline spray.

What is nasal saline irrigation?

Nasal irrigation is used when greater volumes of saline are needed, for example, when large mucus crusts build up or nasal/sinus polyps block mucus clearance.

To irrigate your nasal passages, a bulb syringe (used to clear the nasal passages of babies) can be used.

To make your own nasal irrigation solution, mix:

- 1/4 tsp of kosher or pickling salt;

- 1/4 tsp baking soda;

- 8 oz of warm tap water.

Note: 1 tsp of salt and 1 tsp baking soda per 32 oz of water.

Since tap water may have some bacterial impurities, you may choose to use distilled water instead. Boil the distilled water and store in a refrigerator until you add the salt and baking soda.

Or, you can purchase the "Sinus Rinse" system (available at the University of Michigan Outpatient Pharmacy, Walgreens, and Meijer), which comes with single use salt packets. The Sinus Rinse system may be easier and more comfortable to use than a bulb syringe.

How do I do saline irrigation?

Use 8–16 oz of solution in each nasal cavity one to two times daily, or as often as is prescribed by your health care provider.

- Lower your head over a sink and turn your head so that your left nostril is down.

- Pour solution from the container into your right nostril.

- Water will drain from your left nostril into the sink.

- Gently blow your nose.

- Repeat the same process for other nostril.

To prevent the solution from coming out of your mouth, open your mouth and make a "K" sound, which will close off the mouth and throat. You should use only enough pressure to move the solution to the back of your nose so it comes out though your mouth or nose. This should not cause major discomfort once you are used to it.

Prepare fresh solution each day and clean the Sinus Rinse bottle after each use.

Chapter 41

Medical Therapies for Allergies

Chapter Contents

Section 41.1

Anti Immunoglobulin E Therapy

Over the last few years, doctors have learned many new things about allergy. This new knowledge has led to new treatments for asthma and other allergic diseases.

Specific Allergen Immunotherapy (Allergy Shots)

This treatment has been available since 1911. This treatment decreases sensitivity to the things to which the person is allergic. The treatment is a type of vaccination because it increases the person's resistance to the things causing their allergies.

The allergy vaccines are made from pollens, mold spores, animal dander, dust mites, or bee venom. Allergy shots are helpful for nasal allergy, asthma, and bee sting allergy.

Researchers are trying to find new ways to give allergy vaccines. In the future, vaccines may be nose sprays or drops under the tongue.

Immunoglobulin E (IgE) and Anti-IgE

Our immune system includes cells and proteins. The proteins include antibodies and cytokines. There are many types of antibodies. Immunoglobulin E (IgE) is the type of antibody that causes allergic reactions. IgE is found in the blood and in organs. IgE binds to certain body cells. These cells include mast cells and basophils. After IgE binds to the cells, allergy particles can bind to the IgE. When this happens, the cell releases many chemicals. These chemicals cause allergy symptoms such as itching, sneezing, and wheezing.

If treatment could prevent the release of the chemicals, there would be no itching, sneezing, or wheezing. If IgE could be stopped from binding to the cells, the chemicals would not be released.

Omalizumab is a man-made antibody against IgE (anti-IgE). This treatment is given by injection (shots) once or twice a month. Omalizumab stops IgE from binding to the cells. In 2003, the FDA approved this treatment for teens and adults with uncontrolled asthma.

Some day, people with other allergy problems might be helped by anti-IgE injections. For example, people severely allergic to a food, a medicine, or latex rubber might be helped by injections of anti-IgE.

Cytokines and Cytokine Inhibitors

When the immune system is active, the cells release proteins called cytokines. The cytokines help some parts of the immune response and shut down other parts. Chemists have been making new treatments called cytokine inhibitors. These inhibitors can prevent the cytokines from causing allergy problems. The inhibitors have not yet been approved by the FDA [U.S. Food and Drug Administration]. Some day, cytokine inhibitors might be used to treat asthma and other allergic diseases.

Peptide Immunotherapy (Allergy Shots)

Current allergy shots (immunotherapy) are made from allergenic proteins. However, chemists can make allergy shots from peptides, which are tiny parts of allergenic proteins.

In research, peptide allergy shots have been used to treat people allergic to cats. People who were given peptide allergy shots had fewer allergy problems in their nose and lungs. In the future, peptide immunotherapy may be approved by the FDA.

Section 41.2

Allergy Shots (Immunotherapy) for Kids

Many kids have allergies—in fact, they're the most common cause
of chronic nasal congestion in children.

Allergen immunotherapy (allergy shots) can be an effective treatment for allergies. Here are the basics on allergy shots and how to help
a child deal with them.

Why Allergy Shots Are Used

An allergy occurs when the body's immune system has an exaggerated reaction to a usually harmless substance. The most common allergens (substances that trigger the allergy) are dust mites,
molds, pollen, pets with fur or feathers, stinging insects, and some
kinds of foods.

The body reacts to the trigger by releasing chemicals, one of which
is histamine. Allergic symptoms can include runny nose, congestion,
sneezing, itchy eyes, and ear itching or popping. Asthma also might
occur in some kids.

The best way to prevent or control allergy symptoms is to avoid
triggers. An allergist (a doctor trained to identify and treat allergies)
will look for causes of an allergy by testing a person's reaction to specific allergens with skin or blood tests. Then, based on the test results,
the allergist or another doctor can recommend treatments, including
medications and ways to avoid exposure to allergens.

If environmental control measures and treatment with basic allergy
medications are not successful, allergy shots might be recommended
as the next step.

How Allergy Shots Help

Allergy shots help the body build immunity to specific allergens, thus eventually preventing or lessening reactions from exposure to the allergen. Allergy shots also decrease the risk of developing asthma by 50% and reduce the chance of developing new allergens.

The shots contain a purified form of the allergens that are causing problems. The course of shots is usually given over a 5-year period. The dosage of the allergen is gradually increased over the first 4 to 5 months to a monthly maintenance dose, which is usually given for up to 3 years. After 5 years of getting allergy shots, a patient may no longer seem to be allergic.

If your doctor recommends allergen immunology, your child might begin receiving shots containing very small doses of allergen once or twice a week. The dose is slowly increased with each shot to allow the immune system to safely adjust and build immunity to the allergens. This is called the buildup phase.

Your child might not get symptom relief from allergies until higher doses are achieved at the end of the buildup phase. Once the highest effective and safe dose is reached, the frequency of shots gradually decreases to weekly, then biweekly, and then possibly monthly. This is called maintenance.

Are Allergy Shots Safe?

Allergy shots are really like vaccinations: They boost the defenses of the immune system to help the body reduce the allergic reaction. Given by a well-trained and experienced health professional, allergy shots are safe and effective and can be given to children as young as 4 or 5 years old.

Allergy shots, which are given year-round, work better against some substances than others. Generally, the shots are most effective against insect venoms and allergens that are inhaled, such as pollens, dust, molds, and animal dander.

When your child receives allergy shots, he or she may experience a reaction near the site of the injection. A patch of skin on the arm approximately the size of a quarter may itch and swell. This reaction is a signal that the body is responding to the allergen. You can treat this reaction by applying ice to the area and giving your child an antihistamine.

More serious reactions, such as hives and itching all over the body or wheezing and breathing difficulties, are unusual and occur in less than 2% of patients.

439

Shots might seem like an unusual way to treat allergies, but they're effective at decreasing sensitivity to triggers. The substances in the shots are chosen according to the allergens identified from a person's medical history and by the allergist during the initial testing. The U.S. Food and Drug Administration (FDA) oversees the standards used in preparing the materials for allergy shots given in the United States.

The American College of Allergy, Asthma & Immunology offers these tips to parents to make sure their kids receive allergy shots safely:

- Allergy shots should be administered only under the supervision of an allergist/immunologist or other doctor specifically trained in immunotherapy.

- A child who is ill, especially with asthma or respiratory difficulties, should not receive further allergy shots until a doctor says it's safe.

- To avoid adverse interactions, tell the doctor administering the injections beforehand of any current medications your child is taking.

Allergen immunotherapy isn't necessary for everyone with allergies. Many kids get along fine by living in homes that are as free as possible of allergens or by taking allergy medication during peak allergy season.

But many kids battle allergies year-round, and some can't control their symptoms with medications. For them, allergen immunotherapy can be beneficial.

Side Effects and Reactions

Allergy shots are extremely safe when given properly, but they do have the potential for rare but serious reactions. This is because treatment involves exposure to the substances to which someone is known to be allergic. A qualified allergist/immunologist will have all the medications and equipment necessary at the office to treat a serious reaction immediately.

Every time your child receives an injection, your doctor will have him or her wait 30 minutes in the office to make sure there is no adverse reaction. The doctor's staff will be watching for early signs and symptoms that could require emergency procedures and medications. If a severe reaction occurs, 98% of the time it will occur within 30 minutes of the shot and the reaction will usually respond to treatment with an injection of epinephrine (adrenaline).

In the event of a severe reaction, the doctor will probably reduce the dosage of allergen in the next injection to allow your child's system to build immunity more gradually.

Millions of people each year receive allergy shots without problems; however, to ensure safety, doctors recommend that immunotherapy be given in a controlled environment where the physicians and other health care personnel are trained to respond to an emergency. Board-certified allergists/immunologists have had a minimum of 5 years of training after medical school, which ensures that patients who have problems are cared for according to the highest standards.

In some cases, for convenience, the allergist/immunologist might work together with a child's primary care doctor so that some or most of the shots can be given by the doctor at his or her office.

Finding an Allergist/Immunologist

A primary care doctor can usually recommend a qualified allergist/immunologist. Or ask a family member or friend who is seeing an allergist/immunologist for a recommendation.

And the website of the American Academy of Allergy, Asthma and Immunology, www.aaaai.org, has a listing of allergists by location.

Helping Your Child Cope

An allergy shot is given with a needle that is smaller than those used for most childhood vaccinations, which makes it less painful. Still, for some kids any shot can seem scary. A parent's positive and supportive attitude can go a long way toward helping a child accept the treatment and achieve successful results. Treatment seems to go much better if the parent is confident and committed to the child getting the immunotherapy.

Allergy shots can seem a bit scary at first. But understanding their benefits and how they work will help you and your child accept them as routine.

Section 41.3

Allergy Shots for Adults

Why an allergist? An allergist is a doctor specially trained and experienced in the diagnosis and treatment of allergic diseases and related conditions. These include asthma, hay fever, sinusitis, rashes, hives, and certain kinds of allergic reactions to foods, insect stings, and drugs.

Every board-certified allergist first completes at least 3 years of specialty training in either internal medicine or pediatrics, and then completes an additional training program of 2 or more years studying the diagnosis and treatment of allergic and related diseases. Certification by the American Board of Allergy and Immunology requires not only approved training, but also successful completion of a challenging written examination. Every board-certified allergist thus has credentials in at least two specialties and is qualified to care for both children and adults.

As a result, the board-certified allergist-immunologist has the advanced training and expertise in the techniques of finding out what is causing an allergic reaction and how best to solve the problem.

Step 1: Consultation

Your first step is to see a board-certified allergist-immunologist. You may be sent by your primary care physician, follow the recommendation of a family member or friend who is seeing an allergist, or contact the American College of Allergy, Asthma and Immunology (ACAAI) to receive a list of allergist members in your area. Call 800-842-7777 or go to http://www.acaai.org/Patients/Pages/locate-an-allergist.aspx.

Some health plans and HMOs [health maintenance organizations] require prior approval to see a specialist. If your request is not immediately honored, ask again and be firm.

Step 2: Testing

Your allergist will obtain a detailed medical history, examine you, and evaluate your symptoms. Tests (perhaps lung function tests or x-rays) will be performed to find out the type of your allergic disease. Skin tests or allergy blood tests may be needed to find out the precise causes of your allergic symptoms. Based on the entire clinical evaluation, a diagnosis is made.

If the allergy tests are negative, the allergist can still help find the cause of your symptoms—do not despair. Allergists are also experts in the treatment of nonallergic asthma, rhinitis, food and drug reactions, and other types of problems of your immune system, like frequent infections.

Step 3: Treatment

This is the step where your allergic symptoms and you get better. Allergy treatments are of three types: prevention, medication, and immunotherapy.

Prevention: Once identified, the cause of the symptoms may be avoided or removed from your life. For example, a particular food can be avoided, or a pet can be removed from the home or kept away from sleeping areas.

Some causes of allergic symptoms, such as pollen, molds, and dust mites, cannot be completely eliminated and are difficult to avoid. Exposure can be reduced, however, by environmental control measures prescribed by your allergist.

Medication: Although prevention comes first, more may be needed. Medications are usually used to decrease allergy symptoms and improve the patient's quality of life, recent advances in medications for asthma and other allergic diseases have been phenomenal. Improvements in drugs have eliminated most of the side effects from older drugs.

The allergy specialist is an expert in the latest safe and effective medications for treating allergic illness.

Immunotherapy (allergy shots): If a specific allergy is identified and it cannot be avoided or medications are not sufficient to restore your health, the allergic symptoms may be controlled or eliminated with allergy shots.

Allergy shots have been used since 1911. In the past century, there has been considerable improvement in the effectiveness of this treatment, which decreases a patient's sensitivity (allergy) to a number of allergens, such as cat or ragweed. The treatment is a method for increasing the allergic patient's natural resistance (tolerance) to the things that are triggering the allergic reactions.

This treatment involves injections of small amounts of purified extracts of the substances that are causing allergic reactions. For example, the extracts may be derived from pollens, mold spores, animal dander, dust mites, or insect venom. The U.S. Food and Drug Administration approve them for this use, and over the years they have been improved considerably.

Allergy shots stimulate the immune system to fight allergies safely, effectively, and naturally. Beginning with small doses and increasing them gradually on a weekly or biweekly basis, the therapy continues until a maintenance level is achieved. Then, a maintenance dose is injected every few weeks.

Immunity does not occur immediately, but some patients do begin to feel better quickly. Most patients are continued on monthly injections for 3 to 5 years once they reach the maintenance dose. In some patients, immunity is maintained and treatment can be stopped after several years. For others, treatment may be needed for longer periods of time. Generally the benefits of allergy shots can last for many years, or even a lifetime.

With the immune system restored to good health, few or no medications may be needed. Work or school days are no longer missed. The burden of allergies is lifted, and allergies become something you just don't think about any more. Candidates for allergy shots include most children and adults. Pregnant patients can continue treatment that was started prior to pregnancy.

Allergy shots are prescribed by an allergist and are always given under medical supervision at a location where medical staff and medications are available to handle any serious reaction. Although rare, serious reactions can occur from allergy shots because the treatment involves the substances to which the patient is known to be allergic.

Adverse reactions can occur from allergy shots because treatment involves the injection of substances to which the patient is sensitized. The most common adverse reaction is an immediate red, itching bump at the injection site. In some cases, a similar delayed reaction can occur 6 to 24 hours later. Rare, more severe reactions include generalized itching, chest tightness/wheezing, or dizziness due to a drop in blood pressure. Deaths have been reported from allergy shots at a rate of approximately one in 3 million injections. This is why allergy shots are given under supervision where medical staff and medications are available to handle serious reactions. As allergists, we feel that the benefits far outweigh the extremely small risk of a serious reaction. It is safe for both children and adults, and even pregnant patients may continue treatment started prior to pregnancy.

The Future

Researchers are now studying ways to go beyond today's treatments. We soon may have better and new ways to block the body's allergic response by reducing or inhibiting the release of histamine and other chemicals that cause allergic reactions. Also, a large group of scientific researchers are working in developing the purest, strongest, and safest vaccines for allergy.

When these treatments become available, you can be certain that allergists-immunologists will be at the forefront of their use.

But you don't have to wait for the future. Today, you can put the misery of allergies out of your life with the help of an allergist.

Chapter 42

Complementary and Alternative Medicine (CAM) for Allergies

Chapter Contents

Section 42.1

Types of CAM Used to Treat Allergies

What is alternative medicine?

Any unproven treatment for an illness or disease is considered an alternative medical approach by most American medical doctors. "Unproven" means there is not enough acceptable scientific evidence to show that the treatment works. The term alternative medicine refers to a wide variety of treatments considered outside "mainstream" or "usual" medical approaches in the United States today.

Many people turn to alternative medicine to help alleviate their asthma or allergy symptoms. These treatment approaches may include, but are not limited to, one or more of the following:

- Acupuncture
- Ayurvedic medicine
- Biofeedback, mental imaging, stress reduction, relaxation techniques
- Chiropractic spinal manipulation
- Diet, exercise, yoga, lifestyle changes
- Herbal medicine, vitamin supplements
- Folk medicine from various cultures
- Laser therapy
- Massage
- Hypnosis
- Art or music therapy

Why do people use alternative medicine?

Recent statistics show that nearly 40 percent of Americans try some form of alternative medicine. Medical and scientific experts do believe that some remedies may be worth a try, providing they are not harmful. In some cases, specific alternative medical treatment may improve or relieve symptoms of a specific illness or disease. Risks should not outweigh the potential benefits.

If you believe a particular alternative medical approach might help reduce your asthma or allergy symptoms, talk with your doctor about it, and how you could integrate that treatment into your overall asthma/allergy management plan.

No one should use alternative medicine without first consulting a board-certified physician. Any alternative medical approach should be used in addition to your normal asthma or allergy management plan.

You should not substitute an alternative medical treatment for your regular medications or treatments. Be especially careful about use of alternative medicine on children. Approaches that are harmless for adults may not be harmless for children!

Does health insurance cover alternative medical treatment?

Health plans vary in what alternative medicine expenses they will pay. Many plans provide coverage for some but not all alternative therapies. If your doctor writes you a prescription for a specific treatment such as acupuncture or massage, you may be more likely to get partial or full reimbursement of the expense. Always check with your insurance provider before assuming the coverage is available.

What are cautions or considerations for people who use alternative medicine?

Beware the placebo effect. If you really want an alternative medical treatment to work, you may think it is working, even if it really isn't. This "placebo effect" often occurs for people using alternative medicine. Symptoms of asthma or allergy also may improve on their own as an illness (like a cold or flu) runs its course. If you use prescribed medications for your allergy or asthma symptoms, it may take time for them to "kick in." So you may simply be feeling better because your medications started working—not because the alternative medicine is working.

Read between the label lines. The federal government requires labels to state how an herb or vitamin may affect the body but labels are not required to carry health warnings. Labels also cannot claim any medical or health benefit. Products often are not properly labeled, especially those imported from other countries. Many people experience toxic—and sometimes deadly—effects from improperly using labeled herbs. Some products contain unnamed medicines such as steroids, anti-inflammatories, or sedatives that act to reduce your symptoms. Other "hidden ingredients" in various products can be dangerous or even lethal. Use products tested for safety and effectiveness.

Follow directions. Never increase the amount or frequency of a dose or use a treatment or device in a different way than recommended. Do not use herbs in combinations. Do not take herbs if you are pregnant or breast-feeding.

Beware of developing allergy symptoms. Allergies to specific plants and other substances (such as latex or nickel) can build up over time. Products you've used for years may suddenly cause mild to serious allergy symptoms, especially if you already are allergic to something. Check to see if new herbs, foods, or other products you plan to use are in the same "family" as your known allergens.

Use quality products and services. Lack of quality standards is a serious problem for people who use various alternative medical treatments. Look for products that list the amount of the active ingredient(s). Make sure people giving you any kind of treatment are properly certified. Ask your pharmacist or health product store manager for recommendations. Research the product or service before you use it.

Consult with your physician before starting any new treatment. This point cannot be stressed enough. If you have symptoms of asthma or allergy, but you have not been diagnosed, consult a board-certified doctor for a proper diagnosis. Do not rely on health product store personnel to help treat undiagnosed symptoms. If you know you have asthma or allergies, again, talk with your doctor about the alternative medicine you want to use—before you try it.

Are there useful alternative therapies for people who have asthma or allergies?

Keep in mind: Alternative therapy is medical treatment for which there is no conclusive, supporting scientific evidence. This does not necessarily mean the treatment is useless or ineffective. You simply must be careful in what you choose and how you use it.

- **Acupuncture:** A technique that involves inserting needles into key points of the body. Evidence suggests that acupuncture may signal the brain to release endorphins. These are hormones made by the body. When released, endorphins can help reduce pain and create a sense of well being. People with asthma or allergy may experience more relaxed or calmer breathing. Users should be aware of the risk of contaminated needles or punctured organs.

- **Biofeedback:** A technique that helps people control involuntary physical responses. Results are mixed, with children and teenagers showing the greatest benefit.

- **Chiropractic spinal manipulation:** A technique that emphasizes manipulation of the spine in order to help the body heal itself.

- **Hypnosis:** An artificially induced dream state that leaves the person open to suggestion, hypnosis is a legitimate technique to help people manage various conditions. Hypnosis might give people with asthma or allergies more self-discipline to follow good health practices.

- **Laser treatment:** A technique that uses high intensity light to shrink swollen tissue or unblock sinuses. Laser therapy may provide temporary relief, but it may also cause scarring or other long-term physical problems.

- **Massage, relaxation techniques, art/music therapy, yoga**

Stress and anxiety may cause your airways to constrict more if you have asthma or allergies. Various techniques can help you relax, reduce anxiety, or control your breathing. The results may provide some benefit in helping you cope with asthma or allergy symptoms. However, evidence is not conclusive that these techniques improve lung function.

Health Reference Series Medical Advisor's Notes and Updates

Several well-done trials have found that chiropractic manipulation does not improve asthma or allergy symptoms.

Section 42.2

Can Probiotics Prevent Reactions?

Advertisers often want us to believe that in order to be healthy we must purge bacteria and viruses from our households. Beneficial bacteria, commonly referred to as probiotics, however, may be useful in preventing the onset and perhaps even treating food allergies.

Probiotics, consisting of live bacteria or their components, are reported to have beneficial effects on overall health by improving the balance of bacteria in the intestines, resulting in better digestion. You have probably seen the ads and commercials for Dannon Yogurt's Activa, which claim that the product aids digestion and prevents bloating. Dairy products, including yogurt, that contain the *Lactobacillus* and *Bifidobacterium* species are major sources of probiotics.

People have known of the benefits of probiotics for over a century, but not until recently have researchers performed controlled clinical trials to study the beneficial effects of probiotics in the treatment of food allergies. The following two studies revealed some promising results:

- **Study 1:** In infants and young children with milk allergy, 2-month treatment with probiotics, along with a milk elimination diet, decreased the severity of their eczema.

- **Study 2:** Expectant mothers were given either probiotics or placebo in pregnancy and during breastfeeding, as were their infants for the first 6 months following birth. At 2 years of age, 23 percent of children were reported to have atopic dermatitis (dermatitis caused by food allergy) in the probiotic-treated group compared with 46 percent in the placebo group, indicating that the probiotic had some effect on the prevention of early atopic disease in infants at high risk.

Although the results of these studies show some potential benefit of probiotics, particularly in preventing the onset of food allergies, even their effectiveness as a preventive is yet to be proven. The theory does make sense, however, and warrants some further study.

Many people with food allergies and parents of children with food allergies hear about probiotics and assume it to be the cure they've been waiting for. They want to know which products are best at preventing food allergies or turning off the immune system once the allergy has developed. Unfortunately, the science is so unclear at this stage that I would be skeptical of anyone's recommendations on specific products. Until more conclusive data are available, stick with the standard treatments that your allergist recommends.

Section 42.3

Chinese Herbal Formula May Be Helpful for Peanut Allergies

"Chinese Herbal Formula May Be Helpful for Peanut Allergies," by the National Center for Complementary and Alternative Medicine (NCCAM, www.nccam.nih.gov), part of the National Institutes of Health, 2007.

A study in mice shows that a Chinese herbal formula may help prevent dangerous reactions to peanuts. Peanut allergies affect as many as 6 percent of young children and are a major cause of anaphylaxis—a severe allergic reaction with respiratory symptoms that can be fatal.

Xiu-Min Li and colleagues at Mount Sinai School of Medicine conducted experiments in mice with established peanut allergies to see if a formula of nine Chinese herbs, called FAHF-2, could reduce sensitivity to peanuts. The peanut-sensitive mice received 7 weeks of oral treatment with FAHF-2 or water as a placebo treatment.

The mice were then exposed to peanuts to see if they would have anaphylactic reactions. They were exposed twice—once one day following the conclusion of FAHF-2 treatment and again 4 weeks after treatment finished.

The researchers found that FAHF-2 completely protected the mice from a dangerous reaction on both occasions—showing that protection lasted at least 4 weeks after the treatment finished. The mice treated with the placebo (water) had anaphylactic reactions. The researchers note that the protection of FAHF-2 may result from a shift in the immune balance away from the allergic response.

Reference

C. Qu, K. Srivastava, X.-M. Li, et al. "Induction of tolerance after establishment of peanut allergy by the food allergy herbal formula-2 is associated with up-regulation of interferon-y." *Clinical and Experimental Allergy,* June 2007.

Part Six

Avoiding Allergy Triggers, Preventing Symptoms, and Getting Support

Chapter 43

Improving Indoor Air Quality and Reducing Environmental Triggers

All of us face a variety of risks to our health as we go about our day-to-day lives. Driving in cars, flying in planes, engaging in recreational activities, and being exposed to environmental pollutants all pose varying degrees of risk. Some risks are simply unavoidable. Some we choose to accept because to do otherwise would restrict our ability to lead our lives the way we want. And some are risks we might decide to avoid if we had the opportunity to make informed choices. Indoor air pollution is one risk that you can do something about.

In the last several years, a growing body of scientific evidence has indicated that the air within homes and other buildings can be more seriously polluted than the outdoor air in even the largest and most industrialized cities. Other research indicates that people spend approximately 90 percent of their time indoors. Thus, for many people, the risks to health may be greater due to exposure to air pollution indoors than outdoors.

In addition, people who may be exposed to indoor air pollutants for the longest periods of time are often those most susceptible to the effects of indoor air pollution. Such groups include the young, the elderly, and the chronically ill, especially those suffering from respiratory or cardiovascular disease.

Excerpted from "The Inside Story: A Guide to Indoor Air Quality," by the Environmental Protection Agency (EPA, www.epa.gov), November 24, 2009.

What Causes Indoor Air Problems?

Indoor pollution sources that release gases or particles into the air are the primary cause of indoor air quality problems in homes. Inadequate ventilation can increase indoor pollutant levels by not bringing in enough outdoor air to dilute emissions from indoor sources and by not carrying indoor air pollutants out of the home. High temperature and humidity levels can also increase concentrations of some pollutants.

There are many sources of indoor air pollution in any home. These include combustion sources such as oil, gas, kerosene, coal, wood, and tobacco products; building materials and furnishings as diverse as deteriorated, asbestos-containing insulation, wet or damp carpet, and cabinetry or furniture made of certain pressed wood products; products for household cleaning and maintenance, personal care, or hobbies; central heating and cooling systems and humidification devices; and outdoor sources such as radon, pesticides, and outdoor air pollution.

The relative importance of any single source depends on how much of a given pollutant it emits and how hazardous those emissions are. In some cases, factors such as how old the source is and whether it is properly maintained are significant. For example, an improperly adjusted gas stove can emit significantly more carbon monoxide than one that is properly adjusted.

Some sources, such as building materials, furnishings, and household products like air fresheners, release pollutants more or less continuously. Other sources, related to activities carried out in the home, release pollutants intermittently. These include smoking, the use of unvented or malfunctioning stoves, furnaces, or space heaters, the use of solvents in cleaning and hobby activities, the use of paint strippers in redecorating activities, and the use of cleaning products and pesticides in housekeeping. High pollutant concentrations can remain in the air for long periods after some of these activities.

If too little outdoor air enters a home, pollutants can accumulate to levels that can pose health and comfort problems. Unless they are built with special mechanical means of ventilation, homes that are designed and constructed to minimize the amount of outdoor air that can "leak" into and out of the home may have higher pollutant levels than other homes. However, because some weather conditions can drastically reduce the amount of outdoor air that enters a home, pollutants can build up even in homes that are normally considered "leaky."

How Does Outdoor Air Enter a House?

Outdoor air enters and leaves a house by infiltration, natural ventilation, and mechanical ventilation. In a process known as infiltration, outdoor air flows into the house through openings, joints, and cracks in walls, floors, and ceilings, and around windows and doors. In natural ventilation, air moves through opened windows and doors. Air movement associated with infiltration and natural ventilation is caused by air temperature differences between indoors and outdoors and by wind. Finally, there are a number of mechanical ventilation devices, from outdoor-vented fans that intermittently remove air from a single room, such as bathrooms and kitchen, to air handling systems that use fans and duct work to continuously remove indoor air and distribute filtered and conditioned outdoor air to strategic points throughout the house. The rate at which outdoor air replaces indoor air is described as the air exchange rate. When there is little infiltration, natural ventilation, or mechanical ventilation, the air exchange rate is low and pollutant levels can increase.

What If You Live in an Apartment?

Apartments can have the same indoor air problems as single-family homes because many of the pollution sources, such as the interior building materials, furnishings, and household products, are similar. Indoor air problems similar to those in offices are caused by such sources as contaminated ventilation systems, improperly placed outdoor air intakes, or maintenance activities.

Solutions to air quality problems in apartments, as in homes and offices, involve such actions as eliminating or controlling the sources of pollution, increasing ventilation, and installing air cleaning devices. Often a resident can take the appropriate action to improve the indoor air quality by removing a source, altering an activity, unblocking an air supply vent, or opening a window to temporarily increase the ventilation; in other cases, however, only the building owner or manager is in a position to remedy the problem.

Indoor Air and Your Health

Health effects from indoor air pollutants may be experienced soon after exposure or, possibly, years later.

Immediate effects may show up after a single exposure or repeated exposures. These include irritation of the eyes, nose, and throat, headaches, dizziness, and fatigue. Such immediate effects are usually short-term and treatable. Sometimes the treatment is simply eliminating the person's exposure to the source of the pollution, if it can be identified. Symptoms of some diseases, including asthma, hypersensitivity pneumonitis, and humidifier fever, may also show up soon after exposure to some indoor air pollutants.

The likelihood of immediate reactions to indoor air pollutants depends on several factors. Age and preexisting medical conditions are two important influences. In other cases, whether a person reacts to a pollutant depends on individual sensitivity, which varies tremendously from person to person. Some people can become sensitized to biological pollutants after repeated exposures, and it appears that some people can become sensitized to chemical pollutants as well.

Certain immediate effects are similar to those from colds or other viral diseases, so it is often difficult to determine if the symptoms are a result of exposure to indoor air pollution. For this reason, it is important to pay attention to the time and place the symptoms occur. If the symptoms fade or go away when a person is away from the home and return when the person returns, an effort should be made to identify indoor air sources that may be possible causes. Some effects may be made worse by an inadequate supply of outdoor air or from the heating, cooling, or humidity conditions prevalent in the home.

Other health effects may show up either years after exposure has occurred or only after long or repeated periods of exposure. These effects, which include some respiratory diseases, heart disease, and cancer, can be severely debilitating or fatal. It is prudent to try to improve the indoor air quality in your home even if symptoms are not noticeable.

While pollutants commonly found in indoor air are responsible for many harmful effects, there is considerable uncertainty about what concentrations or periods of exposure are necessary to produce specific health problems. People also react very differently to exposure to indoor air pollutants. Further research is needed to better understand which health effects occur after exposure to the average pollutant concentrations found in homes and which occur from the higher concentrations that occur for short periods of time.

Identifying Air Quality Problems

Some health effects can be useful indicators of an indoor air quality problem, especially if they appear after a person moves to a new residence, remodels or refurnishes a home, or treats a home with pesticides. If you think that you have symptoms that may be related to your home environment, discuss them with your doctor or your local health department to see if they could be caused by indoor air pollution. You may also want to consult a board-certified allergist or an occupational medicine specialist for answers to your questions.

Another way to judge whether your home has or could develop indoor air problems is to identify potential sources of indoor air pollution. Although the presence of such sources does not necessarily mean that you have an indoor air quality problem, being aware of the type and number of potential sources is an important step toward assessing the air quality in your home.

A third way to decide whether your home may have poor indoor air quality is to look at your lifestyle and activities. Human activities can be significant sources of indoor air pollution. Finally, look for signs of problems with the ventilation in your home. Signs that can indicate your home may not have enough ventilation include moisture condensation on windows or walls, smelly or stuffy air, dirty central heating and air cooling equipment, and areas where books, shoes, or other items become moldy. To detect odors in your home, step outside for a few minutes, and then upon reentering your home, note whether odors are noticeable.

Measuring Pollutant Levels

The federal government recommends that you measure the level of radon in your home. Without measurements there is no way to tell whether radon is present because it is a colorless, odorless, radioactive gas. Inexpensive devices are available for measuring radon. EPA provides guidance as to risks associated with different levels of exposure and when the public should consider corrective action. There are specific mitigation techniques that have proven effective in reducing levels of radon in the home.

For pollutants other than radon, measurements are most appropriate when there are either health symptoms or signs of poor ventilation and specific sources or pollutants have been identified as possible causes of indoor air quality problems. Testing for many pollutants can be expensive. Before monitoring your home for pollutants besides radon, consult your state or local health department or professionals who have experience in solving indoor air quality problems in non-industrial buildings.

Weatherizing Your Home

The federal government recommends that homes be weatherized in order to reduce the amount of energy needed for heating and cooling. While weatherization is underway, however, steps should also be taken to minimize pollution from sources inside the home. In addition, residents should be alert to the emergence of signs of inadequate ventilation, such as stuffy air, moisture condensation on cold surfaces, or mold and mildew growth. Additional weatherization measures should not be undertaken until these problems have been corrected.

Weatherization generally does not cause indoor air problems by adding new pollutants to the air. (There are a few exceptions, such as caulking, that can sometimes emit pollutants.) However, measures such as installing storm windows, weather stripping, caulking, and blown-in wall insulation can reduce the amount of outdoor air infiltrating into a home. Consequently, after weatherization, concentrations of indoor air pollutants from sources inside the home can increase.

Source Control

Usually the most effective way to improve indoor air quality is to eliminate individual sources of pollution or to reduce their emissions. Some sources, like those that contain asbestos, can be sealed or enclosed; others, like gas stoves, can be adjusted to decrease the amount of emissions. In many cases, source control is also a more cost-efficient approach to protecting indoor air quality than increasing ventilation because increasing ventilation can increase energy costs.

Ventilation Improvements

Another approach to lowering the concentrations of indoor air pollutants in your home is to increase the amount of outdoor air coming indoors. Most home heating and cooling systems, including forced air heating systems, do not mechanically bring fresh air into the house. Opening windows and doors, operating window or attic fans, when the weather permits, or running a window air conditioner with the vent control open increases the outdoor ventilation rate. Local bathroom or kitchen fans that exhaust outdoors remove contaminants directly from the room where the fan is located and also increase the outdoor air ventilation rate.

It is particularly important to take as many of these steps as possible while you are involved in short-term activities that can generate high levels of pollutants—for example, painting, paint stripping, heating with kerosene heaters, cooking, or engaging in maintenance and hobby activities such as welding, soldering, or sanding. You might also choose to do some of these activities outdoors, if you can and if weather permits.

Advanced designs of new homes are starting to feature mechanical systems that bring outdoor air into the home. Some of these designs include energy-efficient heat recovery ventilators (also known as air-to-air heat exchangers).

Air Cleaners

There are many types and sizes of air cleaners on the market, ranging from relatively inexpensive table-top models to sophisticated and expensive whole-house systems. Some air cleaners are highly effective at particle removal, while others, including most table-top models, are much less so. Air cleaners are generally not designed to remove gaseous pollutants.

The effectiveness of an air cleaner depends on how well it collects pollutants from indoor air (expressed as a percentage efficiency rate) and how much air it draws through the cleaning or filtering element (expressed in cubic feet per minute). A very efficient collector with a low air-circulation rate will not be effective, nor will a cleaner with a high air-circulation rate but a less efficient collector. The long-term performance of any air cleaner depends on maintaining it according to the manufacturer's directions.

Another important factor in determining the effectiveness of an air cleaner is the strength of the pollutant source. Table-top air cleaners, in particular, may not remove satisfactory amounts of pollutants from strong nearby sources. People with a sensitivity to particular sources may find that air cleaners are helpful only in conjunction with concerted efforts to remove the source.

Over the past few years, there has been some publicity suggesting that houseplants have been shown to reduce levels of some chemicals in laboratory experiments. There is currently no evidence, however, that a reasonable number of houseplants remove significant quantities of pollutants in homes and offices. Indoor houseplants should not be overwatered because overly damp soil may promote the growth of microorganisms, which can affect allergic individuals.

At present, EPA does not recommend using air cleaners to reduce levels of radon and its decay products. The effectiveness of these devices is uncertain because they only partially remove the radon decay products and do not diminish the amount of radon entering the home. EPA plans to do additional research on whether air cleaners are, or could become, a reliable means of reducing the health risk from radon.

For most indoor air quality problems in the home, source control is the most effective solution. This section takes a source-by-source look at the most common indoor air pollutants, their potential health effects, and ways to reduce levels in the home.

A Look at Source-Specific Controls

Radon (Rn)

The most common source of indoor radon is uranium in the soil or rock on which homes are built. As uranium naturally breaks down, it releases radon gas, which is a colorless, odorless, radioactive gas. Radon gas enters homes through dirt floors, cracks in concrete walls and floors, floor drains, and sumps. When radon becomes trapped in buildings and concentrations build up indoors, exposure to radon becomes a concern.

Any home may have a radon problem. This means new and old homes, well-sealed and drafty homes, and homes with or without basements.

Sometimes radon enters the home through well water. In a small number of homes, the building materials can give off radon, too. However, building materials rarely cause radon problems by themselves.

The predominant health effect associated with exposure to elevated levels of radon is lung cancer. Research suggests that swallowing water with high radon levels may pose risks, too, although these are believed to be much lower than those from breathing air containing radon. Major health organizations (like the Centers for Disease Control and Prevention, the American Lung Association [ALA], and the American Medical Association) agree with estimates that radon causes thousands of preventable lung cancer deaths each year. EPA estimates that radon causes about 14,000 deaths per year in the United States—however, this number could range from 7,000 to 30,000 deaths per year. If you smoke and your home has high radon levels, your risk of lung cancer is especially high.

Environmental Tobacco Smoke (ETS)

Environmental tobacco smoke (ETS) is the mixture of smoke that comes from the burning end of a cigarette, pipe, or cigar, and smoke exhaled by the smoker. It is a complex mixture of over 4,000 compounds, more than 40 of which are known to cause cancer in humans or animals and many of which are strong irritants. ETS is often referred to as "secondhand smoke" and exposure to ETS is often called "passive smoking."

In 1992, EPA completed a major assessment of the respiratory health risks of ETS. The report concludes that exposure to ETS is responsible for approximately 3,000 lung cancer deaths each year in nonsmoking adults and impairs the respiratory health of hundreds of thousands of children.

Infants and young children whose parents smoke in their presence are at increased risk of lower respiratory tract infections (pneumonia and bronchitis) and are more likely to have symptoms of respiratory irritation like cough, excess phlegm, and wheeze. EPA estimates that passive smoking annually causes between 150,000 and 300,000 lower respiratory tract infections in infants and children under 18 months of age, resulting in between 7,500 and 15,000 hospitalizations each year. These children may also have a build-up of fluid in the middle ear, which can lead to ear infections. Older children who have been exposed to secondhand smoke may have slightly reduced lung function.

Asthmatic children are especially at risk. EPA estimates that exposure to secondhand smoke increases the number of episodes and severity of symptoms in hundreds of thousands of asthmatic children, and may cause thousands of non-asthmatic children to develop the disease each year. EPA estimates that between 200,000 and 1,000,000 asthmatic children have their condition made worse by exposure to secondhand smoke each year. Exposure to secondhand smoke causes eye, nose, and throat irritation. It may affect the cardiovascular system and some studies have linked exposure to secondhand smoke with the onset of chest pain.

To reduce exposure to environmental tobacco smoke, take the following steps:

- **Don't smoke at home or permit others to do so.** Ask smokers to smoke outdoors. The 1986 Surgeon General's report concluded that physical separation of smokers and nonsmokers in a common air space, such as different rooms within the same house, may reduce—but will not eliminate—non-smokers' exposure to environmental tobacco smoke.

- **If smoking indoors cannot be avoided, increase ventilation in the area where smoking takes place.** Open windows or use exhaust fans. Ventilation, a common method of reducing exposure to indoor air pollutants, also will reduce but not eliminate exposure to environmental tobacco smoke. Because smoking produces such large amounts of pollutants, natural or mechanical ventilation techniques do not remove them from the air in your home as quickly as they build up. In addition, the large increases in ventilation it takes to significantly reduce exposure to environmental tobacco smoke can also increase energy costs substantially. Consequently, the most effective way to reduce exposure to environmental tobacco smoke in the home is to eliminate smoking there.

- **Do not smoke if children are present, particularly infants and toddlers.** Children are particularly susceptible to the effects of passive smoking. Do not allow baby-sitters or others who work in your home to smoke indoors. Discourage others from smoking around children. Find out about the smoking policies of the day care center providers, schools, and other care givers for your children. The policy should protect children from exposure to ETS.

Biological Contaminants

Biological contaminants include bacteria, molds, mildew, viruses, animal dander and cat saliva, house dust mites, cockroaches, and pollen. There are many sources of these pollutants. Pollens originate from plants; viruses are transmitted by people and animals; bacteria are carried by people, animals, and soil and plant debris; and household pets are sources of saliva and animal dander. The protein in urine from rats and mice is a potent allergen. When it dries, it can become airborne. Contaminated central air handling systems can become breeding grounds for mold, mildew, and other sources of biological contaminants and can then distribute these contaminants through the home.

By controlling the relative humidity level in a home, the growth of some sources of biologicals can be minimized. A relative humidity of 30–50 percent is generally recommended for homes. Standing water, water-damaged materials, or wet surfaces also serve as a breeding ground for molds, mildews, bacteria, and insects. House dust mites, the source of one of the most powerful biological allergens, grow in damp, warm environments.

Some biological contaminants trigger allergic reactions, including hypersensitivity pneumonitis, allergic rhinitis, and some types of asthma. Infectious illnesses, such as influenza, measles, and chicken pox are transmitted through the air. Molds and mildews release disease-causing toxins.

Symptoms of health problems caused by biological pollutants include sneezing, watery eyes, coughing, shortness of breath, dizziness, lethargy, fever, and digestive problems. Allergic reactions occur only after repeated exposure to a specific biological allergen. However, that reaction may occur immediately upon re-exposure or after multiple exposures over time. As a result, people who have noticed only mild allergic reactions, or no reactions at all, may suddenly find themselves very sensitive to particular allergens. Some diseases, like humidifier fever, are associated with exposure to toxins from microorganisms that can grow in large building ventilation systems. However, these diseases can also be traced to microorganisms that grow in home heating and cooling systems and humidifiers. Children, elderly people, and people with breathing problems, allergies, and lung diseases are particularly susceptible to disease-causing biological agents in the indoor air.

To reduce exposure to biological contaminants, take the following steps:

- **Install and use exhaust fans that are vented to the outdoors in kitchens and bathrooms and vent clothes dryers outdoors.** These actions can eliminate much of the moisture that builds up from everyday activities. There are exhaust fans on the market that produce little noise, an important consideration for some people. Another benefit to using kitchen and bathroom exhaust fans is that they can reduce levels of organic pollutants that vaporize from hot water used in showers and dishwashers.

- **Ventilate the attic and crawl spaces to prevent moisture build-up.** Keeping humidity levels in these areas below 50 percent can prevent water condensation on building materials.

- **If using cool mist or ultrasonic humidifiers, clean appliances according to manufacturer's instructions and refill with fresh water daily.** Because these humidifiers can become breeding grounds for biological contaminants, they have the potential for causing diseases such as hypersensitivity pneumonitis and humidifier fever. Evaporation trays in air conditioners, dehumidifiers, and refrigerators should also be cleaned frequently.

- **Thoroughly clean and dry water-damaged carpets and building materials (within 24 hours if possible) or consider removal and replacement.** Water-damaged carpets and building materials can harbor mold and bacteria. It is very difficult to completely rid such materials of biological contaminants.

- **Keep the house clean.** House dust mites, pollens, animal dander, and other allergy-causing agents can be reduced, although not eliminated, through regular cleaning. People who are allergic to these pollutants should use allergen-proof mattress encasements, wash bedding in hot (130 degree Fahrenheit) water, and avoid room furnishings that accumulate dust, especially if they cannot be washed in hot water. Allergic individuals should also leave the house while it is being vacuumed because vacuuming can actually increase airborne levels of mite allergens and other biological contaminants. Using central vacuum systems that are vented to the outdoors or vacuums with high efficiency filters may also be of help.

- **Take steps to minimize biological pollutants in basements.**
  Clean and disinfect the basement floor drain regularly. Do not
  finish a basement below ground level unless all water leaks are
  patched and outdoor ventilation and adequate heat to prevent condensation are provided. Operate a dehumidifier in the basement if
  needed to keep relative humidity levels between 30–50 percent.

Stoves, Heaters, Fireplaces, and Chimneys

In addition to environmental tobacco smoke, other sources of combustion products are unvented kerosene and gas space heaters, wood
stoves, fireplaces, and gas stoves. The major pollutants released are
carbon monoxide, nitrogen dioxide, and particles. Unvented kerosene
heaters may also generate acid aerosols.

Combustion gases and particles also come from chimneys and flues
that are improperly installed or maintained and cracked furnace heat
exchangers. Pollutants from fireplaces and wood stoves with no dedicated outdoor air supply can be "back-drafted" from the chimney into
the living space, particularly in weatherized homes.

Carbon monoxide (CO) is a colorless, odorless gas that interferes
with the delivery of oxygen throughout the body. At high concentrations it can cause unconsciousness and death. Lower concentrations
can cause a range of symptoms from headaches, dizziness, weakness,
nausea, confusion, and disorientation, to fatigue in healthy people and
episodes of increased chest pain in people with chronic heart disease.
The symptoms of carbon monoxide poisoning are sometimes confused
with the flu or food poisoning. Fetuses, infants, elderly people, and
people with anemia or with a history of heart or respiratory disease
can be especially sensitive to carbon monoxide exposures.

Nitrogen dioxide (NO_2) is a reddish-brown, irritating odor gas that
irritates the mucous membranes in the eye, nose, and throat and causes
shortness of breath after exposure to high concentrations. There is
evidence that high concentrations or continued exposure to low levels
of nitrogen dioxide increases the risk of respiratory infection; there is
also evidence from animal studies that repeated exposures to elevated
nitrogen dioxide levels may lead, or contribute, to the development of
lung disease such as emphysema. People at particular risk from exposure to nitrogen dioxide include children and individuals with asthma
and other respiratory diseases.

Particles, released when fuels are incompletely burned, can lodge in the
lungs and irritate or damage lung tissue. A number of pollutants, including radon and benzo(a)pyrene, both of which can cause cancer, attach to
small particles that are inhaled and then carried deep into the lung.

To reduce exposure to carbon at home, take the following steps:

- **Take special precautions when operating fuel-burning unvented space heaters.** Consider potential effects of indoor air pollution if you use an unvented kerosene or gas space heater. Follow the manufacturer's directions, especially instructions on the proper fuel and keeping the heater properly adjusted. A persistent yellow-tipped flame is generally an indicator of maladjustment and increased pollutant emissions. While a space heater is in use, open a door from the room where the heater is located to the rest of the house and open a window slightly.

- **Install and use exhaust fans over gas cooking stoves and ranges and keep the burners properly adjusted.** Using a stove hood with a fan vented to the outdoors greatly reduces exposure to pollutants during cooking. Improper adjustment, often indicated by a persistent yellow-tipped flame, causes increased pollutant emissions. Ask your gas company to adjust the burner so that the flame tip is blue. If you purchase a new gas stove or range, consider buying one with pilotless ignition because it does not have a pilot light that burns continuously. Never use a gas stove to heat your home. Always make certain the flue in your gas fireplace is open when the fireplace is in use.

- **Keep wood stove emissions to a minimum.** Choose properly sized new stoves that are certified as meeting EPA emission standards. Make certain that doors in old wood stoves are tight-fitting. Use aged or cured (dried) wood only and follow the manufacturer's directions for starting, stoking, and putting out the fire in wood stoves. Chemicals are used to pressure-treat wood; such wood should never be burned indoors.

- **Have central air handling systems, including furnaces, flues, and chimneys, inspected annually and promptly repair cracks or damaged parts.** Blocked, leaking, or damaged chimneys or flues release harmful combustion gases and particles and even fatal concentrations of carbon monoxide. Strictly follow all service and maintenance procedures recommended by the manufacturer, including those that tell you how frequently to change the filter. If manufacturer's instructions are not readily available, change filters once every month or two during periods of use. Proper maintenance is important even for new furnaces because they can also corrode and leak combustion gases, including carbon monoxide.

Household Products

Organic chemicals are widely used as ingredients in household products. Paints, varnishes, and wax all contain organic solvents, as do many cleaning, disinfecting, cosmetic, degreasing, and hobby products. Fuels are made up of organic chemicals. All of these products can release organic compounds while you are using them, and, to some degree, when they are stored.

EPA's Total Exposure Assessment Methodology (TEAM) studies found levels of about a dozen common organic pollutants to be 2 to 5 times higher inside homes than outside, regardless of whether the homes were located in rural or highly industrial areas. Additional TEAM studies indicate that while people are using products containing organic chemicals, they can expose themselves and others to very high pollutant levels, and elevated concentrations can persist in the air long after the activity is completed.

The ability of organic chemicals to cause health effects varies greatly, from those that are highly toxic, to those with no known health effect. As with other pollutants, the extent and nature of the health effect will depend on many factors including level of exposure and length of time exposed. Eye and respiratory tract irritation, headaches, dizziness, visual disorders, and memory impairment are among the immediate symptoms that some people have experienced soon after exposure to some organics. At present, not much is known about what health effects occur from the levels of organics usually found in homes. Many organic compounds are known to cause cancer in animals; some are suspected of causing, or are known to cause, cancer in humans.

To reduce exposure to household chemicals, take the following steps:

- **Follow label instructions carefully.** Potentially hazardous products often have warnings aimed at reducing exposure of the user. For example, if a label says to use the product in a well-ventilated area, go outdoors or in areas equipped with an exhaust fan to use it. Otherwise, open up windows to provide the maximum amount of outdoor air possible.

- **Throw away partially full containers of old or unneeded chemicals safely.** Because gases can leak even from closed containers, this single step could help lower concentrations of organic chemicals in your home. (Be sure that materials you decide to keep are stored not only in a well-ventilated area but are also safely out of reach of children.) Do not simply toss these unwanted products in the garbage can. Find out if your local government or any organization in your community sponsors special days for the collection of toxic household wastes. If such days are available, use them to dispose of the unwanted containers safely. If no such collection days are available, think about organizing one.

- **Buy limited quantities.** If you use products only occasionally or seasonally, such as paints, paint strippers, and kerosene for space heaters or gasoline for lawn mowers, buy only as much as you will use right away.

- **Keep exposure to emissions from products containing methylene chloride to a minimum.** Consumer products that contain methylene chloride include paint strippers, adhesive removers, and aerosol spray paints. Methylene chloride is known to cause cancer in animals. Also, methylene chloride is converted to carbon monoxide in the body and can cause symptoms associated with exposure to carbon monoxide. Carefully read the labels containing health hazard information and cautions on the proper use of these products. Use products that contain methylene chloride outdoors when possible; use indoors only if the area is well ventilated.

- **Keep exposure to benzene to a minimum.** Benzene is a known human carcinogen. The main indoor sources of this chemical are environmental tobacco smoke, stored fuels and paint supplies, and automobile emissions in attached garages. Actions that will reduce benzene exposure include eliminating smoking within the home, providing for maximum ventilation during painting, and discarding paint supplies and special fuels that will not be used immediately.

- **Keep exposure to perchloroethylene emissions from newly dry-cleaned materials to a minimum.** Perchloroethylene is the chemical most widely used in dry cleaning. In laboratory studies, it has been shown to cause cancer in animals. Recent studies indicate that people breathe low levels of this chemical both in homes where dry-cleaned goods are stored and as they wear dry-cleaned clothing. Dry cleaners recapture the perchloroethylene during the dry-cleaning process so they can save money by re-using it, and they remove more of the chemical during the pressing and finishing processes. Some dry cleaners, however, do not remove as much perchloroethylene as possible all of the time. Taking steps to minimize your exposure to this chemical is prudent. If dry-cleaned goods have a strong chemical odor when you pick them up, do not accept them until they have been properly dried. If goods with a chemical odor are returned to you on subsequent visits, try a different dry cleaner.

Formaldehyde

Formaldehyde is an important chemical used widely by industry to manufacture building materials and numerous household products. It is also a byproduct of combustion and certain other natural processes. Thus, it may be present in substantial concentrations both indoors and outdoors.

Sources of formaldehyde in the home include building materials, smoking, household products, and the use of unvented, fuel-burning appliances, like gas stoves or kerosene space heaters. Formaldehyde, by itself or in combination with other chemicals, serves a number of purposes in manufactured products. For example, it is used to add permanent-press qualities to clothing and draperies, as a component of glues and adhesives, and as a preservative in some paints and coating products.

In homes, the most significant sources of formaldehyde are likely to be pressed wood products made using adhesives that contain urea-formaldehyde (UF) resins.

Pressed wood products made for indoor use include particleboard (used as subflooring and shelving and in cabinetry and furniture); hardwood plywood paneling (used for decorative wall covering and used in cabinets and furniture); and medium density fiberboard (used for drawer fronts, cabinets, and furniture tops). Medium density fiberboard contains a higher resin-to-wood ratio than any other UF pressed wood product and is generally recognized as being the highest formaldehyde-emitting pressed wood product.

Other pressed wood products, such as softwood plywood and flake or oriented strandboard, are produced for exterior construction use and contain the dark, or red/black-colored phenol-formaldehyde (PF) resin. Although formaldehyde is present in both types of resins, pressed woods that contain PF resin generally emit formaldehyde at considerably lower rates than those containing UF resin.

Since 1985, the Department of Housing and Urban Development (HUD) has permitted only the use of plywood and particleboard that conform to specified formaldehyde emission limits in the construction of prefabricated and mobile homes. In the past, some of these homes had elevated levels of formaldehyde because of the large amount of high-emitting pressed wood products used in their construction and because of their relatively small interior space.

The rate at which products like pressed wood or textiles release formaldehyde can change. Formaldehyde emissions will generally decrease as products age. When the products are new, high indoor temperatures or humidity can cause increased release of formaldehyde from these products.

During the 1970s, many homeowners had urea-formaldehyde foam insulation (UFFI) installed in the wall cavities of their homes as an energy conservation measure. However, many of these homes were found to have relatively high indoor concentrations of formaldehyde soon after the UFFI installation. Few homes are now being insulated with this product. Studies show that formaldehyde emissions from UFFI decline with time; therefore, homes in which UFFI was installed many years ago are unlikely to have high levels of formaldehyde now.

Formaldehyde, a colorless, pungent-smelling gas, can cause watery eyes, burning sensations in the eyes and throat, nausea, and difficulty in breathing in some humans exposed at elevated levels (above 0.1 parts per million). High concentrations may trigger attacks in people with asthma. There is evidence that some people can develop a sensitivity to formaldehyde. It has also been shown to cause cancer in animals and may cause cancer in humans.

To reduce exposure to formaldehyde, ask about the formaldehyde content of pressed wood products, including building materials, cabinetry, and furniture before you purchase them. If you experience adverse reactions to formaldehyde, you may want to avoid the use of pressed wood products and other formaldehyde-emitting goods. Even if you do not experience such reactions, you may wish to reduce your exposure as much as possible by purchasing exterior-grade products, which emit less formaldehyde.

Some studies suggest that coating pressed wood products with polyurethane may reduce formaldehyde emissions for some period of time. To be effective, any such coating must cover all surfaces and edges and remain intact. Increase the ventilation and carefully follow the manufacturer instructions while applying these coatings. (If you are sensitive to formaldehyde, check the label contents before purchasing coating products to avoid buying products that contain formaldehyde, as they will emit the chemical for a short time after application.) Maintain moderate temperature and humidity levels and provide adequate ventilation. The rate at which formaldehyde is released is accelerated by heat and may also depend somewhat on the humidity level.

Therefore, the use of dehumidifiers and air conditioning to control humidity and to maintain a moderate temperature can help reduce formaldehyde emissions. (Drain and clean dehumidifier collection trays frequently so that they do not become a breeding ground for microorganisms.) Increasing the rate of ventilation in your home will also help in reducing formaldehyde levels.

Pesticides

According to a recent survey, 75 percent of U.S. households used at least one pesticide product indoors during the past year. Products used most often are insecticides and disinfectants. Another study suggests that 80 percent of most people's exposure to pesticides occurs indoors and that measurable levels of up to a dozen pesticides have been found in the air inside homes. The amount of pesticides found in homes appears to be greater than can be explained by recent pesticide use in those households; other possible sources include contaminated soil or dust that floats or is tracked in from outside, stored pesticide containers, and household surfaces that collect and then release the pesticides.

Pesticides used in and around the home include products to control insects (insecticides), termites (termiticides), rodents (rodenticides), fungi (fungicides), and microbes (disinfectants). They are sold as sprays, liquids, sticks, powders, crystals, balls, and foggers.

In 1990, the American Association of Poison Control Centers reported that some 79,000 children were involved in common household pesticide poisonings or exposures. In households with children under 5 years old, almost one half stored at least one pesticide product within reach of children. EPA registers pesticides for use and requires manufacturers to put information on the label about when and how to use the pesticide. It is important to remember that the "-cide" in pesticides means "to kill." These products can be dangerous if not used properly. In addition to the active ingredient, pesticides are also made up of ingredients that are used to carry the active agent. These carrier agents are called "inerts" in pesticides because they are not toxic to the targeted pest; nevertheless, some inerts are capable of causing health problems.

Both the active and inert ingredients in pesticides can be organic compounds; therefore, both could add to the levels of airborne organics inside homes. Both types of ingredients can cause the effects discussed in this document under "Household Products," however, as with other household products, there is insufficient understanding at present about what pesticide concentrations are necessary to produce these effects.

Exposure to high levels of cyclodiene pesticides, commonly associated with misapplication, has produced various symptoms, including headaches, dizziness, muscle twitching, weakness, tingling sensations, and nausea. In addition, EPA is concerned that cyclodienes might cause long-term damage to the liver and the central nervous system, as well as an increased risk of cancer.

There is no further sale or commercial use permitted for the following cyclodiene or related pesticides: Chlordane, aldrin, dieldrin, and heptachlor. The only exception is the use of heptachlor by utility companies to control fire ants in underground cable boxes.

To reduce exposure to pesticides, take the following steps:

- **Read the label and follow the directions.** It is illegal to use any pesticide in any manner inconsistent with the directions on its label. Unless you have had special training and are certified, never use a pesticide that is restricted to use by state-certified pest control operators. Such pesticides are simply too dangerous for application by a non-certified person. Use only the pesticides approved for use by the general public and then only in recommended amounts; increasing the amount does not offer more protection against pests and can be harmful to you and your plants and pets.

- **Ventilate the area well after pesticide use.** Mix or dilute pesticides outdoors or in a well-ventilated area and only in the amounts that will be immediately needed. If possible, take plants and pets outside when applying pesticides to them.

- **Use non-chemical methods of pest control when possible.** Since pesticides can be found far from the site of their original application, it is prudent to reduce the use of chemical pesticides outdoors as well as indoors. Depending on the site and pest to be controlled, one or more of the following steps can be effective: use of biological pesticides, such as *Bacillus thuringiensis,* for the control of gypsy moths; selection of disease-resistant plants; and frequent washing of indoor plants and pets. Termite damage can be reduced or prevented by making certain that wooden building materials do not come into direct contact with the soil and by storing firewood away from the home. By appropriately fertilizing, watering, and aerating lawns, the need for chemical pesticide treatments of lawns can be dramatically reduced.

- **If you decide to use a pest control company, choose one carefully.** Ask for an inspection of your home and get a written control program for evaluation before you sign a contract. The control program should list specific names of pests to be controlled and chemicals to be used; it should also reflect any of your safety concerns. Insist on a proven record of competence and customer satisfaction.

- **Dispose of unwanted pesticides safely.** If you have unused or partially used pesticide containers you want to get rid of, dispose of them according to the directions on the label or on special household hazardous waste collection days. If there are no such collection days in your community, work with others to organize them.

- **Keep exposure to moth repellents to a minimum.** One pesticide often found in the home is paradichlorobenzene, a commonly used active ingredient in moth repellents. This chemical is known to cause cancer in animals, but substantial scientific uncertainty exists over the effects, if any, of long-term human exposure to paradichlorobenzene. EPA requires that products containing paradichlorobenzene bear warnings such as "avoid breathing vapors" to warn users of potential short-term toxic effects. Where possible, paradichlorobenzene, and items to be protected against moths, should be placed in trunks or other containers that can be stored in areas that are separately ventilated from the home, such as attics and detached garages. Paradichlorobenzene is also the key active ingredient in many air fresheners (in fact, some labels for moth repellents recommend that these same products be used as air fresheners or deodorants). Proper ventilation and basic household cleanliness will go a long way toward preventing unpleasant odors.

What about Carpet?

In recent years, a number of consumers have associated a variety of symptoms with the installation of new carpet. Scientists have not been able to determine whether the chemicals emitted by new carpets are responsible. If you are installing new carpet, you may wish to take the following steps:

- Talk to your carpet retailer. Ask for information on emissions from carpet.

- Ask the retailer to unroll and air out the carpet in a well-ventilated area before installation.

- Ask for low-emitting adhesives if adhesives are needed.

- Consider leaving the premises during and immediately after carpet installation. You may wish to schedule the installation when most family members or office workers are out.

- Be sure the retailer requires the installer to follow the Carpet and Rug Institute's installation guidelines.

- Open doors and windows. Increasing the amount of fresh air in the home will reduce exposure to most chemicals released from carpet. During and after installation, use window fans, room air conditioners, or other mechanical ventilation equipment you may have installed in your house, to exhaust fumes to the outdoors. Keep them running for 48 to 72 hours after the new carpet is installed.

- Contact your carpet retailer if objectionable odors persist.

- Follow the manufacturer's instructions for proper carpet maintenance.

Do You Suspect Your Office has an Indoor Air Problem?

Indoor air quality problems are not limited to homes. In fact, many office buildings have significant air pollution sources. Some of these buildings may be inadequately ventilated. For example, mechanical ventilation systems may not be designed or operated to provide adequate amounts of outdoor air. Finally, people generally have less control over the indoor environment in their offices than they do in their homes. As a result, there has been an increase in the incidence of reported health problems.

A number of well-identified illnesses, such as Legionnaire disease, asthma, hypersensitivity pneumonitis, and humidifier fever, have been directly traced to specific building problems. These are called building-related illnesses. Most of these diseases can be treated, nevertheless, some pose serious risks.

Sometimes, however, building occupants experience symptoms that do not fit the pattern of any particular illness and are difficult to trace to any specific source. This phenomenon has been labeled sick building syndrome. People may complain of one or more of the following symptoms: Dry or burning mucous membranes in the nose, eyes, and throat; sneezing; stuffy or runny nose; fatigue or lethargy; headache; dizziness; nausea; irritability and forgetfulness. Poor lighting, noise, vibration, thermal discomfort, and psychological stress may also cause, or contribute to, these symptoms.

There is no single manner in which these health problems appear. In some cases, problems begin as workers enter their offices and diminish as workers leave; other times, symptoms continue until the illness is treated. Sometimes there are outbreaks of illness among many workers in a single building; in other cases, health symptoms show up only in individual workers.

In the opinion of some World Health Organization experts, up to 30 percent of new or remodeled commercial buildings may have unusually

477

high rates of health and comfort complaints from occupants that may potentially be related to indoor air quality.

Three major reasons for poor indoor air quality in office buildings are the presence of indoor air pollution sources; poorly designed, maintained, or operated ventilation systems; and uses of the building that were unanticipated or poorly planned for when the building was designed or renovated.

As with homes, the most important factor influencing indoor air quality is the presence of pollutant sources. Commonly found office pollutants and their sources include environmental tobacco smoke; asbestos from insulating and fire-retardant building supplies; formaldehyde from pressed wood products; other organics from building materials, carpet, and other office furnishings, cleaning materials and activities, restroom air fresheners, paints, adhesives, copying machines, and photography and print shops; biological contaminants from dirty ventilation systems or water-damaged walls, ceilings, and carpets; and pesticides from pest management practices.

Ventilation Systems

Mechanical ventilation systems in large buildings are designed and operated not only to heat and cool the air, but also to draw in and circulate outdoor air. If they are poorly designed, operated, or maintained, however, ventilation systems can contribute to indoor air problems in several ways.

For example, problems arise when, in an effort to save energy, ventilation systems are not used to bring in adequate amounts of outdoor air. Inadequate ventilation also occurs if the air supply and return vents within each room are blocked or placed in such a way that outdoor air does not actually reach the breathing zone of building occupants. Improperly located outdoor air intake vents can also bring in air contaminated with automobile and truck exhaust, boiler emissions, fumes from dumpsters, or air vented from restrooms.

Finally, ventilation systems can be a source of in door pollution themselves by spreading biological contaminants that have multiplied in cooling towers, humidifiers, dehumidifiers, air conditioners, or the inside surfaces of ventilation duct work.

Use of the Building

Indoor air pollutants can be circulated from portions of the building used for specialized purposes, such as restaurants, print shops, and dry-cleaning stores, into offices in the same building. Carbon monoxide and other components of automobile exhaust can be drawn from underground parking garages through stairwells and elevator shafts into office spaces.

In addition, buildings originally designed for one purpose may end up being converted to use as office space. If not properly modified during building renovations, the room partitions and ventilation system can contribute to indoor air quality problems by restricting air recirculation or by providing an inadequate supply of outdoor air.

What to Do If You Suspect a Problem

If you or others at your office are experiencing health or comfort problems that you suspect may be caused by indoor air pollution, you can do the following:

- Talk with other workers, your supervisor, and union representatives to see if the problems are being experienced by others and urge that a record of reported health complaints be kept by management, if one has not already been established.

- Talk with your own physician and report your problems to the company physician, nurse, or health and safety officer.

- Call your state or local health department or air pollution control agency to talk over the symptoms and possible causes.

- Frequently, indoor air quality problems in large commercial buildings cannot be effectively identified or remedied without a comprehensive building investigation. These investigations may start with written questionnaires and telephone consultations in which building investigators assess the history of occupant symptoms and building operation procedures. In some cases, these inquiries may quickly uncover the problem and on-site visits are unnecessary. More often, however, investigators will need to come to the building to conduct personal interviews with occupants, to look for possible sources of the problems, and to inspect the design and operation of the ventilation system and other building features. Because taking measurements of pollutants at the very low levels often found in office buildings is expensive and may not yield information readily useful in identifying problem sources, investigators may not take many measurements. The process of solving indoor air quality problems that result in health and comfort complaints can be a slow one, involving several trial solutions before successful remedial actions are identified.

- If a professional company is hired to conduct a building investigation, select a company on the basis of its experience in identifying and solving indoor air quality problems in non-industrial buildings.

- Work with others to establish a smoking policy that eliminates involuntary nonsmoker exposure to environmental tobacco smoke.

Call the National Institute for Occupational Safety and Health (NIOSH) for information on obtaining a health hazard evaluation of your office (800-35NIOSH), or contact the Occupational Safety and Health Administration at 202-219-8151.

Chapter 44

Guide to Air Cleaners in the Home

Indoor air pollutants are unwanted, sometimes harmful materials in the air. Indoor air pollution is among the top five environmental health risks. Usually the best way to address this risk is to control or eliminate the sources of pollutants, and to ventilate a home with clean outdoor air. The ventilation method may, however, be limited by weather conditions or undesirable levels of contaminants contained in outdoor air. If these measures are insufficient, an air cleaning device may be useful. Air cleaning devices are intended to remove pollutants from indoor air. Some air cleaning devices are designed to be installed in the ductwork of a home's central heating, ventilating, and air-conditioning (HVAC) system to clean the air in the whole house. Portable room air cleaners can be used to clean the air in a single room or specific areas, but they are not intended for whole-house filtration.

Indoor Air Pollutants

Pollutants that can affect air quality in a home fall into the following categories:

- Particulate matter includes dust, smoke, pollen, animal dander, tobacco smoke, particles generated from combustion appliances such as cooking stoves, and particles associated with tiny organisms such as dust mites, molds, bacteria, and viruses.

Excerpted from "Guide to Air Cleaners in the Home," by the Environmental Protection Agency (EPA, www.epa.gov), May 2008.

- Gaseous pollutants come from combustion processes. Sources include gas cooking stoves, vehicle exhaust, and tobacco smoke. They also come from building materials, furnishings, and the use of products such as adhesives, paints, varnishes, cleaning products, and pesticides.

Understanding the Types of Air Cleaning Devices

Before deciding whether to use an air cleaning device, several questions should be considered:

- What types of pollutants can an air cleaner remove?
- How is the performance of an air cleaner measured?
- Will air cleaning reduce adverse health effects?
- What other factors should I consider?

What Types of Pollutants Can an Air Cleaner Remove?

There are several types of air cleaning devices available, each designed to remove certain types of pollutants.

Particle Removal

Two types of air cleaning devices can remove particles from the air—mechanical air filters and electronic air cleaners. Mechanical air filters remove particles by capturing them on filter materials. High efficiency particulate air (HEPA) filters are in this category. Electronic air cleaners such as electrostatic precipitators use a process called electrostatic attraction to trap charged particles. They draw air through an ionization section where particles obtain an electrical charge. The charged particles then accumulate on a series of flat plates called a collector that is oppositely charged. Ion generators, or ionizers, disperse charged ions into the air, similar to the electronic air cleaners but without a collector. These ions attach to airborne particles, giving them a charge so that they attach to nearby surfaces such as walls or furniture, or attach to one another and settle faster.

Gaseous Pollutant Removal

Gas-phase air filters remove gases and odors by using a material called a sorbent, such as activated carbon, which adsorbs the pollutants. These filters are typically intended to remove one or more gaseous

482

pollutants from the airstream that passes through them. Because gas-phase filters are specific to one or a limited number of gaseous pollutants, they will not reduce concentrations of pollutants for which they were not designed. Some air cleaning devices with gas-phase filters may remove a portion of the gaseous pollutants and some of the related hazards, at least on a temporary basis. However, none are expected to remove all of the gaseous pollutants present in the air of a typical home. For example, carbon monoxide is a dangerous gaseous pollutant that is produced whenever any fuel such as gas, oil, kerosene, wood, or charcoal is burned, and it is not readily captured using currently available residential gas-phase filtration products.

Pollutant Destruction

Some air cleaners use ultraviolet (UV) light technology intended to destroy pollutants in indoor air. These air cleaners are called ultraviolet germicidal irradiation (UVGI) cleaners and photocatalytic oxidation (PCO) cleaners. Ozone generators that are sold as air cleaners intentionally produce ozone gas, a lung irritant, to destroy pollutants.

- UVGI cleaners use ultraviolet radiation from UV lamps that may destroy biological pollutants such as viruses, bacteria, allergens, and molds that are airborne or growing on HVAC surfaces (e.g., found on cooling coils, drain pans, or ductwork). If used, they should be applied with, but not as a replacement for, filtration systems.

- PCO cleaners use a UV lamp along with a substance, called a catalyst, that reacts with the light. They are intended to destroy gaseous pollutants by converting them into harmless products, but are not designed to remove particulate pollutants.

- Ozone generators use UV light or an electrical discharge to intentionally produce ozone. Ozone is a lung irritant that can cause adverse health effects. At concentrations that do not exceed public health standards, ozone has little effect in removing most indoor air contaminants. Thus, ozone generators are not always safe and effective in controlling indoor air pollutants. Consumers should instead use methods proven to be both safe and effective to reduce pollutant concentrations, which include eliminating or controlling pollutant sources and increasing outdoor air ventilation.

In addition to understanding the different types of air cleaning devices, consumers should consider their performance, as explained in the following text.

How Is the Performance of an Air Cleaner Measured?

There are different ways to measure how well air cleaning devices work, which depend on the type of device and the basic configuration. Air cleaning devices are configured either in the ductwork of HVAC systems (i.e., in-duct) or as portable air cleaners.

In-Duct Particle Removal

Most mechanical air filters are good at capturing larger airborne particles, such as dust, pollen, dust mite and cockroach allergens, some molds, and animal dander. However, because these particles settle rather quickly, air filters are not very good at removing them completely from indoor areas. Although human activities such as walking and vacuuming can stir up particles, most of the larger particles will resettle before an air filter can remove them.

Consumers can select a particle removal air filter by looking at its efficiency in removing airborne particles from the air stream that passes through it. This efficiency is measured by the minimum efficiency reporting value (MERV) for air filters installed in the ductwork of HVAC systems. The American Society of Heating, Refrigerating and Air-Conditioning Engineers, or ASHRAE developed this measurement method. MERV ratings (ranging from a low of 1 to a high of 20) also allow comparison of air filters made by different companies.

- **Flat or panel air filters with a MERV of 1 to 4 are commonly used in residential furnaces and air conditioners:** For the most part, such filters are used to protect the HVAC equipment from the buildup of unwanted materials on the surfaces such as fan motors and heating or cooling coils, and not for direct indoor air quality reasons. They have low efficiency on smaller airborne particles and medium efficiency on larger particles, as long as they remain airborne and pass through the filter. Some smaller particles found within a house include viruses, bacteria, some mold spores, a significant fraction of cat and dog allergens, and a small portion of dust mite allergens.

- **Pleated or extended surface filters:** Medium efficiency filters with a MERV of 5 to 13 are reasonably efficient at removing small to large airborne particles. Filters with a MERV between 7 and 13 are likely to be nearly as effective as true HEPA filters at controlling most airborne indoor particles. Medium efficiency air filters are generally less expensive than

HEPA filters, and allow quieter HVAC fan operation and higher airflow rates than HEPA filters since they have less airflow resistance. Higher efficiency filters with a MERV of 14 to 16, sometimes misidentified as HEPA filters, are similar in appearance to true HEPA filters, which have MERV values of 17 to 20. True HEPA filters are normally not installed in residential HVAC systems; installation of a HEPA filter in an existing HVAC system would probably require professional modification of the system. A typical residential air handling unit and the associated ductwork would not be able to accommodate such filters because of their physical dimensions and increase in airflow resistance.

Some residential HVAC systems may not have enough fan or motor capacity to accommodate higher efficiency filters. Therefore, the HVAC manufacturer's information should be checked prior to upgrading filters to determine whether it is feasible to use more efficient filters. Specially built high performance homes may occasionally be equipped with true HEPA filters installed in a properly designed HVAC system.

There is no standard measurement for the effectiveness of electronic air cleaners. While they may remove small particles, they may be ineffective in removing large particles. Electronic air cleaners can produce ozone—a lung irritant. The amount of ozone produced varies among models. Electronic air cleaners may also produce ultrafine particles resulting from reaction of ozone with indoor chemicals such as those coming from household cleaning products, air fresheners, certain paints, wood flooring, or carpets. Ultrafine particles may be linked with adverse health effects in some sensitive populations.

In-Duct Gaseous Pollutant Removal

Although there is no standard measurement for the effectiveness of gas-phase air filters, ASHRAE is developing a standard method to be used in choosing gas-phase filters installed in home HVAC systems. Gas-phase filters are much less commonly used in homes than particle air filters. The useful lifetime of gas-phase filters can be short because the filter material can quickly become overloaded and may need to be replaced often. There is also concern that, when full, these filters may release trapped pollutants back into the air. Finally, a properly designed and built gas-phase filtration system would be unlikely to fit in a typical home HVAC system or portable air cleaner.

In-Duct Pollutant Destruction

There is no standard measurement for the effectiveness of UVGI cleaners. Typical UVGI cleaners used in homes have limited effectiveness in killing bacteria and molds. Effective destruction of some viruses and most mold and bacterial spores usually requires much higher UV exposure than is provided in a typical home unit. Furthermore, dead mold spores can still produce allergic reactions, so UVGI cleaners may not be effective in reducing allergy and asthma symptoms.

There is no standard measurement for the effectiveness of PCO cleaners. The use of PCO cleaners in homes is limited because currently available catalysts are ineffective in destroying gaseous pollutants from indoor air. Some PCO cleaners fail to destroy pollutants completely and instead produce new indoor pollutants that may cause irritation of the eyes, throat, and nose.

Portable Air Cleaners

Portable air cleaners generally contain a fan to circulate the air and use one or more of the air cleaning devices already discussed. Portable air cleaners may be moved from room to room and used when continuous and localized air cleaning is needed. They may be an option if a home is not equipped with a central HVAC system or forced air heating system.

Portable air cleaners can be evaluated by their effectiveness in reducing airborne pollutants. This effectiveness is measured by the clean air delivery rate, or CADR, developed by the Association of Home Appliance Manufacturers, or AHAM. The CADR is a measure of a portable air cleaner's delivery of contaminant-free air, expressed in cubic feet per minute. For example, if an air cleaner has a CADR of 250 for dust particles, it may reduce dust particle levels to the same concentration as would be achieved by adding 250 cubic feet of clean air each minute. While a portable air cleaner may not achieve its rated CADR under all circumstances, the CADR value does allow comparison across different portable air cleaners.

Many of the portable air cleaners tested by AHAM have moderate to large CADR ratings for small particles. However, for typical room sizes, most portable air cleaners currently on the market do not have high enough CADR values to effectively remove large particles such as pollen, dust mite, and cockroach allergens. Some portable air cleaners using electronic air cleaners might produce ozone, which is a lung irritant. AHAM has a portable air cleaner certification program, and provides a complete listing of all certified cleaners with their CADR values on its website at www.cadr.org.

Will Air Cleaning Reduce Adverse Health Effects?

The ability to remove particles, including microorganisms, is not, in itself, an indication of the ability of an air cleaning device to reduce adverse health effects from indoor pollutants. The use of air cleaning devices may help to reduce levels of smaller airborne allergens or particles. However, air cleaners may not reduce adverse health effects completely in sensitive population such as children, the elderly, and people with asthma and allergies. For example, the evidence is weak that air cleaning devices are effective in reducing asthma symptoms associated with small particles that remain in the air, such as those from some airborne cat dander and dust mite allergens. Larger particles, which may contain allergens, settle rapidly before they can be removed by filtration, so effective allergen control measures require washing sheets weekly, frequent vacuuming of carpets and furniture, and dusting and cleaning of hard surfaces. There are no studies to date linking gas-phase filtration, UVGI, and PCO systems in homes to reduced health symptoms in sensitive populations.

Additional Factors to Consider

When making decisions about using air cleaning devices, consumers should also consider the following:

- **Installation:** In-duct air cleaning devices have certain installation requirements that must be met, such as sufficient access for inspection during use, repairs, or maintenance.

- **Major costs:** These include the initial purchase, maintenance (such as cleaning or replacing filters and parts), and operation (such as electricity).

- **Odors:** Air cleaning devices designed for particle removal are incapable of controlling gases and some odors. The odor and many of the carcinogenic gas-phase pollutants from tobacco smoke will still remain.

- **Soiling of walls and other surfaces:** Ion generators generally are not designed to remove the charged particles that they generate from the air. These charged particles may deposit on room surfaces, soiling walls and other surfaces.

- **Noise:** Noise may be a problem with portable air cleaners containing a fan. Portable air cleaners without a fan are typically much less effective than units with a fan.

Conclusion

Indoor air pollution is among the top five environmental health risks. The best way to address this risk is to control or eliminate the sources of pollutants, and to ventilate a home with clean outdoor air. The ventilation method may, however, be limited by weather conditions or undesirable levels of contaminants in outdoor air. If these measures are insufficient, an air cleaning device may be useful. While air cleaning devices may help to control the levels of airborne allergens, particles, or, in some cases, gaseous pollutants in a home, they may not decrease adverse health effects from indoor air pollutants.

Chapter 45

Cleaning up Mold in Your Home

Why is mold growing in my home?

Molds are part of the natural environment. Outdoors, molds play a part in nature by breaking down dead organic matter such as fallen leaves and dead trees, but indoors, mold growth should be avoided. Molds reproduce by means of tiny spores; the spores are invisible to the naked eye and float through outdoor and indoor air. Mold may begin growing indoors when mold spores land on surfaces that are wet. There are many types of mold, and none of them will grow without water or moisture.

Can mold cause health problems?

Molds are usually not a problem indoors, unless mold spores land on a wet or damp spot and begin growing. Molds have the potential to cause health problems. Molds produce allergens (substances that can cause allergic reactions), irritants, and in some cases, potentially toxic substances (mycotoxins).

Inhaling or touching mold or mold spores may cause allergic reactions in sensitive individuals. Allergic responses include hay fever-type symptoms, such as sneezing, runny nose, red eyes, and skin rash (dermatitis). Allergic reactions to mold are common. They can be immediate

From "A Brief Guide to Mold, Moisture, and Your Home," by the Environmental Protection Agency (EPA, www.epa.gov), 2002. Reviewed by David A. Cooke, MD, FACP, August 10, 2010.

or delayed. Molds can also cause asthma attacks in people with asthma who are allergic to mold. In addition, mold exposure can irritate the eyes, skin, nose, throat, and lungs of both mold-allergic and non-allergic people. Symptoms other than the allergic and irritant types are not commonly reported as a result of inhaling mold.

Research on mold and health effects is ongoing. This text provides a brief overview; it does not describe all potential health effects related to mold exposure. For more detailed information consult a health professional. You may also wish to consult your state or local health department.

How do I get rid of mold?

It is impossible to get rid of all mold and mold spores indoors; some mold spores will be found floating through the air and in house dust. The mold spores will not grow if moisture is not present. Indoor mold growth can and should be prevented or controlled by controlling moisture indoors. If there is mold growth in your home, you must clean up the mold and fix the water problem. If you clean up the mold, but don't fix the water problem, then, most likely, the mold problem will come back.

Who should do the cleanup?

Who should do the cleanup depends on a number of factors. One consideration is the size of the mold problem. If the moldy area is less than about 10 square feet (less than roughly a 3-foot by 3-foot patch), in most cases, you can handle the job yourself, following the guidelines below. However:

- If there has been a lot of water damage, and/or mold growth covers more than 10 square feet, consult the U.S. Environmental Protection Agency (EPA) for information.

- If you choose to hire a contractor (or other professional service provider) to do the cleanup, make sure the contractor has experience cleaning up mold. Check references and ask the contractor to follow the recommendations in EPA's Mold Remediation in Schools and Commercial Buildings, the guidelines of the American Conference of Governmental Industrial Hygienists (ACGIH), or other guidelines from professional or government organizations.

- If you suspect that the heating/ventilation/air conditioning (HVAC) system may be contaminated with mold (it is part of an identified moisture problem, for instance, or there is mold near the intake to the system), do not run the HVAC system if you know or suspect that it is contaminated with mold—it could spread mold throughout the building.

- If the water and/or mold damage was caused by sewage or other contaminated water, then call in a professional who has experience cleaning and fixing buildings damaged by contaminated water.

- If you have health concerns, consult a health professional before starting cleanup.

What are some tips and techniques?

The tips and techniques presented here will help you clean up your mold problem. Professional cleaners or remediators may use methods not covered in this publication. Please note that mold may cause staining and cosmetic damage. It may not be possible to clean an item so that its original appearance is restored.

- Fix plumbing leaks and other water problems as soon as possible. Dry all items completely.

- Scrub mold off hard surfaces with detergent and water, and dry completely.

- Absorbent or porous materials, such as ceiling tiles and carpet, may have to be thrown away if they become moldy. Mold can grow on or fill in the empty spaces or crevices of porous materials, so the mold may be difficult or impossible to remove completely.

- Avoid exposing yourself or others to mold.

- Do not paint or caulk moldy surfaces. Clean up the mold and dry the surfaces before painting. Paint applied over moldy surfaces is likely to peel.

- If you are unsure about how to clean an item, or if the item is expensive or of sentimental value, you may wish to consult a specialist. Specialists in furniture repair, restoration, painting, art restoration and conservation, carpet and rug cleaning, water damage, and fire or water restoration are commonly listed in phone books. Be sure to ask for and check references. Look for specialists who are affiliated with professional organizations.

- Avoid breathing in mold or mold spores. In order to limit your exposure to airborne mold, you may want to wear an N-95 respirator, available at many hardware stores and from companies that advertise on the internet. (They cost about $12 to $25.) Some N-95 respirators resemble a paper dust mask with a nozzle on the front, others are made primarily of plastic or rubber and have removable cartridges that trap most of the mold spores from entering. In order to be effective, the respirator or mask must fit properly, so carefully follow the instructions supplied with the respirator.

- Wear gloves. Long gloves that extend to the middle of the forearm are recommended. When working with water and a mild detergent, ordinary household rubber gloves may be used. If you are using a disinfectant, a biocide such as chlorine bleach, or a strong cleaning solution, you should select gloves made from natural rubber, neoprene, nitrile, polyurethane, or PVC. Avoid touching mold or moldy items with your bare hands.

- Wear goggles. Goggles that do not have ventilation holes are recommended. Avoid getting mold or mold spores in your eyes.

How do I know when the remediation or cleanup is finished?

You must have completely fixed the water or moisture problem before the cleanup or remediation can be considered finished.

- You should have completed mold removal. Visible mold and moldy odors should not be present. Please note that mold may cause staining and cosmetic damage.

- You should have revisited the site(s) shortly after cleanup and it should show no signs of water damage or mold growth.

- People should have been able to occupy or re-occupy the area without health complaints or physical symptoms.

- Ultimately, this is a judgment call; there is no easy answer. If you have concerns or questions call the EPA Indoor Air Quality Information Clearinghouse at 800-438-4318.

How can I control moisture?

- When water leaks or spills occur indoors, act quickly. If wet or damp materials or areas are dried 24–48 hours after a leak or spill happens, in most cases mold will not grow.

- Clean and repair roof gutters regularly.

- Make sure the ground slopes away from the building foundation, so that water does not enter or collect around the foundation.

- Keep air conditioning drip pans clean and the drain lines unobstructed and flowing properly.

- Keep indoor humidity low. If possible, keep indoor humidity below 60 percent (ideally between 30 and 50 percent) relative humidity. Relative humidity can be measured with a moisture or humidity meter, a small, inexpensive ($10–$50) instrument available at many hardware stores.

- If you see condensation or moisture collecting on windows, walls, or pipes—act quickly to dry the wet surface and reduce the moisture/water source.

Condensation can be a sign of high humidity. Actions that will help to reduce humidity include the following:

- Vent appliances that produce moisture, such as clothes dryers, stoves, and kerosene heaters to the outside where possible. (Combustion appliances such as stoves and kerosene heaters produce water vapor and will increase the humidity unless vented to the outside.)

- Use air conditioners and/or dehumidifiers when needed.

- Run the bathroom fan or open the window when showering. Use exhaust fans or open windows whenever cooking, running the dishwasher, or dishwashing, etc.

Actions that will help prevent condensation include the following:

- Reduce the humidity.

- Increase ventilation or air movement by opening doors and/or windows, when practical. Use fans as needed.

- Cover cold surfaces, such as cold water pipes, with insulation.

- Increase air temperature.

Renters: Report all plumbing leaks and moisture problems immediately to your building owner, manager, or superintendent. In cases where persistent water problems are not addressed, you may want to contact local, state, or federal health or housing authorities.

How do I test for mold?

In most cases, if visible mold growth is present, sampling is unnecessary. Since no EPA or other federal limits have been set for mold or mold spores, sampling cannot be used to check a building's compliance with federal mold standards. Surface sampling may be useful to determine if an area has been adequately cleaned or remediated. Sampling

493

for mold should be conducted by professionals who have specific experience in designing mold sampling protocols, sampling methods, and interpreting results. Sample analysis should follow analytical methods recommended by the American Industrial Hygiene Association (AIHA), the American Conference of Governmental Industrial Hygienists (ACGIH), or other professional organizations.

What if I suspect hidden mold?

You may suspect hidden mold if a building smells moldy, but you cannot see the source, or if you know there has been water damage and residents are reporting health problems. Mold may be hidden in places such as the backside of dry wall, wallpaper, or paneling, the top side of ceiling tiles, the underside of carpets and pads, etc. Other possible locations of hidden mold include areas inside walls around pipes (with leaking or condensing pipes), the surface of walls behind furniture (where condensation forms), inside ductwork, and in roof materials above ceiling tiles (due to roof leaks or insufficient insulation).

Investigating hidden mold problems may be difficult and will require caution when the investigation involves disturbing potential sites of mold growth. For example, removal of wallpaper can lead to a massive release of spores if there is mold growing on the underside of the paper. If you believe that you may have a hidden mold problem, consider hiring an experienced professional.

How do I clean up with biocides?

Biocides are substances that can destroy living organisms. The use of a chemical or biocide that kills organisms such as mold (chlorine bleach, for example) is not recommended as a routine practice during mold cleanup. There may be instances, however, when professional judgment may indicate its use (for example, when immune-compromised individuals are present). In most cases, it is not possible or desirable to sterilize an area; a background level of mold spores will remain—these spores will not grow if the moisture problem has been resolved. If you choose to use disinfectants or biocides, always ventilate the area and exhaust the air to the outdoors. Never mix chlorine bleach solution with other cleaning solutions or detergents that contain ammonia because toxic fumes could be produced.

Please note: Dead mold may still cause allergic reactions in some people, so it is not enough to simply kill the mold, it must also be removed.

Chapter 46

Avoiding Skin Allergies: Choosing Safe Cosmetics

What are cosmetics? How are they different from over-the-counter (OTC) drugs?

Cosmetics are products people use to cleanse or change the look of the face or body.

Cosmetic products include the following:

- Skin creams
- Lotions
- Perfumes
- Lipsticks
- Fingernail polishes
- Eye and face makeup products
- Permanent waves
- Hair dyes
- Toothpastes
- Deodorants

Unlike drugs, which are used to treat or prevent disease in the body, cosmetics do not change or affect the body's structure or functions.

Excerpted from "Cosmetics and Your Health," by the Office on Women's Health (www.womenshealth.gov), November 1, 2004. Reviewed by David A. Cooke, MD, FACP, August 10, 2010.

What's in cosmetics?

Fragrances and preservatives are the main ingredients in cosmetics. Fragrances are the most common cause of skin problems. More than 5,000 different kinds are used in products. Products marked "fragrance-free" or "without perfume" means that no fragrances have been added to make the product smell good.

Preservatives in cosmetics are the second most common cause of skin problems. They prevent bacteria and fungus from growing in the product and protect products from damage caused by air or light. But preservatives can also cause the skin to become irritated and infected. Some examples of preservatives are the following:

- Paraben
- Imidazolidinyl urea
- Quaternium-15
- DMDM [dimethylimidazolidine-2,4-dione] hydantoin
- Phenoxyethanol
- Formaldehyde

The ingredients below cannot be used, or their use is limited, in cosmetics. They may cause cancer or other serious health problems.

- Bithionol
- Mercury compounds
- Vinyl chloride
- Halogenated salicylanilides
- Zirconium complexes in aerosol sprays
- Chloroform
- Methylene chloride
- Chlorofluorocarbon propellants
- Hexachlorophene

Are cosmetics safe?

Yes, for the most part. Serious problems from cosmetics are rare. But sometimes problems can happen.

The most common injury from cosmetics is from scratching the eye with a mascara wand. Eye infections can result if the scratches go untreated. These infections can lead to ulcers on the cornea (clear covering of the eye), loss of lashes, or even blindness. To play it safe, never try to apply mascara while riding in a car, bus, train, or plane.

Sharing makeup can also lead to serious problems. Cosmetic brushes and sponges pick up bacteria from the skin. And if you moisten brushes with saliva, the problem can be worse. Washing your hands before using makeup will help prevent this problem.

Sleeping while wearing eye makeup can cause problems, too. If mascara flakes into your eyes while you sleep, you might wake up with itching, bloodshot eyes, infections, or eye scratches. So be sure to remove all makeup before going to bed.

Cosmetic products that come in aerosol containers also can be a hazard. For example, it is dangerous to use aerosol hairspray near heat, fire, or while smoking. Until hairspray is fully dry, it can catch on fire and cause serious burns. Fires related to hairsprays have caused injuries and death. Aerosol sprays or powders also can cause lung damage if they are deeply inhaled into the lungs.

How can I protect myself against the dangers of cosmetics?

- Never drive and put on makeup. Not only does this make driving a danger, hitting a bump in the road and scratching your eyeball can cause serious eye injury.

- Never share makeup. Always use a new sponge when trying products at a store. Insist that salespersons clean container openings with alcohol before applying to your skin.

- Keep makeup containers closed tight when not in use.

- Keep makeup out of the sun and heat. Light and heat can kill the preservatives that help to fight bacteria. Don't keep cosmetics in a hot car for a long time.

- Don't use cosmetics if you have an eye infection, such as pinkeye.

- Throw away any makeup you were using when you first found the problem.

- Never add liquid to a product unless the label tells you to do so.

- Throw away any makeup if the color changes, or it starts to smell.

- Never use aerosol sprays near heat or while smoking, because they can catch on fire.

- Don't deeply inhale hairsprays or powders. This can cause lung damage.

• Avoid color additives that are not approved for use in the eye area, such as "permanent" eyelash tints and kohl (color additive that contains lead salts and is still used in eye cosmetics in other countries). Be sure to keep kohl away from children. It may cause lead poisoning.

What are "cosmeceuticals?"

Some products can be both cosmetics and drugs. This may happen when a product has two uses. For example, a shampoo is a cosmetic because it's used to clean the hair. But an anti-dandruff treatment is a drug because it's used to treat dandruff. So an antidandruff shampoo is both a cosmetic and a drug. Other examples are the following:

• Toothpastes that contain fluoride

• Deodorants that are also antiperspirants

• Moisturizers and makeup that provide sun protection

These products must meet the standards for both cosmetics (color additives) and drugs.

Some cosmetic makers use the term "cosmeceutical" to refer to products that have drug-like benefits. The U.S. Food and Drug Administration (FDA) does not recognize this term. A product can be a drug, a cosmetic, or a combination of both. But the term "cosmeceutical" has no meaning under the law.

While drugs are reviewed and approved by FDA, FDA does not approve cosmetics. If a product acts like a drug, FDA must approve it as a drug.

What are hypoallergenic cosmetics?

Hypoallergenic cosmetics are products that makers claim cause fewer allergic reactions than other products.

Women with sensitive skin, and even those with "normal" skin, may think these products will be gentler. But there are no federal standards for using the term hypoallergenic. The term can mean whatever a company wants it to mean. Cosmetic makers do not have to prove their claims to the FDA.

Some products that have "natural" ingredients can cause allergic reactions. If you have an allergy to certain plants or animals, you could have an allergic reaction to cosmetics with those things in them. For example, lanolin from sheep wool is found in many lotions. But it's a common cause of allergies, too.

Are tattoos and permanent makeup safe?

FDA is looking into the safety of tattoos and permanent makeup since they are now more popular. The inks, or dyes, used for tattoos are color additives. Right now, no color additives have been approved for tattoos, including those used in permanent makeup.

You should be aware of these risks of tattoos and permanent makeup:

- Tattoo needles and supplies can transmit diseases, such as hepatitis C and HIV [human immunodeficiency virus]. Be sure all needles and supplies are sterile before they are used on you.

- Tattoos and permanent makeup are not easy to take off. Removal may cause a permanent change in color.

- Think carefully before getting a tattoo. You could have an allergic reaction.

- You cannot make blood donations for a year after getting a tattoo or permanent makeup.

Are cosmetic products with alpha hydroxy acids safe?

Alpha hydroxy acids (AHAs) come from fruit and milk sugars. They are found in many creams and lotions. Many people buy products with AHAs, because they claim to reduce wrinkles, spots, sun-damaged skin, and other signs of aging. Some studies suggest they may work.

But are these products safe? FDA has received reports of reactions in people using AHA products. Their complaints include the following:

- Severe redness
- Swelling (especially in the area of the eyes)
- Burning
- Blistering
- Bleeding
- Rash
- Itching
- Skin discoloration

AHAs may also increase your skin's risk of sunburn. To find out if a product contains an AHA, look on the list of ingredients. By law, all cosmetics have ingredients on their outer label. AHAs may be called other names, like glycolic acid and lactic acid.

What precautions should I follow when using AHA products?

If you want to use AHA products, follow these safety tips:

- Always protect your skin before going out during the day. Use a sunscreen with a SPF (sun protection factor) of at least 15. Wear a hat with a brim. Cover up with lightweight, loose-fitting, long-sleeved shirts, and pants.

- Buy products with good label information, including the following:

  - A list of ingredients to see which AHA or other chemical acids are in the product

  - The name and address of the maker

  - A statement about the product's AHA and pH levels

- Buy only products with an AHA level of 10 percent or less and a pH of 3.5 or more.

- Test a small area of skin to see if it is sensitive to any AHA product before using a lot of it.

- Stop using the product right away if you have a reaction, such as stinging, redness, or bleeding.

- Talk with your doctor or dermatologist (a doctor that treats skin problems) if you have a problem.

Are hair dyes safe?

The decision to change your hair color may be a hard one. Some studies have linked hair dyes with a higher risk of certain cancers, while other studies have not found this link. Most hair dyes also don't have to go through safety testing that other cosmetic color additives do before hitting store shelves. Women are often on their own trying to figure out whether hair dyes are safe.

When hair dyes first came out, the main ingredient in coal-tar hair dye caused allergic reactions in some people. Most hair dyes are now made from petroleum sources. But FDA still considers them to be coal-tar dyes. This is because they have some of the same compounds found in these older dyes.

Cosmetic makers have stopped using things known to cause cancer in animals. For example, 4-methoxy-m-phenylenediamine (4MMPD) or 4-methoxy-m-phenylenediamine sulfate (4MMPD sulfate) is no longer used. But chemicals made almost the same way have replaced some of the cancer-causing compounds. Some experts feel that these newer ingredients aren't very different from the things they're replacing.

Experts suggest that you may reduce your risk of cancer by using less hair dye over time. You may also reduce you risk by not dyeing your hair until it starts to gray.

What precautions should I take when I dye my hair?

You should follow these safety tips when dyeing your hair:

- Don't leave the dye on your head any longer than needed.

- Rinse your scalp thoroughly with water after use.

- Wear gloves when applying hair dye.

- Carefully follow the directions in the hair dye package.

- Never mix different hair dye products.

- Be sure to do a patch test for allergic reactions before applying the dye to your hair. Almost all hair dye products include instructions for doing a patch test. It's important to do this each time you dye your hair. Your hairdresser should also do the patch test before dyeing your hair. To test, put a dab of hair dye behind your ear, and don't wash it off for two days. If you don't have any signs of allergic reaction, such as itching, burning, or redness at the test spot, you can be somewhat sure that you won't have a reaction to the dye applied to your hair. If you do react to the patch test, do the same test with different brands or colors until you find one to which you're not allergic.

- Never dye your eyebrows or eyelashes. An allergic reaction to dye could cause swelling or increase risk of infection in the eye area. This can harm the eye and even cause blindness. Spilling dye into the eye by accident could also cause permanent damage. FDA bans the use of hair dyes for eyelash and eyebrow tinting or dyeing even in beauty salons.

Are lead acetates safe in hair dyes?

Lead acetate is used as a color additive in "progressive" hair dye products. These products are put on over a period of time to produce a gradual coloring effect. You can safely use these products if you follow the directions carefully. This warning statement must appear on the product labels of lead acetate hair dyes: "Caution: Contains lead acetate. For external use only. Keep this product out of children's reach.

Do not use on cut or abraded scalp. If skin irritation develops, discontinue use. Do not use to color mustaches, eyelashes, eyebrows, or hair on parts of the body other than the scalp. Do not get in eyes. Follow instructions carefully and wash hands thoroughly after use."

Chapter 47

Exercising with Allergies

Chapter Contents

Section 47.1

Tips to Prevent Reactions during Exercise

Exercise is an important activity for everyone. Exercise will help people with asthma and other allergy problems.

Is exercise recommended for patients with allergies and asthma?

In general, a person with allergies or asthma is usually able to exercise. However, exercise should not be done during times of sickness. Also, no person should push beyond his or her capabilities.

An exercise program should begin carefully. It is a good idea to discuss such a program with your physician before starting.

How can symptoms during exercise be prevented?

Patients can often prevent symptoms by taking medication prior to exercising. The type of medication used depends on several factors. For example, people with hay fever might take an antihistamine tablet before exercise.

For people with asthma, an inhaler can be used before exercise to prevent asthma problems. Your physician can recommend the best medication for you to use before exercise.

If you have dust mite allergy, you may want to exercise outdoors to avoid breathing indoor dust. If you are allergic to grasses and weeds, you may want to exercise in an indoor location during certain seasons.

Exercising should be avoided in areas where there are large amounts of chemicals. For example, you should not exercise outdoors near heavy traffic areas with high levels of exhaust fumes from cars and trucks. Indoor areas with irritating odors or fumes, also, should be avoided.

What form of exercise is best for people with asthma?

For people with asthma, exercise that has stop-and-go activity tends to cause less trouble than exercise involving long periods of running. Swimming seems to be the easiest form of exercise for people with asthma.

Weather conditions also are important. Cold air and very dry air can be quite irritating to the bronchial tubes. Warm, moist air generally allows people with asthma to exercise successfully.

Special precautions: Special precautions should be taken by people with allergy problems from insect stings. If exercising is done outdoors, people with bee-sting allergy should not wear bright-colored clothing, cologne, perfume, or lotion. They should avoid areas such as flowerbeds and trash cans where bees and wasps like to hide.

In addition, people with severe bee-sting allergy should:

- wear a medical warning bracelet;

- carry a syringe filled with adrenaline for emergency treatment;

- avoid exercise locations far away from hospitals and doctors.

Section 47.2

Gardening with Allergies

"Allergies and Gardening," by Leonard P. Perry, PhD, Extension
Professor, University of Vermont © 2002. Reprinted with permission.
Reviewed by David A. Cooke, MD, FACP, August 3, 2010.

If you're like one in six Americans, you get some sort of seasonal
allergies each year. If you're a gardener, this doesn't mean you have
to suffer. Or you don't have to give up gardening during part of the
season. Or you don't have to convert your landscape into silk flowers,
gravel beds, and garden gnomes or plastic flamingos. Perhaps changing some gardening practices, or some of your plants, may be all that's
needed to lessen the grief.

Most see the yellow pollen on their car in spring or summer and
think, that's it. But this relatively big, showy pollen you see from trees
and flowers really isn't the culprit. It's the microscopic pollen you don't
see that causes allergies. This can be from deciduous trees in the spring
such as oak, elm, birch, maple, ash, alder, some pines, box elder, and
willow. The hardwoods especially are the culprits. Other trees, especially in warmer parts of the country (whether you live there, or may
be traveling there to visit gardens) include cedar, cottonwood, hickory,
mulberry, olive, palm, and pecan.

Trees with showy flowers, just as with flowers, tend to be pol-
linated by bees, butterflies, or similar, so have larger pollen which
doesn't blow around and cause allergies. Examples of low or no allergen trees include many of the fruit trees such as apples, crabapples,
cherries, pear, plum, and others in warmer climates such as dogwoods
and magnolias.

Shrubs to avoid include many junipers, and in warmer climates
cypress and privet. Hydrangea, azaleas, and viburnum are okay, as
are in warmer climates the boxwood and hibiscus.

In his book *Allergy-Free Gardening*, author Thomas Ogren attri-
butes many of our allergies to recent changes in our landscapes, particularly the planting of male trees and shrubs. We often do this to
avoid messy fruit from female trees, but end up as a result with more
pollen. He even advocates sex changes in trees—grafting a female top

onto existing trunks of male trees. He has also developed and advocates using the Ogren Plant Allergy Scale, rating plants from 1 (low) to 10 (high) for pollen and allergies.

As with the woody plants, those herbaceous plants with showy flowers are generally okay and include many such as daffodil, tulip, daisies, geranium impatiens, iris, lilies, pansies, petunias, roses, sunflowers, zinnias, and many more. Some flowers with strong scents may also aggravate allergies, even if they normally have larger pollen.

Most lawn grasses don't cause problems as they are mowed often and not allowed to set seed. But they can cause problems if allowed to go to seed including perennial rye, fescue, and Bermuda in warmer climates.

Of course weeds are often the most allergenic plants. One ragweed plant can produce up to one billion pollen grains, and they have been tracked over 400 miles away! Others include pigweed and Russian thistle. A couple perennials are falsely accused of allergies, as they bloom at the same time as ragweed. You see the goldenrod and Helen's flower (alias "sneezeweed") and think these are the enemy, while it is really the ragweed lurking in the background.

Plants and pollen are the only allergy producers in the garden. Molds cause allergies in some people and children, and can be produced from composts and decomposing bark mulch. If you or family members are allergic to molds, consider buying finished compost, not making it at home. And you may want to replace bark mulch, shredded leaves, cocoa hulls, or similar organic material with pebbles or even just clean cultivation. I prefer to quickly get plants established, so they cover the bed and leave no room or light for weed seeds to germinate (well, at least fewer seeds).

Here are 13 gardening practices you might change to reduce sneezing, itchy, and runny noses and still be able to garden:

- Limiting gardening in the afternoon in spring, and early mornings in fall, when pollen counts tend to be highest.

- Remain indoors during windy days, during allergic pollen times as pollen can blow in from far away (even though it is otherwise quite local in nature, such as from a tree in your yard).

- Once done working outdoors, wash well or shower, and wash clothes.

- Don't hang laundry on the line during high pollen periods. (I learned this hanging bed sheets on the line to dry, then wondering why I keep sneezing all night even indoors with the windows closed.)

- Use an air conditioner if you have one, particularly at night, or while driving, and set on recirculate if possible.

- Beware of, and wash, pets that might pick up pollen outdoors and share with you!

- Cover bodies with clothing, even caps for hair, and breathing masks especially if mowing. Best is to have someone not allergic do the mowing!

- Keep windows closed during, and a few hours after, mowing.

- Begin allergy medication prior to your normal allergy season, follow directions through the season, and if severe consult a doctor or allergist.

- Choose low allergen producing plants to begin with, or to replace others in your landscape. Remember in general to avoid wind-pollinated plants, choosing insect-pollinated plants instead.

- Choose those with showy flowers, whether woody or herbaceous.

- Possibly avoid strongly scented flowers, as these may aggravate allergies.

- Beware of molds from compost and bark mulches, possibly substituting the latter with gravel.

- Avoid hedges which can trap dust, pollen, and mold. Keep existing ones thinned.

For more information, you may wish to consult the book *Allergy-Free Gardening* by Thomas Ogren. Websites with useful information are those of the American Lung Association, the American Academy of Allergy, Asthma and Immunology, and the Intellicast weather site among others. These any more can be found through a search on an internet search engine such as Google. Also keep watch in your local daily broadcast and print media during the season for pollen counts, and garden when the counts are lower.

Chapter 48

Preventing Allergy Symptoms during Travel

Gillian loves to travel, and she's determined not to let her food allergies stop her. Sure, sometimes she feels like she's standing under the "Look at me, I'm not like everyone else" spotlight. But she says feelings of awkwardness and worry about her food allergy have faded as she gets older. Now she doesn't hesitate to ask questions about food, no matter where she is. She knows that ignoring her food allergy could lead to a bad reaction—and draw a lot more attention to her, not to mention put her in some serious (and vacation-wrecking) danger.

Yes, people with life-threatening food allergies really can take off on weekend road trips, spend a summer abroad, or vacation in the wilderness. It just takes confidence and planning.

Get Your Mind Ready

Planning a trip can be stressful for anyone. But people with food allergies may feel particularly anxious about leaving their familiar home environments. It's easy to understand why: Not only do people have to stay safe in a new place, but they also have to handle any social concerns that arise, like asking for special accommodations, avoiding certain activities or places, or explaining the need to prepare and eat their own food.

"Food Allergies and Travel," June 2008, reprinted with permission from www .kidshealth.org. Copyright © 2008 The Nemours Foundation. This information was provided by KidsHealth, one of the largest resources online for medically reviewed health information written for parents, kids, and teens. For more articles like this one, visit www.KidsHealth.org, or www.TeensHealth.org.

Even among friends, people can sometimes feel embarrassed or un-comfortable raising food allergy concerns. So it's natural to worry that it might feel even more awkward in a new environment or culture.

Perhaps the best way to boost confidence and calm nerves is to re-search and plan your trip thoroughly. Think ahead. Instead of trying to push worries aside, use them as a guide to prepare yourself for the kinds of situations you might face in a new place. Remind yourself that your anxiety is real—and understandable.

You already know how to manage your food allergies—you do it every day. The strategies that help you cope at home can work well on trips too.

Think about what kinds of situations might come up and how to deal with them. Talk through any worries with supportive friends and family who will be joining you on the trip. Not only can they help you avoid risky situations, they can also be your emotional support system. If you're traveling overseas, talk to someone who understands the country's traditions and culture to get tips on how to manage your allergy and still fit in.

If someone other than you or your family (like a teacher or friend's parent) is organizing your trip, be sure that person is clear on what your needs are. Be sure that he or she understands enough about food allergies to look out for you.

Get Your Plan Ready

Planning ahead can help you feel less anxious about what could go wrong and more excited about the adventure ahead. Start a couple of weeks to a month in advance by making a detailed to-do list. List each of the tasks below—along with any others your doctor or nurse educator recommends—starting with the one that needs to be done farthest in advance.

Choose where to go: For people with food allergies, deciding on a destination might take some extra thought. For example, if you have a peanut allergy, some places, like a remote village in Thailand, might be more risky than others. It's wise to discuss travel options with your doctor before making any final decisions.

Check prescriptions: Discuss travel plans ahead of time with your allergist to be sure you have all the medicines you need, from antihistamines and inhalers to epinephrine injectors. Don't plan to rely on local pharmacies for your prescriptions—medications may not be the same overseas. Instead, take your meds with you.

If your insurance company or pharmacy limits how much of a prescription you can fill at once, a letter from a doctor explaining the situation may allow an exception to their policy. Also, if you're traveling by airplane or train, ask your doctor to write a letter authorizing you to carry your medicine to prevent potential confusion/delays at security checkpoints.

Research local hospitals and medical care: Before you go, find out where local emergency medical help is and how long it will take you to get there. That way, if you need emergency care, you'll know your options.

Research grocery stores, restaurants, and accommodations: Well ahead of your visit, find out which grocery stores (if any) at your destination carry allergen-free products, which restaurants seem to be "allergy-aware," and which hotels offer rooms with a kitchen. Support groups and food allergy websites can often be helpful, whether you're traveling within the country or internationally.

If you're going abroad and speak the language, talk directly to grocery store, restaurant, and hotel managers. If language is a barrier, or you just need more answers, seek help from food allergy organizations, travel agents, trip coordinators, or local friends and relatives. Prepare a list of questions before making your calls and take careful notes.

Research transportation: If you're sharing a car, let your traveling companions know about your food allergy. If you're traveling by train, bus, or plane, find out about their policies and services. Do they serve snacks that contain ingredients you're allergic to? Can you board early or get a seat by yourself? Is emergency medical help available?

For air travel, research airlines in advance. Some airlines are more accommodating than others when it comes to food allergies. Call and discuss your needs well before you make reservations. Ask for a safe snack, but bring your own food along just in case. Ask if you can board early so you can wipe down your seating area without holding other travelers up. When you board, remind the flight crew of your needs. If it helps you feel more comfortable, ask that they alert other passengers to your allergy.

Carry enough medicine: Keep your meds in your hand luggage so they're easily available. Also keep your food allergy emergency action plan in your bag. It should be signed by your doctor and describe the allergies you have and the treatment you need. Wrap and pack your meds carefully so they don't get crushed or leak.

Carry hand wipes: Washing your hands frequently and keeping them away from your mouth, nose, and eyes is a great way to prevent accidentally coming into contact with allergens. But when you're traveling you can't count on having access to soap and running water. A good supply of hand wipes ensures that you can clean your hands as well as wipe around seating areas on planes, trains, buses, and other forms of transportation where contact with allergens is likely.

Pack safe food: If you can, bring enough safe food to see you through at least the beginning of your trip. Of course, how much you bring will depend on where you're going and how long you'll be traveling: If you're in an area where you cannot easily purchase or order allergen-free food, stock up on your food supply. If you're someplace where you can buy and prepare what you need, pack less. If you're traveling internationally, you may not be able to read labels at local grocery stores. Again, it's best to bring a sizeable supply of safe food with you.

Alert others to your allergy: You don't have to wear a T-shirt that screams, "Hey, everyone, I have a food allergy!" But it's a good idea to wear a medical ID bracelet when you travel, so that people can help you get proper emergency medical help if you need it. You may also wish to carry a medical release form, signed by your doctor, which authorizes others to give you emergency medicine, such as epinephrine.

If you will be eating out, carry a personalized "chef card." These cards detail your allergies and help kitchen staff understand how to prepare a safe meal for you. Chef card forms are readily available, in many different languages, through food allergy websites. But the card is not a substitute for direct communication. It's best to speak directly with your waiter and possibly the chef when you eat out.

Staying alert, taking precautions, and carrying meds are just part of normal life for someone who has a food allergy. Once you've done it once or twice, traveling with food allergies feels perfectly routine also. You feel less like you're "traveling with food allergies" and more like you're simply "traveling."

With careful planning, travel can be liberating and help you feel more independent. You'll learn just how good you are at taking care of yourself.

Chapter 49

Preventing Allergy Symptoms during Pregnancy

Asthma is the most common potentially serious medical condition to complicate pregnancy. In fact, asthma affects approximately 8 percent of women in their childbearing years. Well-controlled asthma is not associated with significant risk to mother or fetus. Uncontrolled asthma can cause serious complications to the mother, including high blood pressure, toxemia, premature delivery, and rarely death. For the baby, complications of uncontrolled asthma include increased risk of stillbirth, fetal growth retardation, premature birth, low birth weight, and a low Apgar score at birth.

Asthma can be controlled by careful medical management and avoidance of known triggers, so asthma need not be a reason for avoiding pregnancy. Most measures used to control asthma are not harmful to the developing fetus and do not appear to contribute to either miscarriage or birth defects.

Although the outcome of any pregnancy can never be guaranteed, most women with asthma and allergies do well with proper medical management by physicians familiar with these disorders and the changes that occur during pregnancy.

What Is Asthma and What Are Its Symptoms?

Asthma is a condition characterized by obstruction in the airways of the lungs caused by spasm of surrounding muscles, accumulation of mucus, and swelling of the airway walls due to the gathering of inflammatory cells. Unlike individuals with emphysema who have irreversible destruction of their lung cells, asthmatic patients usually have a condition that can be reversed with vigorous treatment.

Individuals with asthma most often describe what they feel in their airways as a "tightness." They also describe wheezing, shortness of breath, chest pain, and cough. Symptoms of asthma can be triggered by allergens (including pollen, mold, animals, feathers, house dust mites, and cockroaches), other environmental factors, exercise, infections, and stress.

What Are the Effects of Pregnancy on Asthma?

When women with asthma become pregnant, one third of the patients improve, one third worsen, and the last third remain unchanged. Although studies vary widely on the overall effect of pregnancy on asthma, several reviews find the following similar trends:

- Women with severe asthma are more likely to worsen, while those with mild asthma are more likely to improve or remain unchanged.

- The change in the course of asthma in an individual woman during pregnancy tends to be similar on successive pregnancies.

- Asthma exacerbations are most likely to appear during the weeks 24 to 36 of gestation, with only occasional patients (10 percent or fewer) becoming symptomatic during labor and delivery.

- The changes in asthma noted during pregnancy usually return to prepregnancy status within 3 months of delivery.

Pregnancy may affect asthmatic patients in several ways. Hormonal changes that occur during pregnancy may affect both the nose and sinuses, as well as the lungs. An increase in the hormone estrogen contributes to congestion of the capillaries (tiny blood vessels) in the lining of the nose, which in turn leads to a "stuffy" nose in pregnancy (especially during the third trimester). A rise in progesterone causes increased respiratory drive, and a feeling of shortness of breath may be experienced as a result of this hormonal increase. These events may be confused with or add to allergic or other triggers of asthma.

Spirometry and peak flow are measurements of airflow obstruction (a marker of asthma) that help your physician determine if asthma is the cause of shortness of breath during pregnancy.

Fetal Monitoring

For pregnant women with asthma, the type and frequency of fetal evaluation is based on gestational age and maternal risk factors. Ultrasound can be performed before 12 weeks if there is concern about the accuracy of an estimated due date and repeated later if a slowing of fetal growth is suspected. Electronic heart rate monitoring, called "non-stress testing" or "contraction stress testing," and ultrasonic determinations in the third trimester may be used to assess fetal well being. For third trimester patients with significant asthma symptoms, the frequency of fetal assessment should be increased if problems are suspected. Asthma patients should record fetal activity or kick counts daily to help monitor their baby according to their physician's instructions.

During a severe asthma attack in which symptoms do not quickly improve, there is risk for significant maternal hypoxemia, a low oxygen state. This is an important time for fetal assessment; continuous electronic fetal heart rate monitoring may be necessary along with measurements of the mother's lung function.

Fortunately during labor and delivery, the majority of asthma patients do well, although careful fetal monitoring remains very important. In low risk patients whose asthma is well-controlled, fetal assessment can be accomplished by 20 minutes of electronic monitoring (the admission test). Intensive fetal monitoring with careful observation is recommended for patients who enter labor and delivery with severe asthma, have a non-reassuring admission test, or other risk factors.

Avoidance and Control

The connection between asthma and allergies is common. Most asthmatic patients (75 percent to 85 percent) will be allergic to one or more substances such as pollens, molds, animals, house dust mites, and cockroaches. Pet allergies are caused by protein found in animal dander, urine, and saliva. These allergens may trigger asthma symptoms or make existing symptoms worse.

Other non-allergic substances may also worsen asthma and allergies. These include tobacco smoke, paint and chemical fumes, strong odors, environmental pollutants (including ozone and smog), and drugs, such as aspirin or beta-blockers (used to treat high blood pressure, migraine headache, and heart disorders).

Avoidance of specific triggers should lessen the frequency and intensity of asthmatic and allergic symptoms. Allergist-immunologists recommend the following methods:

- Remove allergy causing pets from the house, or at the least keep them out of the bedroom at all times.

- Seal pillows, mattresses, and box springs in special dust mite-proof casings (your allergist should be able to give you information regarding comfortable cases).

- If possible, wash bedding weekly in 130-degree Fahrenheit water (comforters may be dry-cleaned periodically) to kill dust mites. However, keeping the hot water tank at this temperature may not be advisable if there are small children or others at risk of scalding at home.

- Keep home humidity under 50 percent to control dust mite and mold growth.

- Use filtering vacuums or "filter vacuum bags" to control airborne dust when cleaning.

- Close windows, use air conditioning, and limit outdoor activity between 5 a.m. and 10 a.m., when pollen and pollution are at their highest.

- Limit exposure to chemical fumes and, most importantly, tobacco smoke.

Can Asthma Medications Safely Be Used during Pregnancy?

Though no medication has been proven entirely safe for use during pregnancy, your doctor will carefully balance medication use and symptom control. Your treatment plan will be individualized so that potential benefits of medications outweigh the potential risks of these medications or of uncontrolled asthma.

Asthma is a disease in which intensity of symptoms can vary from day to day, month to month, or season to season regardless of pregnancy. Therefore, a treatment plan should be chosen based both on asthma severity and experience during pregnancy with those medications.

Remember that the use of medications should not replace avoidance of allergens or irritants, as avoidance will potentially reduce medication needs.

In general, asthma medications used in pregnancy are chosen based on the following criteria:

- Inhaled medications are generally preferred because they have a more localized effect with only small amounts entering the bloodstream.

- When appropriate, time-tested older medications are preferred since there is more experience with their use during pregnancy.

- Medication use is limited in the first trimester as much as possible when the fetus is forming. Birth defects from medications are rare (no more than 1 percent of all birth defects are attributable to all medications.

- In general, the same medications used during pregnancy are appropriate during labor and delivery and when nursing.

Bronchodilator Medication

Short-acting inhaled beta$_2$-agonists, often called "asthma relievers" or "rescue medications," are used as necessary to control acute symptoms. Albuterol is the preferred short-acting inhaled beta$_2$-agonist for use during pregnancy since there are more available reassuring human gestational safety data.

Two long-acting inhaled beta agonists, salmeterol (Serevent®) and formoterol (Foradil®), are available. No large-scale trials of these medications in pregnancy have been performed. However, because of their inhaled route, chemical relation to albuterol, and efficacy data, long-acting beta agonists are recommended during pregnancy for patients not controlled on inhaled corticosteroids.

Theophylline has extensive human experience without evidence of significant abnormalities. Newborns can have jitteriness, vomiting, and fast pulse if the maternal blood level is too high. Therefore, patients who receive theophylline should have blood levels checked during pregnancy.

Ipratropium (Atrovent®), an anticholinergic bronchodilator medication, does not cause problems in animals; however, there is no published experience in humans. Ipratropium is absorbed less than similar medications in this class, such as atropine.

Anti-Inflammatory Medication

The anti-inflammatory medications are preventive, or "asthma controllers," and include inhaled cromolyn (Intal®), corticosteroids, and leukotriene modifiers. Patients requiring the use of beta$_2$-agonists more often than three times a week, or who have reduced peak flow readings or spirometry (lung function studies), usually need daily anti-inflammatory medication. Inhaled cromolyn sodium is virtually devoid of side effects but is less effective than inhaled corticosteroids.

Budesonide (Pulmicort®) is recommended as the inhaled corticosteroid of choice for use during pregnancy due to a large amount of reassuring human gestational safety data. However, other inhaled corticosteroids (such as beclomethasone [Qvar®], fluticasone [Flovent®], flunisolide [AeroBid®], mometasone [Asmanex®], and triamcinolone [Azmacort®] have not been proven to be unsafe during pregnancy and can be continued in patients well-controlled by them prior to pregnancy.

In some cases oral or injectable corticosteroids, such as prednisone, prednisolone, or methylprednisolone may be necessary for a few days in patients with severe asthma exacerbations or throughout pregnancy in women with severe asthma. Some studies have demonstrated a slight increase in the incidence of pre-eclampsia, premature deliveries, or low-birth-weight infants with chronic use of corticosteroids. However, they are the most effective drugs for the treatment of patients with more severe asthma and other allergic disorders. Therefore, their significant benefit usually far exceeds their minimal risk.

Three leukotriene modifiers, montelukast (Singulair®), zafirlukast (Accolate®), and zileuton (Zyflo®) are available. Results of animal studies are reassuring for montelukast and zafirlukast , but there are minimal data in human pregnancy with this new class of anti-inflammatory drugs.

Can Allergy Medications Safely Be Used during Pregnancy?

Antihistamines may be useful during pregnancy to treat the nasal and eye symptoms of seasonal or perennial allergic rhinitis, allergic conjunctivitis, the itching of urticaria (hives) or eczema, and as an adjunct to the treatment of serious allergic reactions, including anaphylaxis (allergic shock). With the exception of life-threatening anaphylaxis, the benefits from their use must be weighed against any risk to the fetus. Because symptoms may be of such severity to affect maternal eating, sleeping, or emotional well-being, and because un-controlled rhinitis may predispose to sinusitis or may worsen asthma, antihistamines may provide definite benefit during pregnancy.

Chlorpheniramine (Chlor-Trimeton®) and diphenhydramine (Benadryl®) have been used for many years during pregnancy with reassuring animal studies. Generally, chlorpheniramine would be the preferred choice, but a major drawback of these medications is drowsiness and performance impairment in some patients. Two of the newer less sedating antihistamines loratadine (Claritin®) and cetiriz-ine (Zyrtec®) have reassuring animal and human study data and are currently recommended when indicated for use during pregnancy.

The use of decongestants is more problematic. The nasal spray oxymetazoline (Afrin®, Neo-Synephrine® Long-Acting, etc.) appears to be the safest product because there is minimal, if any, absorption into the bloodstream. However, these and other over-the-counter nasal sprays can cause rebound congestion and actually worsen the condi-tion for which they are used. Their use is generally limited to very intermittent use or regular use for only 3 consecutive days.

Although pseudoephedrine (Sudafed®) has been used for years, and studies have been reassuring, there have been recent reports of a slight increase in abdominal wall defects in newborns. Use of decon-gestants during the first trimester should only be entertained after consideration of the severity of maternal symptoms unrelieved by other medications. Phenylephrine and phenylpropanolamine are less desir-able than pseudoephedrine based on the information available.

A corticosteroid nasal spray should be considered in any patient whose allergic nasal symptoms are more than mild and last for more than a few days. These medications prevent symptoms and lessen the need for oral medications. There are few specific data regarding the safety of intranasal corticosteroids during pregnancy. However, based on the data for the same medications used in an inhaled form (for asthma), budesonide (Rhinocort®) would be considered the intranasal corticosteroid of choice, but other intranasal corticosteroids could be continued if they were providing effective control prior to pregnancy.

Immunotherapy and Influenza Vaccine

Allergen immunotherapy (allergy shots) is often effective for those patients in whom symptoms persist despite optimal environmental control and proper drug therapy. Allergen immunotherapy can be carefully continued during pregnancy in patients who are benefiting and not experiencing adverse reactions. Due to the greater risk of anaphylaxis with increasing doses of immunotherapy and a delay of several months before it becomes effective, it is generally recommended that this therapy not be started during pregnancy.

Patients receiving immunotherapy during pregnancy should be carefully evaluated. It may be appropriate to lower the dosage in order to further reduce the chance of an allergic reaction to the injections.

Influenza (flu) vaccine is recommended for all patients with moderate and severe asthma. There is no evidence of associated risk to the mother or fetus.

Can Asthma Medications Safely Be Used while Nursing?

Nearly all medications enter breast milk, though infants are generally exposed to very low concentrations of the drugs. Hence, the medications described above rarely present problems for the infant during breastfeeding. Specifically, very little of the inhaled beta agonists, inhaled or oral steroids, and theophylline will appear in mother's milk. Some infants can have irritability and insomnia if exposed to higher doses of medication or to theophylline. In general, the lowest drug concentration in mother's milk can be obtained by taking theophylline 15 minutes after nursing or 3 to 4 hours before the next feeding.

Summary

It is important to remember that the risks of asthma medications are lower than the risks of uncontrolled asthma, which can be harmful to both mother and child. The use of asthma or allergy medication needs to be discussed with your doctor, ideally before pregnancy. Therefore, the doctor should be notified whenever you are planning to discontinue birth control methods or as soon as you know that you are pregnant. Regular follow up for evaluation of asthma symptoms and medications is necessary throughout the pregnancy to maximize asthma control and to minimize medication risks.

This article has been prepared by members of the Pregnancy Committee of the American College of Allergy, Asthma and Immunology, an organization whose members are dedicated to providing optimal care to all patients with asthma, including those who are pregnant.

Chapter 50

Support at School and Work: The Americans with Disabilities Act and Allergies

Americans with Disabilities Act: How It Affects You

Has your child been rejected by a preschool or excluded from a field trip because a teacher was afraid to use his or her EpiPen? Does a moldy carpet at work or school make you sick? Does stale smoke in offices, hotel rooms, or conference centers make it hard for you to take part in routine business activities?

The Americans with Disabilities Act (ADA) is a civil rights law that gives you the right to ask for changes where policies, practices, or conditions exclude or disadvantage you. As of January 26, 1992, public entities and public accommodations must ensure that individuals with disabilities have full access to and equal enjoyment of all facilities, programs, goods, and services.

The ADA borrows from Section 504 of the Rehabilitation Act of 1973. Section 504 prohibits discrimination on the basis of disability in employment and education in agencies, programs, and services that receive federal money. The ADA extends many of the rights and duties of Section 504 to public accommodations such as restaurants, hotels, theaters, stores, doctors' offices, museums, private schools, and child care programs. They must be readily accessible to and usable by individuals with disabilities. No one can be excluded or denied services just because he/she is disabled or based on ignorance, attitudes, or stereotypes.

"Americans with Disabilities Act," reprinted with permission from the Asthma and Allergy Foundation of America, © 2005. All rights reserved. Reviewed by David A. Cooke, MD, FACP, August 3, 2010.

Does the ADA Apply to People with Asthma and Allergies?

Yes. In both the ADA and Section 504, a person with a disability is described as someone who has a physical or mental impairment that substantially limits one or more major life activities, or is regarded as having such impairments. Breathing, eating, working, and going to school are "major life activities." Asthma and allergies are still considered disabilities under the ADA, even if symptoms are controlled by medication.

The ADA can help people with asthma and allergies obtain safer, healthier environments where they work, shop, eat, and go to school. The ADA also affects employment policies. For example, a private preschool can not refuse to enroll children because giving medication to or adapting snacks for students with allergies requires special staff training or because insurance rates might go up. A firm can not refuse to hire an otherwise qualified person solely because of the potential time or insurance needs of a family member.

In public schools where policies and practices do not comply with Section 504, the ADA should stimulate significant changes. In contrast, the ADA will cause few changes in schools where students have reliable access to medication, options for physical education, and classrooms that are free of allergens and irritants.

How Will the ADA Work?

In most cases, employees and employers, consumers and businesses, and administrators and students will work together to improve conditions and remove barriers to promote equal access and full inclusion.

Marie Trottier, Harvard University's Administrator of Disability Services, explains that her role includes educating nonallergic managers, colleagues, and coworkers about the needs of people with environmental sensitivities. She also trains staff in education and employment policies, benefits, and procedures.

"Changes depend as much on interpersonal consideration as they do on legal rights," she says. "It shouldn't be uncommon for people with asthma and allergies to get the same respect for their needs as people with more visible disabilities."

When Ms. Trottier arranges for accommodations in offices, classrooms, and student housing, she considers the nature of the disability and the specifics of each situation. She might install an air conditioner or arrange for an office with a window that opens. She has relocated a microwave oven and reorganized office spaces to help people with allergies avoid cooking odors.

Employees might need prior notice of renovation or lawn care projects so they can modify their schedules to avoid the irritants and allergens.

Professors may ask students not to wear scented products to class. Students affected by dust, paper fibers, or ink can have someone borrow library materials for them or they can use an online computer system. Ms. Trottier says that "all of these options for students and employees require time and energy, flexibility and creativity, more so than money." A sign in her office underscores her point, "Attitudes are the real disabilities."

Making the ADA Work for You

If you or your child would like consideration due to asthma or allergies, speak with a school administrator, manager, employer, human specialist, or disabilities service coordinator. He or she should know the procedure for collecting necessary information and planning appropriate changes, aids or services. You can call on a variety of sources for advice and creative practical ideas.

Under Section 504, public schools and programs cannot avoid their responsibility by claiming to have limited funds or resources. Nor can they impose a "disparate impact" on people with disabilities. The ADA requires public accommodations to make changes, except in cases where an "undue burden" would result.

The law does not define "undue burden." It depends on the organization's size and the real costs of the changes. The business or program must show that it properly assessed the individual's needs and tried to find the necessary.

Don't Be Afraid to Speak Up

The ADA prohibits retaliation, harassment, or coercion against individuals who exercise their rights or assist others in doing so. If you feel you have been treated unfairly, you may file a complaint with the U.S. Attorney General who refers complaints to the appropriate agency. The Attorney General can bring lawsuits to seek money damages and civil penalties in cases of general public importance, or where there is a "pattern or practice" of discrimination.

Individuals can also file a private suit to get a court order requiring a business or program to make necessary changes and to pay attorney's fees. Other remedies may include reinstatement in your job and back pay.

The ADA Is Evolving

Court decisions and rulings will slowly define how the ADA will affect us. The real momentum for change will come as we work creatively together to promote the inclusive attitudes and environments that fulfill the promise of the ADA for ourselves and our children.

Chapter 51

Starting an Allergy Support Group

If at all possible, join or start a local support group for parents of children with severe food allergies. Caring for a child with life-threatening food allergies is very difficult. A support group can provide emotional support from other parents who are facing similar challenges, and provides a forum for sharing resources, ideas, and experiences. It is truly wonderful to be able to meet face-to-face with other parents who really "get it."

How to Get a Group Started

Arrange for a meeting room. Make arrangements for a room in which to hold your group's meetings. A local community center room or meeting room in a local restaurant is ideal. Many hospitals have meeting rooms that are available as well. It is best to avoid meeting in members' homes, so that the meeting is not affected by that person's availability.

You will probably want to plan to hold your meetings without the children, so that the members will be able to speak freely. Your children should not hear you complain about how difficult it is to care for them, and they may be frightened by some of the subjects that are discussed (such as accounts of other children's anaphylactic episodes).

Adapted from *How To Manage Your Child's Life-Threatening Food Allergies: Practical Tips for Everyday Life* by Linda Marienhoff Coss (Plumtree Press, May 2004). © 2004 Linda Marienhoff Coss. All rights reserved. For additional information, visit www.foodallergybooks.com. Reviewed by David A. Cooke, MD, FACP, August 3, 2010.

Advertise your new group. Create a simple flyer with a brief description of your group and information about your first meeting. See http://www.kidswithfoodallergies.org/sampleflyer.html for a sample flyer.

Talk to everyone you can think of who might know of other area parents of food-allergic children. Don't forget to call local:

- allergists;
- pediatricians;
- school nurses;
- mothers' groups;
- daycare centers;
- La Leche League chapters;
- hospitals;
- churches and synagogues.

Ask all of the above contacts to help you distribute and/or post your flyer.

Post a notice on the "Geographic—Local Support" forum at Kids With Food Allergies (http://www.kidswithfoodallergies.com) announcing the formation of your new group. Contact the Food Allergy & Anaphylaxis Network (www.foodallergy.org) to add your support group to their list of local groups. Contact websites that list local food allergy support groups and ask to be added to their lists as well.

Spread the news through word of mouth; network with friends, neighbors, acquaintances. There are bound to be others in your area who would be interested in joining. Your job is to find them!

Even if only one guest shows up for your first meeting, don't despair. A support group of two is much better than no support group at all. Once you get started your group is bound to grow.

Plan Your Group's First Meeting

At your first meeting you should:

- Have each person fill out a nametag and sign a sign-in sheet upon arrival. Be sure to obtain detailed contact information (including name, address, phone number, e-mail address, and children's names, ages, and allergies) for each person present.

- Have each person introduce herself and tell about her child's-allergies.

- Discuss the purpose and goals of the group.

- Determine who will be the group's leader; this person will lead meetings and be the group's contact person.

- Divide responsibilities and encourage active involvement. People will be more supportive of an organization which they help create.

- Have others suggest topics and speakers, take responsibility for member communications, do research, offer sample recipes or products, and bring up issues.

- Discuss how the members want to structure the meetings: free form vs. formal vs. something in between. Some groups are very informal and focus on free-form discussions of allergy-related issues and questions raised by individual members; other groups regularly feature guest speakers (such as doctors, nutritionists, psychologists, chefs, and school nurses) at their meetings. Many groups plan topics for each meeting.

- Your group may choose to devote its energies to outreach efforts such as fundraising or legislative advocacy.

- Set up a method for communicating with each other, such as distribution of the group's roster and creation of an e-mail distribution list.

- Set up a time and place for the next meeting. If possible, set a 6- or 12-month meeting calendar.

Support Group Social Events

Support group family social events are a great opportunity for your child to meet other children with food allergies. Children like to see that they are not alone, that there is a whole group of children in their area who also must be careful about what they eat, carry medication, and wear MedicAlert® bracelets.

Family parties: Imagine taking your child to the buffet table at a party and telling him that all of the food is "safe" and he can eat whatever he wants. And then imagine letting your child wander off on his own at that same party, with you only supervising him to the same degree that most parents keep an eye on their children at a party—no trailing along right next to him, no worrying about what his playmates are eating or what he's touching. With the help of your support group, you can make this fantasy come true.

Your support group can create family parties at which every child in attendance can eat every food item served. Here's how. In order to ensure that the party menu takes all of the attendees' needs into account, have a policy requiring that those who wish to attend the party either attend the party-planning meeting or RSVP (with a complete list of their family's allergens) prior to this meeting.

At the planning meeting, start by determining the general menu "ground rules" based on the common allergies that you're dealing with (such as no dairy, egg, nut, wheat, or citrus fruits). Then brainstorm food ideas, with each party attendee having veto power over any food idea that is put forth.

If your support group is particularly large you may want to create several parties. For example, you can split the group up by allergens or by the children's ages.

Of course, don't forget to plan non-food activities, too. Ideas include:

- arts and crafts;

- party games;

- relay races;

- carnival-type games (such as a bean bag toss);

- holiday-themed activities (such as a Halloween Costume Parade);

- for older kids, try a "food allergy quiz game" where the kids and the parents square off to test their food allergy knowledge;

- filling goody bags with non-food treats (such as pencils, small plastic toys, etc.).

Other family activity ideas: Ideas for family activities include parties and picnics, children's play groups, bowling or miniature golf outings, family camping trips, fundraising events, and babysitting co-ops. Be sure to include siblings, too.

Baked goods exchanges: Another popular event that your support group might want to consider is a Baked Goods Exchange. For this parents only meeting, each member bakes up a large batch of something that is safe for their child and that meets the event's basic ground rules (for example, you might want to agree in advance that everything will be nut-free). The member comes to the meeting with a tray of individually wrapped baked goods, a "tasting tray" of the item made, copies of the recipe, and information about all of the ingredients.

At the meeting each attendee distributes her recipe, describes in detail exactly what is in the dish (i.e., the ingredients of the margarine, the sprinkles, etc.), and passes the tasting tray. Everyone has a great time sampling each item, and then each member fills a bakery box with a few of each treat that is safe for her children. Because kids with food allergies usually cannot eat things from bakeries, dessert buffets, and so forth, this is a fabulous opportunity for them to get the thrill of enjoying a whole assortment of baked goods at once.

Part Seven

Additional Help
and Information

Chapter 52

Glossary of Terms Related to Allergies and the Immune System

allergen: A substance that causes an allergic reaction.

amino acids: Any of the 26 building blocks of proteins.

anaphylaxis: A severe reaction to an allergen that can cause itching, fainting, and in some cases, death.

antibody: A molecule tailor-made by the immune system to lock onto and destroy specific foreign substances such as allergens.

antigen: A substance or molecule that is recognized by the immune system. The antigen can be from foreign material such as bacteria or viruses.

assay: A laboratory method of measuring a substance such as immunoglobulin.

asthma: A respiratory disease of the lungs characterized by episodes of inflammation and narrowing of the lower airways in response to asthma triggers, such as infectious agents, stress, pollutants such as cigarette smoke, and common allergens such as cat dander, dust mites, and pollen.

autoantibody: An antibody that reacts against a person's own tissue.

Definitions in this chapter were compiled from documents published by the National Institute of Allergy and Infectious Diseases (NIAID, www.niaid.nih.gov), part of the National Institutes of Health.

autoimmune disease: A disease that results when the immune system mistakenly attacks the body's own tissues. Examples include multiple sclerosis, type 1 diabetes, rheumatoid arthritis, and systemic lupus erythematosus.

B cell or B lymphocyte: A small white blood cell crucial to the immune defenses. B cells come from bone marrow and develop into blood cells called plasma cells, which are the source of antibodies.

bacteria: Microscopic organisms composed of a single cell. Some cause disease.

basophil: A white blood cell that contributes to inflammatory reactions. Along with mast cells, basophils are responsible for the symptoms of allergy.

celiac disease: A disease of the digestive system that damages the small intestine and interferes with absorption of nutritional contents of food.

cells: The smallest units of life; the basic living things that make up tissues.

challenge: Process of assessing the immune system's response to a food allergen.

complement: A complex series of blood proteins whose action "complements" the work of antibodies. Complement destroys bacteria, produces inflammation, and regulates immune reactions.

conjunctivitis: Inflammation of the lining of the eyelid, causing red-rimmed, swollen eyes, and crusting of the eyelids.

cytotoxicity testing: An unproven laboratory method of diagnosing allergies by examining blood samples under a microscope to see if white blood cells "die."

elimination diet: Certain foods are removed from a person's diet and a substitute food of the same type, such as another source of protein in place of eggs, is introduced.

enzyme: A protein produced by living cells that promotes the chemical processes of life without itself being altered.

eosinophil: A white blood cell containing granules filled with chemicals damaging to parasites and enzymes that affect inflammatory reactions.

epinephrine: A drug form of adrenaline (a natural hormone in the body) that stimulates nerves.

extract: A concentrated liquid preparation containing minute parts of specific foods.

fungus: A member of a class of relatively primitive vegetable organisms. Fungi include mushrooms, yeasts, rusts, molds, and smuts.

gastrointestinal (GI) tract: An area of the body that includes the stomach and intestines.

gene: A unit of genetic material (DNA) inherited from a parent that controls specific characteristics. Genes carry coded directions a cell uses to make specific proteins that perform specific functions.

glucocorticoid: A type of steroid drug that reduces inflammation.

granule: A grain-like part of a cell.

histamine toxicity: An allergic-like reaction to eating foods containing high levels of histamine.

histamine: A chemical released by mast cells and basophils.

immune response: A reaction of the immune system to foreign substances. Although normal immune responses are designed to protect the body from pathogens, immune dysregulation can damage normal cells and tissues, as in the case of autoimmune diseases.

immune system: A complex network of specialized cells, tissues, and organs that defends the body against attacks by disease-causing organisms.

immunoglobulin: One of a large family of proteins, also known as antibody.

inflammation: An immune system reaction to "foreign" invaders such as microbes or allergens. Signs include redness, swelling, pain, or heat.

inflammatory response: Redness, warmth, and swelling produced in response to infection; the result of increased blood flow and an influx of immune cells and their secretions.

lactose intolerance: The inability to digest lactose, a kind of sugar found in milk and other food products. Lactose intolerance is caused by a shortage of the enzyme lactase, which is produced by the cells that line the small intestine.

lymphocytes: Small white blood cells that are important parts of the immune system.

** st cell:** A granulocyte found in tissue. The contents of mast cells, along with those of basophils, are responsible for the symptoms of allergy.

microbes: Tiny life forms, such as bacteria, viruses, and fungi, which may cause disease.

molecules: The building blocks of a cell. Some examples are proteins, fats, and carbohydrates.

organism: An individual living thing.

perennial: Describes something that occurs throughout.

provocative challenge: An unproven test in which diluted food allergen is placed under the tongue or injected under the skin to find out whether symptoms get worse.

rhinitis: Inflammation of the nasal passages, which can cause a runny nose.

sinuses: Hollow air spaces located within the bones of the skull surrounding the nose.

sinusitis: When sinuses are infected or inflamed.

sputum: Matter ejected from the lungs and windpipe through the mouth.

tissues: Groups of similar cells joined to perform the same function.

tonsils and adenoids: Prominent oval masses of lymphoid tissues on either side of the throat.

toxin: An agent produced in plants and bacteria, normally very damaging to cells.

upper respiratory tract: Area of the body that includes the nasal passages, mouth, and throat.

vaccine: A preparation that stimulates an immune response that can prevent an infection or create resistance to an infection. Vaccines do not cause disease.

Chapter 53

Directory of Organizations That Provide Information about Allergies

Government Agencies That Provide Information about Allergies

Agency for Healthcare Research and Quality (AHRQ)
Office of Communications and Knowledge Transfer
540 Gaither Road, Suite 2000
Rockville, MD 20850
Phone: 301-427-1364
Fax: 301-427-1873
Website: www.ahrq.gov

Centers for Disease Control and Prevention (CDC)
1600 Clifton Road
Atlanta, GA 30333
Toll-Free: 800-CDC-INFO
(232-4636)
Toll-Free TTY: 888-232-6348
Phone: 404-639-3311
Websites: www.cdc.gov
E-mail: cdcinfo@cdc.gov

Environmental Protection Agency (EPA)
Ariel Rios Building
1200 Pennsylvania Avenue, NW
Washington, DC 20460
Phone: 202-272-0167
TTY: 202-272-0165
Website: www.epa.gov

Healthfinder®
National Health Information Center
P.O. Box 1133
Washington, DC 20013-1133
Toll-Free: 800-336-4797
Phone: 301-565-4167
Fax: 301-984-4256
Website: www.healthfinder.gov
E-mail: healthfinder@nhic.org

Resources in this chapter were compiled from several sources deemed reliable; all contact information was verified and updated in August 2010.

National Center for Complementary and Alternative Medicine (NCCAM)
National Institutes of Health
NCCAM Clearinghouse
P.O. 7923
Gaithersburg, MD 20898-7923
Toll-Free: 888-644-6226
TTY: 866-464-3615
Fax: 866-464-3616
Website: nccam.nih.gov
E-mail: info@nccam.nih.gov

National Digestive Diseases Information Clearinghouse (NDDIC)
2 Information Way
Bethesda, MD 20892-3570
Toll-Free: 800-891-5389
TTY: 866–569–1162
Fax: 703-738-4929
Website: digestive.niddk.nih.gov
E-mail: nddic@info.niddk.nih.gov

National Heart, Lung, and Blood Institute (NHLBI)
P.O. Box 30105
Bethesda, MD 20824-0105
Phone: 301-592-8573
TTY: 240-629-3255
Fax: 301-592-8563
Website: www.nhlbi.nih.gov
E-mail: nhlbiinfo@nhlbi.nih.gov

National Human Genome Research Institute (NHGRI)
Building 31
Room 4B09
31 Center Drive, MSC 2152
9000 Rockville Pike
Bethesda, MD 20892-2152
Phone: 301-402-0911
Fax: 301-402-2218
Website: www.genome.gov

National Institute of Allergy and Infectious Diseases (NIAID)
6610 Rockledge Drive, MSC 6612
Bethesda, MD 20892-6612
Toll-Free: 866-284-4107
TDD: 800-877-8339
Fax: 301-402-3573
Website: www.niaid.nih.gov
E-mail: ocpostoffice@niaid.nih.gov

National Institute of Arthritis and Musculo-skeletal and Skin Diseases (NIAMS)
Information Clearinghouse
National Institutes of Health
1 AMS Circle
Bethesda, MD 20892-3675
Toll Free: 877-22-NIAMS
(226-4267)
Phone: 301-495-4484
TTY: 301–565–2966
Fax: 301-718-6366
Website: www.niams.nih.gov
E-mail: NIAMSinfo@mail.nih.gov

National Institute of Environmental Health Sciences (NIEHS)
P.O. Box 12233, MD K3-16
Research Triangle Park, NC 27709-2233
Website: www.niehs.nih.gov
E-mail: webcenter@niehs.nih.gov

National Institutes of Health (NIH)
9000 Rockville Pike
Bethesda, MD 20892
Phone: 301-496-4000
TTY: 301-402-9612
Website: www.nih.gov
E-mail: NIHinfo@od.nih.gov

National Women's Health Information Center (NWHIC)
Office on Women's Health
8270 Willow Oaks Corporate Drive
Fairfax, VA 22031
Washington, DC 20201
Toll-Free: 800-994-9662
Toll-Free TTY: 888-220-5446
Website: www.womenshealth.gov

U.S. Food and Drug Administration (FDA)
10903 New Hampshire Avenue
Silver Spring, MD 20993
Toll-Free: 888-INFO-FDA (463-6332)
Website: www.fda.gov

U.S. National Library of Medicine (NLM)
8600 Rockville Pike
Bethesda, MD 20894
Toll-Free: 888-FIND-NLM (346-3656)
Toll-Free TDD: 800-735-2258
Phone: 301-594-5983
Fax: 301-402-1384
Website: www.nlm.nih.gov
E-mail: custserv@nlm.nih.gov

United States Department of Agriculture (USDA)
1400 Independence Avenue, SW
Washington, DC 20250
Phone: 202-720-2791
Website: www.usda.gov

Private Agencies That Provide Information about Allergies

AllergicChild.com
425 W Rockrimmon Blvd.
Suite 202
Colorado Springs, CO 80919
Website: www.allergicchild.com

Allergic Living *Magazine*
2100 Bloor Street West
Suite 6-168
Toronto, Ontario M6S 5A5
Toll-Free: 888-771-7747
Phone: 416-604-0110
Website: www.allergicliving.com
E-mail: info@allergicliving.com

Allergy and Asthma Information Association
295 The West Mall,
Suite 118
Toronto, Ontario M9C 4Z4
Phone: 416-621-4571
Fax: 416-621-5034
Website: www.aaia.ca
E-mail: admin@aaia.ca

Allergy and Asthma Network Mothers of Asthmatics
8201 Greenboro Drive,
Suite 300
McLean, VA 22102
Toll-Free: 800-878-4403
Fax: 703-288-5271
Website: www.aanma.org

Allergy UK
Planwell House
LEFA Business Park
Edgington Way
Sidcup, Kent
DA14 5BH
United Kingdom
Helpline: +13 22 619898
Fax: +13 22 663480
Website: www.allergyuk.org
E-mail: info@allergyuk.org

American Academy of Asthma, Allergy, and Immunology
555 East Wells Street,
Suite 1100
Milwaukee, WI 53202-3823
Phone: 414-272-6071
E-mail: info@aaaai.org
Websites: www.aaaai.org;
www.aaaai.org/nab

American Academy of Dermatology
P.O. Box 4014
Schaumburg, IL 60168
Toll-Free: 866-503-SKIN
(503-7546)
Phone: 847-330-0230
Fax: 847-240-1859
Website: www.aad.org

American Academy of Family Physicians
P.O. Box 11210
Shawnee Mission, KS 66207-1210
Toll-Free: 800-274-2237
Phone: 913-906-6000
Fax: 913-906-6075
Website: www.aafp.org

American Academy of Otolaryngic Allergy
1990 M Street, NW, Suite 680
Washington, DC 20036
Phone: 202-955-5010
Fax: 202-955-5016
Website: www.aaoaf.org

American Academy of Otolaryngology-Head and Neck Surgery
1650 Diagonal Road
Alexandria, VA 22314-2857
Phone: 703-836-4444
Website: www.entnet.org

American Academy of Pediatrics
141 Northwest Point Boulevard
Elk Grove Village, IL 60007-1098
Phone: 847-434-4000
Fax: 847-434-8000
Website: www.aap.org
E-mail: kidsdocs@aap.org

American Association for Respiratory Care
9425 N. MacArthur Boulevard, Suite 100
Irving, TX 75063-4706
Phone: 972-243-2272
Fax: 972-484-2720
Website: www.aarc.org
E-mail: info@aarc.org

American Association of Immunologists
9650 Rockville Pike
Bethesda, MD 20814
Phone: 301-634-7178
Fax: 301-634-7887
Website: www.aai.org
E-mail: infoaai@aai.org

American Board of Allergy and Immunology
111 S. Independence Mall East
Suite 701
Philadelphia, PA 19106
Toll-Free: 866-264-5568
Phone: 215-592-9466
Fax: 215-592-9411
Website: www.abai.org
E-mail: abai@abai.org

American Celiac Disease Alliance
2504 Duxbury Place
Alexandria, VA 22308
Phone: 703-622-3331
Website: www.americanceliac.org
E-mail: info@americanceliac.org

American College of Allergy, Asthma and Immunology
85 West Algonquin Road
Suite 550
Arlington Heights, IL 60005
Phone: 847-427-1200
Fax: 847-427-1294
Website: www.acaai.org
E-mail: info@acaai.org

541

American College of Chest Physicians
3300 Dundee Road
Northbrook, IL 60062-2348
Toll-Free: 800-343-2227
Phone: 847-498-1400
Fax: 847-498-5460
Website: www.chestnet.org

American College of Emergency Physicians
1125 Executive Circle
Irving, TX 75038-2522
Toll-Free: 800-798-1822
Phone: 972-550-0911
Fax: 972-580-2816
Website: www.acep.org

American Dietetic Association
120 South Riverside Plaza,
Suite 2000
Chicago, IL 60606-6995
Toll-Free: 800-877-1600
Phone: 312-899-0040
Website: www.eatright.org

American Latex Allergy Association
P.O. Box 198
Slinger, WI 53086
Toll-Free: 888-972-5378
Phone: 262-677-9707
Website:
www.latexallergyresources.org
E-mail:
alert@latexallergyresources.org

American Lung Association
1301 Pennsylvania Avenue, NW,
Suite 800
Washington, DC 20004
Toll-Free: 800-LUNGUSA
(586-4872)
Website: www.lungusa.org

American Osteopathic College of Dermatology
1501 East Illinois Street
P.O. Box 7525
Kirksville, MO 63501
Toll-Free: 800-449-2623
Phone: 660-665-2184
Fax: 660-627-2623
Website: www.aocd.org
E-mail: ExecDirector@AOCD.org

American Medical Association
515 North State Street
Chicago, IL 60654
Toll-Free: 800-621-8335
Website: www.ama-assn.org

American Partnership for Eosinophilic Disorders
P.O. Box 29545
Atlanta, GA 30359
Phone: 713-493-7749
Website: www.apfed.org
E-mail: mail@apfed.org

American Rhinologic Society
P.O. Box 495
Warwick, NY 10990-0495
Phone: 845-988-1631
Fax: 845-986-1527
Website:
www.american-rhinologic.org
E-mail:
arsinfo@american-rhinologic.org

Anaphylaxis Canada
2005 Sheppard Avenue East,
Suite 800
Toronto, Ontario M2J 5B4
Toll-Free: 866-785-5660
Telephone: 416-785-5666
Fax: 416-785-0458
Websites: www.anaphylaxis.ca,
www.whyriskit.ca
E-mail: info@anaphylaxis.ca

Association of Camp Nurses
8630 Thorsonveien NE
Bemidji, MN 56601
Phone: 218-586-2633
Website: www.acn.org
E-mail: acn@campnurse.org

Asthma and Allergy Foundation of America
8201 Corporate Drive,
Suite 1000
Landover, MD 20785
Toll-Free: 800-727-8462
Website: www.aafa.org
E-mail: info@aafa.org

Celiac Disease Foundation
13251 Ventura Boulevard
Suite 1
Studio City, CA 91604
Phone: 818-990-2354
Fax: 818-990-2379
Website: www.celiac.org
E-mail: cdf@celiac.org

Cleveland Clinic
9500 Euclid Avenue
Cleveland, OH 44195
Toll-Free: 800-223-2273
TTY: 216-444-0261
Website: my.clevelandclinic.org

Food Allergy & Anaphylaxis Network
11781 Lee Jackson Highway
Suite 160
Fairfax, VA 22033-3309
Toll-Free: 800-929-4040
Phone: 703-691-2713
Websites: www.foodallergy.org;
www.fankids.org;
www.faanteen.org

Food Allergy Initiative
1414 Avenue of the Americas
Suite 1804
New York, NY 10019-2514
Phone: 212-207-1974
Fax: 917-338-5130
Website: www.faiusa.org
E-mail: info@faiusa.org

Food Allergy Research & Resource Program
University of Nebraska-Lincoln
143 Food Industry Complex
University of Nebraska
Lincoln, NE 68583-0919
Phone: 402-472-2833
Website: www.farrp.org

Inflammatory Skin Disease Institute
P.O. Box 1074
Newport News, VA 23601
Phone: 757-223-0795
Fax: 757-595-1842
Website: www.isdionline.org

International Food Information Council
1100 Connecticut Avenue NW
Suite 430
Washington, DC 20036
Phone: 202-296-6540
Website: www.foodinsight.org
E-mail: info@foodinsight.org

Job Accommodation Network
P.O. Box 6080
Morgantown, WV 26506-6080
Toll-Free: 800-526-7234
TTY: 877-781-9403
Fax: 304-293-5407
Website: www.askjan.org

Kids with Food Allergies
73 Old Dublin Pike, Suite 10, #163
Doylestown, PA 18901
Phone: 215-230-5394
Fax: 215-340-7674
Website:
www.kidswithfoodallergies.org

National Association of School Nurses
8484 Georgia Avenue, Suite 420
Silver Spring, MD 20910
Toll-Free: 866-627-6767
Phone: 240-821-1130
Fax: 301-585-1791
Website: www.nasn.org
E-mail: nasn@nasn.org

National Coalition for Food Safe Schools
Website:
www.foodsafeschools.org
E-mail: info@foodsafeschools.org

National Eczema Association
4460 Redwood Highway
Suite 16D
San Rafael, CA 94903-1953
Toll-Free: 800-818-7546
Phone: 415-499-3474
Website:
www.nationaleczema.org
E-mail: info@nationaleczema.org

National Jewish Medical and Research Center
1400 Jackson Street
Denver, CO 80206
Toll-Free: 800-423-8891
Phone: 303-388-4461
Website: www.njc.org

Nemours Foundation Center for Children's Health Media
1600 Rockland Road
Wilmington, DE 19803
Phone: 302-651-4000
Website: www.kidshealth.org
E-mail: info@kidshealth.org

New Zealand Dermatological Society
c/o Tristram Clinic
6 Knox Street
Hamilton, New Zealand
Phone: +64 7 838-1035
Fax: +64 7 838-2032
Website: www.dermnetnz.org

PeanutAllergy.com
Website: www.peanutallergy.com

Pollen.com
220 West Germantown Pike
Plymouth Meeting, PA 19462
Phone: 610-834-0800
Website: www.pollen.com

World Allergy Organization
555 East Wells Street
Suite 1100
Milwaukee, WI 53202-3823
Phone: 414-276-1791
Fax: 414-276-3349
Website: www.worldallergy.org
E-mail: info@worldallergy.org

Chapter 54

Resources for People with Food Allergies

Chapter Contents

Section 54.1

Directory of Companies That Market Food Products as a Service to People with Food Allergies

"Helpful Food Products," © 2010 Food Allergy Initiative
(www.faiusa.org). Reprinted with permission.

As this list shows, a growing number of companies are serving the needs of food-allergic customers. Please note that some or all of the products offered by companies marked with a [K] are kosher. A few companies do not have websites; in these cases, we've provided their address and phone number.

Baked Goods, Mixes, Candies, and Snacks

A & J Bakery
Website: www.aandjbakery.net

Amanda's Own Confections
Website: www.amandasown.com

Chocolate Emporium[K]
Website: www.choclat.com

Chocolate Gelt[K]
Website: www.chocolategelt.com

Caroline's Cakes
Website: www.carolinescakes.com

Cherrybrook Kitchen[K]
Website: www.cherrybrookkitchen.com

Dare Foods[K]
Website: www.darefoods.com

Divvies[K]
Website: www.divvies.com

The Donut Pub (New York City)
203 West 14th St.
New York, NY
Phone: 212-929-0126

Enjoy Life Foods[K]
Website: www.enjoylifefoods.com

Gimbal's Fine Candy[K]
Website: www.gimbalscandy.com

Grandma's Kitchen (New Jersey)
125 Paris Avenue
Northvale, NJ 07647
Phone: 201-750-2301
Website: www.grandmaskitchennj.com

HomeFree[K]
Website: www.homefreetreats.com

Nonuttin' Foods[K]
Website: www.nonuttin.com

Peanut-Free Planet[K]
Website: www.peanutfreeplanet.com

Sweet Alexis
Website: www.sweetalexis.com

Tootsie Roll Industries
Website: www.tootsie.com

Vermont Nut Free Chocolates
Website: www.vermontnutfree.com

Wheyout Chocolate
Website: www.wheyoutchocolate.com

Yummy Earth[K]
Website: www.yummyearth.com

General

Allergy Grocer[K]
Website: www.allergygrocer.com

AllerNeeds[K]
Website: www.allerneeds.com

Ener-G Foods[K]
Website: www.ener-g.com

Free From Market[K]
Website: www.freefrommarket.com

Ice Cream and Ices

PhillySwirl
Website: www.phillyswirl.com

Turtle Mountain
Website: www.turtlemountain.com

Nutrition Bars

AllerEnergy[K]
Website: www.allerenergy.com

Peanut Butter Substitutes

Simple Food[K]
Website: www.simplefood.com

SoyNut Butter Company[K]
Website: www.soynutbutter.com

Recipes, Cooking Lessons, and Cooking Tips

Food Allergy Kitchen
Website: www.foodallergykitchen.com

Kids with Food Allergies
Website: www.kidswithfoodallergies.com

Lovebites Kitchen
Website: www.lovebiteskitchen.com

Section 54.2

Directory of Websites and Cookbooks for People with Food Allergies

Resources in this chapter were compiled from several
sources deemed reliable, August 2010.

Recipe Books for People with Food Allergies

8 Degrees of Ingredients. By Melisa K. Priem. CreateSpace: 2008. ISBN: 1451582617.

Allergy-Free Desserts. By Elizabeth Gordon. Wiley: 2010. ISBN: 0470448466.

The Allergy Self-Help Cookbook. By Marjorie Hurt Jones. Rodale: 2001. ISBN: 157954276X.

The Allergen-Free Baker's Handbook. By Cybele Pascal. Celestial Arts: 2009. ISBN: 1587613484.

Amazing Dairy-Free Desserts. By Penny Wantuck Eisenberg. Surris Books: 2006. ISBN: 0977961796.

Bakin' Without Eggs. By Rosemarie Emro. St. Martin's Griffin: 1999. ISBN: 0312206356.

The Food Allergy Mama's Baking Book. By Kelly Rudnicki. Agate Surrey: 2009. ISBN: 1572841028.

Food Allergy News Cookbook. By Anne Munoz-Furlong. Wiley: 1998. ISBN: 0471346926.

Kid-Friendly Food Allergy Cookbook. By Leslie Hammond and Lynne Marie Rominger. Fair Winds Press: 2004. ISBN: 1592330541.

Wheat-Free Recipes and Menus. By Carol Fenster. Avery Trade: 2004. ISBN: 1583331913.

The Whole Foods Allergy Cookbook. By Cybele Pascal. Square One Publishers: 2005. 1890612456.

Go Dairy Free. By Alisa Marie Fleming. Fleming Ink: 2008. ISBN: 0979128625.

The Everything Food Allergy Cookbook. By Linda Larsen. Adams Media: 2008. ISBN: 1598695606.

Online Allergy Tools and Applications for Mobile Devices

Allergy Alert
Website: www.pollen.com/iphone.asp

Allergy Companion No Peanut
Website: allergycompanion.com

Cook IT Allergy Free
Website: www.cookitallergyfree.com

EMNet findER™
Website: itunes.apple.com/app/emnet-finder/id376928203?mt=8

Food Content Alerts
Website: www.foodcontentalerts.com

iCanEatOnTheGo Gluten & Allergen Free
Website: www.allergyfreepassport.com

Polka Close Call
Website: blog.polka.com/?p=170

Pollen Journal
Website: www.ringfulhealth.com/apps/pollen

WebArtisan Food Additives
Website: webartisan.com.au/apps/index.php/iphone-apps/food-additives

Zyrtec® Allergy Cast
Website: itunes.apple.com/us/app/zyrtec-allergycast/id320298020?mt=8

Section 54.3

Allergen-Free Recipes for People with Food Allergies

"Allergy Free Birthday Cake," "Allergy Free Ice Cream," "Allergy Free Mashed Potatoes," "Chicken Pot Pies," and "Dairy Free Hot Chocolate Mix," by Kristi Winkels, RD. © 2010 EatingWithFoodAllergies.com. Reprinted with permission.

Allergy Free Birthday Cake

Ingredients

- 1 cup white rice flour
- 1/3 cup potato starch
- 3 tablespoons tapioca starch
- 1/2 teaspoon xanthan gum
- 1 cup sugar
- 1/4 cup cocoa powder
- 1/2 teaspoon salt
- 1 teaspoon baking soda
- 1 teaspoon pure vanilla extract
- 1 tablespoon vinegar (any variety will do)
- 5 tablespoons canola oil
- 1 1/4 cup cold water

Directions

1. Preheat oven to 350 degrees.
2. Combine the rice flour, potato starch, tapioca starch, xanthan gum, sugar, cocoa powder, salt, and baking soda in a mixing bowl. Add the vanilla extract, vinegar, canola oil, and water. Mix well.

3. For cake: Pour batter into an ungreased square cake pan. Bake at 350 degrees for 30–35 minutes or until a toothpick inserted in the middle comes out clean. For cupcakes: Pour batter into a muffin tin with paper liners. Bake at 350 degrees for 20–25 minutes or until a toothpick inserted in the middle of a cupcake comes out clean. Remove from the pan immediately and place on a cooling rack. Makes 12 cupcakes.

Allergy Free Ice Cream

Ingredients

- 4 cups vanilla rice milk
- 3 tablespoons arrowroot starch flour
- 15 large marshmallows
- 1/3 cup sugar
- dash of salt
- 1/2 cup canola oil
- 1/2 teaspoon xanthan gum
- 1 1/2 teaspoons vanilla extract

Directions

1. In a large mixing bowl, combine the amaranth [arrowroot starch] flour with 1/4 cup of the rice milk; set aside. In a large saucepan, combine the remaining rice milk, marshmallows, sugar, and salt. Bring mixture to a boil and immediately remove from the heat. Pour the hot mixture over the amaranth flour and milk mixture and stir well. Add the oil, xanthan gum, and vanilla extract and whisk mixture together until blended. Place in the refrigerator until completely cooled.

2. Pour cooled mixture into an ice cream maker and freeze according to the manufacturer's instructions. Makes about 1 quart.

Allergy Free Mashed Potatoes

Ingredients

- 6 medium Yukon Gold potatoes, peeled and cubed
- 1/2 cup chicken broth
- 3/4 cup rice milk
- 2 tablespoons butter-flavored grapeseed oil, olive oil, or dairy free margarine
- Salt and pepper to taste

Directions

Place the potatoes in a large stock pot and cover with water. Bring to a boil. Reduce heat, cover, and simmer for 20–25 minutes or until potatoes are tender. Drain the potatoes and add the broth, rice milk, oil or margarine, and salt and pepper. Mash until light and fluffy. For lump free potatoes, put them in a food mill or ricer before adding the other ingredients. Makes 12 (1/2 cup) servings.

Chicken Pot Pies

Ingredients

- 1-single pie crust
- cooking spray
- salt
- 2 tablespoons white rice flour
- 1 teaspoon rubbed sage
- 1/4 teaspoon salt
- 1/4 teaspoon black pepper
- 1 14-ounce package chicken breast tenders, cut into bite size pieces
- 2 tablespoons "safe" margarine or extra virgin olive oil
- 2 tablespoons white rice flour
- 1 cup "safe" milk (soy, rice, or potato)
- 1/4 cup gluten free chicken broth (I use Kitchen Basics)
- 1 1/4 cups water
- 1 1/2 cups frozen mixed vegetables
- 1 small can of sliced mushrooms

Directions

1. For the pie crust toppers: Preheat oven to 425 degrees. With a round cookie cutter or using a bowl or large cup as a guide, cut 4 (3–4 inch) circles out of the dough. Place the dough circles on a baking sheet coated with cooking spray. Lightly coat dough with cooking spray and sprinkle with salt. Pierce top of dough with a fork. Bake at 425 for 8 minutes.

2. For the sauce: In a small saucepan, add the margarine or olive oil and cook on medium high until margarine is melted or oil is hot. Add the flour and whisk together until mixture is smooth. Add the milk and chicken broth while stirring. Cook, stirring frequently, until the mixture bubbles and becomes thick.

3. In a freezer bag, combine flour, sage, salt, pepper, and chicken. Seal the bag and toss to coat the chicken. Heat a non-stick skillet coated with cooking spray over medium high heat. Add the chicken and brown on all sides. Add the water and scrape the pan to loosen the bits of chicken. Stir in the vegetables, mushrooms, and sauce; bring to a boil. Reduce heat and simmer for about 10 minutes. Ladle 1 cup of the chicken mixture into bowls; top each serving with 1 pie crust round. Makes 4 servings.

Dairy Free Hot Chocolate Mix

Ingredients

- 1 tablespoon Vance's DariFree Powder
- 2 tablespoons cocoa powder
- 2 tablespoons sugar or sugar substitute
- 1 cup boiling water
- dash of cinnamon
- 2 small or 1 large candy cane (optional)
- mini marshmallows

Directions

1. In a mug, combine the potato milk [DariFree Powder], cocoa powder, sugar, and cinnamon.

2. If desired, place candy canes in a sandwich bag and crush with a rolling pin (you could also finely chop with a food processor). Add crushed candy cane to mix.

3. Add boiling water and stir until powder is dissolved. Top with marshmallows.

Index

Index

Health Reference Series
Complete Catalog
List price $93 per volume. School and library price $84 per volume.

Adolescent Health Sourcebook, 3rd Edition

Basic Consumer Health Information about Adolescent Growth and Development, Puberty, Sexuality, Reproductive Health, and Physical, Emotional, Social, and Mental Health Concerns of Teens and Their Parents, Including Facts about Nutrition, Physical Activity, Weight Management, Acne, Allergies, Cancer, Diabetes, Growth Disorders, Juvenile Arthritis, Infections, Substance Abuse, and More

Along with Information about Adolescent Safety Concerns, Youth Violence, a Glossary of Related Terms, and a Directory of Resources

Edited by Amy L. Sutton. 600 pages. 2010. 978-0-7808-1140-9.

Adult Health Concerns Sourcebook

Basic Consumer Health Information about Medical and Mental Concerns of Adults, Including Facts about Choosing Healthcare Providers, Navigating Insurance Options, Maintaining Wellness, Preventing Cancer, Heart Disease, Stroke, Diabetes, and Osteoporosis, and Understanding Aging-Related Health Concerns, Including Menopause, Cognitive Changes, and Changes in the Coronary and Vascular Systems

Along with Tips on Caring for Aging Parents and Dealing with Health-Related Work and Travel Issues, a Glossary, and a Directory of Resources for Additional Help and Information

Edited by Sandra J. Judd. 648 pages. 2008. 978-0-7808-0999-4.

"Provides a thorough list of topics that are important to adult health and for caregivers."
—*CHOICE*, Nov '08

"Written in easy-to-understand language... the content is well-organized and is intended to aid adults in making health care-related decisions."
—*AORN Journal*, Dec '08

AIDS Sourcebook, 4th Edition

Basic Consumer Health Information about Human Immunodeficiency Virus (HIV) and Acquired Immunodeficiency Syndrome (AIDS), Featuring Updated Statistics and Facts about Risks, Prevention, Screening, Diagnosis, Treatments, Side Effects, and Complications, and Including a Section about the Impact of HIV/AIDS on the Health of Women, Children, and Adolescents

Along with Tips on Managing Life with AIDS, Reports on Current Research Initiatives and Clinical Trials, a Glossary of Related Terms, and Resource Directories for Further Help and Information

Edited by Ivy L. Alexander. 680 pages. 2008. 978-0-7808-0997-0.

SEE ALSO *Contagious Diseases Sourcebook, 2nd Edition*

Alcoholism Sourcebook, 3rd Edition

Basic Consumer Health Information about Alcohol Use, Abuse, and Dependence, Featuring Facts about the Physical, Mental, and Social Health Effects of Alcohol Addiction, Including Alcoholic Liver Disease, Pancreatic Disease, Cardiovascular Disease, Neurological Disorders, and the Effects of Drinking during Pregnancy

Along with Information about Alcohol Treatment, Medications, and Recovery Programs, in Addition to Tips for Reducing the Prevalence of Underage Drinking, Statistics about Alcohol Use, a Glossary of Related Terms, and Directories of Resources for More Help and Information

Edited by Joyce Brennfleck Shannon. 600 pages. 2010. 978-0-7808-1141-6.

SEE ALSO *Drug Abuse Sourcebook, 3rd Edition*

Allergies Sourcebook, 3rd Edition

Basic Consumer Health Information about Allergic Disorders, Such as Anaphylaxis, Hives,

Eczema, Rhinitis, Sinusitis, and Conjunctivitis, and Their Triggers, Including Pollen, Mold, Dust Mites, Animal Dander, Insects, Chemicals, Food, Food Additives, and Medications

Along with Advice about the Diagnosis and Treatment of Allergy Symptoms, a Glossary of Related Terms, a Directory of Resources for Help and Information, and Suggestions for Additional Reading

Edited by Amy L. Sutton. 588 pages. 2007. 978-0-7808-0950-5.

SEE ALSO Asthma Sourcebook, 2nd Edition

Alzheimer Disease Sourcebook, 4th Edition

Basic Consumer Health Information about Alzheimer Disease, Other Dementias, and Related Disorders, Including Multi-Infarct Dementia, Dementia with Lewy Bodies, Frontotemporal Dementia (Pick Disease), Wernicke-Korsakoff Syndrome (Alcohol-Related Dementia), AIDS Dementia Complex, Huntington Disease, Creutzfeldt-Jacob Disease, and Delirium

Along with Information about Coping with Memory Loss and Forgetfulness, Maintaining Skills, and Long-Term Planning for People with Dementia, and Suggestions Addressing Common Caregiver Concerns, Updated Information about Current Research Efforts, a Glossary of Related Terms, and Directories of Sources for Additional Help and Information

Edited by Karen Bellenir. 603 pages. 2008. 978-0-7808-1001-3.

"An invaluable resource for persons who have received a diagnosis, for caregivers, and for family members dealing with this insidious disease. It is recommended for public, community college, and ready-reference sections in academic libraries."
—*American Reference Books Annual, 2009*

SEE ALSO Brain Disorders Sourcebook, 3rd Edition

Arthritis Sourcebook, 3rd Edition

Basic Consumer Health Information about the Risk Factors, Symptoms, Diagnosis, and Treatment of Osteoarthritis, Rheumatoid Arthritis, Juvenile Arthritis, Gout, Infectious Arthritis, and Autoimmune Disorders Associated with Arthritis

Along with Facts about Medications, Surgeries, and Self-Care Techniques to Manage Pain and Disability, Tips on Living with Arthritis, a Glossary of Related Terms, and Resources for Additional Help and Information

Edited by Amy L. Sutton. 600 pages. 2010. 978-0-7808-1077-8.

Asthma Sourcebook, 2nd Edition

Basic Consumer Health Information about the Causes, Symptoms, Diagnosis, and Treatment of Asthma in Infants, Children, Teenagers, and Adults, Including Facts about Different Types of Asthma, Common Co-Occurring Conditions, Asthma Management Plans, Triggers, Medications, and Medication Delivery Devices

Along with Asthma Statistics, Research Updates, a Glossary, a Directory of Asthma-Related Resources, and More

Edited by Karen Bellenir. 581 pages. 2006. 978-0-7808-0866-9.

SEE ALSO Lung Disorders Sourcebook; Respiratory Disorders Sourcebook, 2nd Edition

Attention Deficit Disorder Sourcebook

Basic Consumer Health Information about Attention Deficit/Hyperactivity Disorder in Children and Adults, Including Facts about Causes, Symptoms, Diagnostic Criteria, and Treatment Options Such as Medications, Behavior Therapy, Coaching, and Homeopathy

Along with Reports on Current Research Initiatives, Legal Issues, and Government Regulations, and Featuring a Glossary of Related Terms, Internet Resources, and a List of Additional Reading Material

Edited by Dawn D. Matthews. 447 pages. 2002. 978-0-7808-0624-5.

"Recommended reference source."
—*Booklist, Jan '03*

SEE ALSO Learning Disabilities Sourcebook, 3rd Edition

Autism and Pervasive Developmental Disorders Sourcebook

Basic Consumer Health Information about Autism Spectrum and Pervasive Developmental Disorders, Such as Classical Autism, Asperger Syndrome, Rett Syndrome, and Childhood Disintegrative Disorder, Including Information about Related Genetic Disorders and Medical Problems and Facts about Causes, Screening Methods, Diagnostic Criteria, Treatments and Interventions, and Family and Education Issues

Along with a Glossary of Related Terms, Tips for Evaluating the Validity of Health Claims, and a Directory of Resources for Additional Help and Information

Edited by Sandra J. Judd. 603 pages. 2007. 978-0-7808-0953-6.

"This book provides a current overview of disorders on the autism spectrum and information about various therapies, educational resources, and help for families with practical issues such as workplace adjustments, living arrangements, and estate planning. It is a useful resource for public and consumer health libraries."
—*American Reference Books Annual, 2009*

SEE ALSO *Learning Disabilities Sourcebook, 3rd Edition*

Back and Neck Disorders Sourcebook, 2nd Edition

Basic Consumer Health Information about Spinal Pain, Spinal Cord Injuries, and Related Disorders, Such as Degenerative Disk Disease, Osteoarthritis, Scoliosis, Sciatica, Spina Bifida, and Spinal Stenosis, and Featuring Facts about Maintaining Spinal Health, Self-Care, Pain Management, Rehabilitative Care, Chiropractic Care, Spinal Surgeries, and Complementary Therapies

Along with Suggestions for Preventing Back and Neck Pain, a Glossary of Related Terms, and a Directory of Resources

Edited by Amy L. Sutton. 607 pages. 2004. 978-0-7808-0738-9.

"Recommended... An easy to use, comprehensive medical reference book."
—*E-Streams, Sep '05*

"For anyone who has back or neck problems, this book is ideal. Its easy-to-understand language and variety of topics makes this sourcebook a worthwhile read. The price... is reasonable for the amount of information contained in the book"
—*Occupational Therapy in Health Care, 2007*

Blood & Circulatory Disorders Sourcebook, 3rd Edition

Basic Consumer Health Information about Blood and Circulatory System Disorders, Such as Anemia, Leukemia, Lymphoma, Rh Disease, Hemophilia, Thrombophilia, Other Bleeding and Clotting Deficiencies, and Artery, Vascular, and Venous Diseases, Including Facts about Blood Types, Blood Donation, Bone Marrow and Stem Cell Transplants, Tests and Medications, and Tips for Maintaining Circulatory Health

Along with a Glossary of Related Terms and a List of Resources for Additional Help and Information

Edited by Sandra J. Judd. 600 pages. 2010. 978-0-7808-1081-5.

SEE ALSO *Leukemia Sourcebook*

Brain Disorders Sourcebook, 3rd Edition

Basic Consumer Health Information about Acquired and Traumatic Brain Injuries, Brain Tumors, Cerebral Palsy and Other Genetic and Congenital Brain Disorders, Infections of the Brain, Epilepsy, and Degenerative Neurological Disorders Such as Dementia, Huntington Disease, and Amyotrophic Lateral Sclerosis (ALS)

Along with Information on Brain Structure and Function, Treatment and Rehabilitation Options, a Glossary of Terms Related to Brain Disorders, and a Directory of Resources for More Information

Edited by Joyce Brennfleck Shannon. 600 pages. 2010. 978-0-7808-1083-9.

SEE ALSO *Alzheimer Disease Sourcebook, 4th Edition*

Breast Cancer Sourcebook, 3rd Edition

Basic Consumer Health Information about Breast Health and Breast Cancer, Including Facts about Environmental, Genetic, and Other Risk Factors, Prevention Efforts, Screening and Diagnostic Methods, Surgical Treatment Options and Other Care Choices, Complementary and Alternative Therapies, and Post-Treatment Concerns

Along with Statistical Data, News about Research Advances, a Glossary of Related Terms, and Directories of Resources for Additional Information and Support

Edited by Karen Bellenir. 606 pages. 2009. 978-0-7808-1030-3.

"A very useful reference for people wanting to learn more about breast cancer and how to negotiate their care or the care of a loved one. The third edition is necessary as information/treatment options continue to evolve."
— *Doody's Review Service, 2009*

SEE ALSO Cancer Sourcebook for Women, 3rd Edition, Women's Health Concerns Sourcebook, 3rd Edition

Breastfeeding Sourcebook

Basic Consumer Health Information about the Benefits of Breastmilk, Preparing to Breastfeed, Breastfeeding as a Baby Grows, Nutrition, and More, Including Information on Special Situations and Concerns Such as Mastitis, Illness, Medications, Allergies, Multiple Births, Prematurity, Special Needs, and Adoption

Along with a Glossary and Resources for Additional Help and Information

Edited by Jenni Lynn Colson. 367 pages. 2002. 978-0-7808-0332-9.

SEE ALSO Pregnancy and Birth Sourcebook, 3rd Edition

Burns Sourcebook

Basic Consumer Health Information about Various Types of Burns and Scalds, Including Flame, Heat, Cold, Electrical, Chemical, and Sun Burns

Along with Information on Short-Term and Long-Term Treatments, Tissue Reconstruction, Plastic Surgery, Prevention Suggestions, and First Aid

Edited by Allan R. Cook. 604 pages. 1999. 978-0-7808-0204-9.

"This is an exceptional addition to the series and is highly recommended for all consumer health collections, hospital libraries, and academic medical centers."
— *E-Streams, Mar '00*

"This key reference guide is an invaluable addition to all health care and public libraries in confronting this ongoing health issue."
— *American Reference Books Annual, 2000*

SEE ALSO Dermatological Disorders Sourcebook, 2nd Edition

Cancer Sourcebook, 5th Edition

Basic Consumer Health Information about Major Forms and Stages of Cancer, Featuring Facts about Head and Neck Cancers, Lung Cancers, Gastrointestinal Cancers, Genitourinary Cancers, Lymphomas, Blood Cell Cancers, Endocrine Cancers, Skin Cancers, Bone Cancers, Metastatic Cancers, and More

Along with Facts about Cancer Treatments, Cancer Risks and Prevention, a Glossary of Related Terms, Statistical Data, and a Directory of Resources for Additional Information

Edited by Karen Bellenir. 1105 pages. 2007. 978-0-7808-0947-5.

"The 5th, updated edition of Cancer Sourcebook should be in every public and health lending library collection... An unparalleled discussion essential for any health collections considering an all-in-one basic general reference."
— *California Bookwatch, Aug '07*

SEE ALSO Breast Cancer Sourcebook, 3rd Edition, Cancer Survivorship Sourcebook, Leukemia Sourcebook

Cancer Sourcebook for Women, 4th Edition

Basic Consumer Health Information about Gynecologic Cancers and Other Cancers of Special Concern to Women, Including Cancers of the Breast, Cervix, Colon, Lung, Ovaries, Thyroid, and Uterus

Along with Facts about Benign Conditions of the Female Reproductive System, Cancer Risk

Factors, Diagnostic and Treatment Procedures, Side Effects of Cancer and Cancer Treatments, Women's Issues in Cancer Survivorship, a Glossary of Related Terms, and a Directory of Resources for Additional Help and Information

Edited by Karen Bellenir. 600 pages. 2010. 978-0-7808-1139-3.

SEE ALSO Breast Cancer Sourcebook, 3rd Edition, Women's Health Concerns Sourcebook, 3rd Edition

Cancer Survivorship Sourcebook
Basic Consumer Health Information about the Physical, Educational, Emotional, Social, and Financial Needs of Cancer Patients from Diagnosis, through Cancer Treatment, and Beyond, Including Facts about Researching Specific Types of Cancer and Learning about Clinical Trials and Treatment Options, and Featuring Tips for Coping with the Side Effects of Cancer Treatments and Adjusting to Life after Cancer Treatment Concludes

Along with Suggestions for Caregivers, Friends, and Family Members of Cancer Patients, a Glossary of Cancer Care Terms, and Directories of Related Resources

Edited by Karen Bellenir. 633 pages. 2007. 978-0-7808-0985-7.

"Well organized and comprehensive in coverage, the book speaks to issues encountered both during and after cancer treatment. Recommended for consumer health and public libraries."
—*Library Journal, Aug 1 '07*

"Cancer Survivorship Sourcebook will be useful to anyone who has a friend or loved one with a cancer diagnosis."
—*American Reference Books Annual, 2008*

SEE ALSO *Cancer Sourcebook, 5th Edition, Disease Management Sourcebook*

Cardiovascular Disorders Sourcebook, 4th Edition
Basic Consumer Health Information about Heart and Blood Vessel Diseases and Disorders, Such as Angina, Heart Attack, Heart Failure, Cardiomyopathy, Arrhythmias, Valve Disease, Atherosclerosis, Aneurysms, and

Congenital Heart Defects, Including Information about Cardiovascular Disease in Women, Men, Children, Adolescents, and Minorities

Along with Facts about Diagnosing, Managing, and Preventing Cardiovascular Disease, a Glossary of Related Medical Terms, and a Directory of Resources for Additional Information

Edited by Amy L. Sutton. 600 pages. 2010. 978-0-7808-1080-8.

Caregiving Sourcebook
Basic Consumer Health Information for Caregivers, Including a Profile of Caregivers, Caregiving Responsibilities and Concerns, Tips for Specific Conditions, Care Environments, and the Effects of Caregiving

Along with Facts about Legal Issues, Financial Information, and Future Planning, a Glossary, and a Listing of Additional Resources

Edited by Joyce Brennfleck Shannon. 583 pages. 2001. 978-0-7808-0331-2.

"Essential for most collections."
—*Library Journal, Apr 1 '02*

"An ideal addition to the reference collection of any public library. Health sciences information professionals may also want to acquire the Caregiving Sourcebook for their hospital or academic library for use as a ready reference tool by health care workers interested in aging and caregiving."
—*E-Streams, Jan '02*

Child Abuse Sourcebook, 2nd Edition
Basic Consumer Health Information about the Physical, Sexual, and Emotional Abuse of Children, Neglect, Münchhausen Syndrome by Proxy (MSBP), and Shaken Baby Syndrome, and Featuring Facts about Withholding Medical Care, Corporal Punishment, Child Maltreatment in Youth Sports, and Parental Substance Abuse

Along with Information about Child Protective Services, Foster Care, Adoption, Parenting Challenges, Abuse Prevention Programs, and Intervention, Treatment, and Recovery Guidelines, a Glossary of Related Terms, and Resources for Additional Help and Information

Edited by Joyce Brennfleck Shannon. 600 pages. 2009. 978-0-7808-1037-2.

SEE ALSO Domestic Violence Sourcebook, 3rd Edition

Childhood Diseases and Disorders Sourcebook, 2nd Edition

Basic Consumer Health Information about the Physical, Mental, and Developmental Health of Pre-Adolescent Children, Including Facts about Infectious Diseases, Asthma, Allergies, Diabetes, and Other Acute and Chronic Conditions Affecting the Gastrointestinal Tract, Ears, Nose, Throat, Liver, Kidneys, Heart, Blood, Brain, Muscles, Bones, and Skin

Along with Reports on Recommended Childhood Vaccinations, Wellness Guidelines, a Glossary of Related Medical Terms, and a List of Resources for Parents

Edited by Sandra J. Judd. 694 pages. 2009. 978-0-7808-1031-0.

"The strength of this source is the wide range of information given about childhood health issues... It is most appropriate for public libraries and academic libraries that field medical questions."
—American Reference Books Annual, 2009

SEE ALSO Healthy Children Sourcebook

Colds, Flu and Other Common Ailments Sourcebook

Basic Consumer Health Information about Common Ailments and Injuries, Including Colds, Coughs, the Flu, Sinus Problems, Headaches, Fever, Nausea and Vomiting, Menstrual Cramps, Diarrhea, Constipation, Hemorrhoids, Back Pain, Dandruff, Dry and Itchy Skin, Cuts, Scrapes, Sprains, Bruises, and More

Along with Information about Prevention, Self-Care, Choosing a Doctor, Over-the-Counter Medications, Folk Remedies, and Alternative Therapies, and Including a Glossary of Important Terms and a Directory of Resources for Further Help and Information

Edited by Chad T. Kimball. 622 pages. 2001. 978-0-7808-0435-7.

"A good starting point for research on common illnesses. It will be a useful addition to public and consumer health library collections."
—American Reference Books Annual, 2002

"Will prove valuable to any library seeking to maintain a current, comprehensive reference collection of health resources... Excellent reference."
—The Bookwatch, Aug '01

SEE ALSO Contagious Diseases Sourcebook, 2nd Edition

Communication Disorders Sourcebook

Basic Information about Deafness and Hearing Loss, Speech and Language Disorders, Voice Disorders, Balance and Vestibular Disorders, and Disorders of Smell, Taste, and Touch

Edited by Linda M. Ross. 533 pages. 1996. 978-0-7808-0077-9.

"This is skillfully edited and is a welcome resource for the layperson. It should be found in every public and medical library."
—Booklist Health Sciences Supplement, Oct '97

Complementary & Alternative Medicine Sourcebook, 4th Edition

Basic Consumer Health Information about Ayurveda, Acupuncture, Aromatherapy, Chiropractic Care, Diet-Based Therapies, Guided Imagery, Herbal and Vitamin Supplements, Homeopathy, Hypnosis, Massage, Meditation, Naturopathy, Pilates, Reflexology, Reiki, Shiatsu, Tai Chi, Traditional Chinese Medicine, Yoga, and Other Complementary and Alternative Medical Therapies

Along with Statistics, Tips for Selecting a Practitioner, Treatments for Specific Health Conditions, a Glossary of Related Terms, and a Directory of Resources for Additional Help and Information

Edited by Amy L. Sutton. 600 pages. 2010. 978-0-7808-1082-2.

Congenital Disorders Sourcebook, 2nd Edition

Basic Consumer Health Information about Nonhereditary Birth Defects and Disorders

Related to Prematurity, Gestational Injuries, Congenital Infections, and Birth Complications, Including Heart Defects, Hydrocephalus, Spina Bifida, Cleft Lip and Palate, Cerebral Palsy, and More

Along with Facts about the Prevention of Birth Defects, Fetal Surgery and Other Treatment Options, Research Initiatives, a Glossary of Related Terms, and Resources for Additional Information and Support

Edited by Sandra J. Judd. 619 pages. 2007. 978-0-7808-0945-1.

"Congenital Disorders Sourcebook provides an excellent, non-technical overview of many aspects of pregnancy with the focus on congenital disorders."
—*American Reference Books Annual, 2008*

"An excellent readable reference aimed at the lay public for difficult to understand medical problems. An excellent starting point for the interested parent or family member who may then be motivated to seek more information."
—*Doody's Review Service, 2007*

SEE ALSO *Pregnancy and Birth Sourcebook, 3rd Edition*

Contagious Diseases Sourcebook, 2nd Edition

Basic Consumer Health Information about Diseases Spread from Person to Person through Direct Physical Contact, Airborne Transmissions, Sexual Contact, or Contact with Blood or Other Body Fluids, Including Pneumococcal, Staphylococcal, and Streptococcal Diseases, Colds, Influenza, Lice, Measles, Mumps, Tuberculosis, and Others

Along with Facts about Self-Care and Over-the-Counter Medications, Antibiotics and Drug Resistance, Disease Prevention, Vaccines, and Bioterrorism, a Glossary, and a Directory of Resources for More Information

Edited by Joyce Brennfleck Shannon. 600 pages. 2010. 978-0-7808-1075-4.

SEE ALSO *AIDS Sourcebook, 4th Edition, Hepatitis Sourcebook*

Cosmetic and Reconstructive Surgery Sourcebook, 2nd Edition

Basic Consumer Information about Plastic Surgery and Non-Surgical Appearance-Enhancing Procedures, Including Facts about Botulinum Toxin, Collagen Replacement, Dermabrasion, Chemical Peels, Eyelid Surgery, Nose Reshaping, Lip Augmentation, Liposuction, Breast Enlargement and Reduction, Tummy Tucking, and Other Skin, Hair, Facial, and Body Shaping Procedures

Along with Information about Reconstructive Procedures for Congenital Disorders, Disfiguring Diseases, Burns, and Traumatic Injuries, a Glossary of Related Terms, and a Directory of Additional Resources

Edited by Karen Bellenir. 483 pages. 2007. 978-0-7808-0951-2.

"A comprehensive source for people considering cosmetic surgery... also recommended for medical students who will perform these procedures later in their careers; and public librarians and academic medical librarians who may assist patrons interested in this information."
—*Medical Reference Services Quarterly, Fall '08*

"A practical guide for health care consumers and health care workers... This easy-to-read reference guide would be useful for novice and veteran health care consumers, surgical technology students, nursing students, and perioperative nurses new to plastic and reconstructive surgery. It also may be helpful for medical-surgical nurses as a guide for patient teaching in their practices."
—*AORN Journal, Aug '08*

SEE ALSO *Surgery Sourcebook, 2nd Edition*

Death and Dying Sourcebook, 2nd Edition

Basic Consumer Health Information about End-of-Life Care and Related Perspectives and Ethical Issues, Including End-of-Life Symptoms and Treatments, Pain Management, Quality-of-Life Concerns, the Use of Life Support, Patients' Rights and Privacy Issues, Advance Directives, Physician-Assisted Suicide, Caregiving, Organ and Tissue Donation, Autopsies, Funeral Arrangements, and Grief

Along with Statistical Data, Information about the Leading Causes of Death, a Glossary, and Directories of Support Groups and Other Resources

Edited by Joyce Brennfleck Shannon. 626 pages. 2006. 978-0-7808-0871-3.

Dental Care and Oral Health Sourcebook, 3rd Edition

Basic Consumer Health Information about Dental Care and Oral Health Throughout the Lifespan, Including Facts about Cavities, Bad Breath, Cold and Canker Sores, Dry Mouth, Toothaches, Gum Disease, Malocclusion, Temporomandibular Joint and Muscle Disorders, Oral Cancers, and Dental Emergencies

Along with Information about Mouth Hygiene, Crowns, Bridges, Implants, and Fillings, Surgical, Orthodontic, and Cosmetic Dental Procedures, Pain Management, Health Conditions that Impact Oral Care, a Glossary of Related Terms, and a Directory of Additional Resources

Edited by Amy L. Sutton. 619 pages. 2008. 978-0-7808-1032-7.

"Could serve as turning point in the battle to educate consumers in issues concerning oral health. Tightly written in terms the average person can understand, yet comprehensive in scope and authoritative in tone, it is another excellent sourcebook in the Health Reference Series... Should be in the reference department of all public libraries, and in academic libraries that have a public constituency."
—*American Reference Books Annual, 2009*

Depression Sourcebook, 2nd Edition

Basic Consumer Health Information about Unipolar Depression, Bipolar Disorder, Dysthymia, Seasonal Affective Disorder, Postpartum Depression, and Other Depressive Disorders, Including Facts about Populations at Special Risk, Coexisting Medical Conditions, Symptoms, Treatment Options, and Suicide Prevention

Along with Statistical Data, a Glossary of Related Terms, and a Directory of Resources for Additional Help and Information

Edited by Sandra J. Judd. 646 pages. 2008. 978-0-7808-1003-7.

"Recommended for public libraries."
—*American Reference Books Annual, 2009*

SEE ALSO *Mental Health Disorders Sourcebook, 4th Edition*

Dermatological Disorders Sourcebook, 2nd Edition

Basic Consumer Health Information about Conditions and Disorders Affecting the Skin, Hair, and Nails, Such as Acne, Rosacea, Rashes, Dermatitis, Pigmentation Disorders, Birthmarks, Skin Cancer, Skin Injuries, Psoriasis, Scleroderma, and Hair Loss, Including Facts about Medications and Treatments for Dermatological Disorders and Tips for Maintaining Healthy Skin, Hair, and Nails

Along with Information about How Aging Affects the Skin, a Glossary of Related Terms, and a Directory of Resources for Additional Help and Information

Edited by Amy L. Sutton. 617 pages. 2006. 978-0-7808-0795-2.

"Well organized... presents a plethora of information in a manner that is appropriate in style and readability for the intended audience."
—*Physical Therapy, Nov '06*

"Helpfully brings together... sources in one convenient place, saving the user hours of research time."
—*American Reference Books Annual, 2006*

SEE ALSO *Burns Sourcebook*

Diabetes Sourcebook, 4th Edition

Basic Consumer Health Information about Type 1 and Type 2 Diabetes Mellitus, Gestational Diabetes, Monogenic Forms of Diabetes, and Insulin Resistance, with Guidelines for Lifestyle Modifications and the Medical Management of Diabetes, Including Facts about Insulin, Insulin Delivery Devices, Oral Diabetes Medications, Self-Monitoring of Blood Glucose, Meal Planning, Physical Activity Recommendations, Foot Care, and Treatment Options for People with Kidney Failure

Along with a Section about Diabetes Complications and Co-Occurring Conditions, a Glossary of Related Terms, and Directories of Resources for Additional Help and Information

Edited by Karen Bellenir. 627 pages. 2008. 978-0-7808-1005-1.

"Completely and comprehensively covering almost everything a student or physician would need to know... well worth the investment."
— Internet Bookwatch, Dec '08

SEE ALSO Endocrine and Metabolic Disorders Sourcebook, 2nd Edition

---

Diet and Nutrition Sourcebook, 3rd Edition

Basic Consumer Health Information about Dietary Guidelines and the Food Guidance System, Recommended Daily Nutrient Intakes, Serving Proportions, Weight Control, Vitamins and Supplements, Nutrition Issues for Different Life Stages and Lifestyles, and the Needs of People with Specific Medical Concerns, Including Cancer, Celiac Disease, Diabetes, Eating Disorders, Food Allergies, and Cardiovascular Disease

Along with Facts about Federal Nutrition Support Programs, a Glossary of Nutrition and Dietary Terms, and Directories of Additional Resources for More Information about Nutrition

Edited by Joyce Brennfleck Shannon. 605 pages. 2006. 978-0-7808-0800-3.

"A valuable resource tool for any individual."
— Journal of Dental Hygiene, Apr '07

"From different recommended eating habits to reduce disease and common ailments to nutrition advice for those with specific conditions, Diet and Nutrition Sourcebook is especially important because so much is changing in this area, and so rapidly."
— California Bookwatch, Jun '06

SEE ALSO Eating Disorders Sourcebook, 2nd Edition, Vegetarian Sourcebook

---

Digestive Diseases and Disorders Sourcebook

Basic Consumer Health Information about Diseases and Disorders that Impact the Upper and Lower Digestive System, Including Celiac

Disease, Constipation, Crohn's Disease, Cyclic Vomiting Syndrome, Diarrhea, Diverticulosis and Diverticulitis, Gallstones, Heartburn, Hemorrhoids, Hernias, Indigestion (Dyspepsia), Irritable Bowel Syndrome, Lactose Intolerance, Ulcers, and More

Along with Information about Medications and Other Treatments, Tips for Maintaining a Healthy Digestive Tract, a Glossary, and Directory of Digestive Diseases Organizations

Edited by Karen Bellenir. 323 pages. 2000. 978-0-7808-0327-5.

"An excellent addition to all public or patient-research libraries."
— American Reference Books Annual, 2001

"Recommended reference source."
— Booklist, May '00

SEE ALSO Gastrointestinal Diseases and Disorders Sourcebook, 2nd Edition

---

Disabilities Sourcebook

Basic Consumer Health Information about Physical and Psychiatric Disabilities, Including Descriptions of Major Causes of Disability, Assistive and Adaptive Aids, Workplace Issues, and Accessibility Concerns

Along with Information about the Americans with Disabilities Act, a Glossary, and Resources for Additional Help and Information

Edited by Dawn D. Matthews. 602 pages. 2000. 978-0-7808-0389-3.

"A must for libraries with a consumer health section."
— American Reference Books Annual, 2002

"A much needed addition to the Omnigraphics Health Reference Series. A current reference work to provide people with disabilities, their families, caregivers or those who work with them, a broad range of information in one volume, has not been available until now... It is recommended for all public and academic library reference collections."
— E-Streams, May '01

"An excellent source book in easy-to-read format covering many current topics; highly recommended for all libraries."
— CHOICE, Jan '01

Disease Management Sourcebook

Basic Consumer Health Information about Coping with Chronic and Serious Illnesses, Navigating the Health Care System, Communicating with Health Care Providers, Assessing Health Care Quality, and Making Informed Health Care Decisions, Including Facts about Second Opinions, Hospitalization, Surgery, and Medications

Along with a Section about Children with Chronic Conditions, Information about Legal, Financial, and Insurance Issues, a Glossary of Related Terms, and Directories of Additional Resources

Edited by Joyce Brennfleck Shannon. 621 pages. 2008. 978-0-7808-1002-0.

"Consumers need to know how to manage their health care the same way they manage anything else in their lives. The text is very readable and is written for the layperson and consumer. The cost is not prohibitive. This book should be in all collections of health care libraries and public libraries."
— American Reference Books Annual, 2009

"The information is very current, and the selection of font and layout make the book easy to read. A hardback that will stand up to much usage, this is an excellent resource for consumers... Recommended. General readers."
—CHOICE, Nov '08

"Intended for lay readers, this resource clarifies the many confusing and overwhelming details associated with chronic disease care. Meticulous and clearly explained, the book even includes diagrams intended to ease comprehension of over-the-counter medication labels. An essential guide to navigating the health-care rapids."
—Library Journal, Aug '08

Domestic Violence Sourcebook, 3rd Edition

Basic Consumer Health Information about Warning Signs, Risk Factors, and Health Consequences of Intimate Partner Violence, Sexual Violence and Rape, Stalking, Human Trafficking, Child Maltreatment, Teen Dating Violence, and Elder Abuse

Along with Facts about Victims and Perpetrators, Strategies for Violence Prevention, and Emergency Interventions, Safety Plans, and Financial and Legal Tips for Victims, a Glossary of Related Terms, and Directories of Resources for Additional Information and Support

Edited by Joyce Brennfleck Shannon. 634 pages. 2009. 978-0-7808-1038-9.

"A recommended pick for any library interested in consumer health and social issues... A 'must' for any serious health collection."
—California Bookwatch, Jul '09

SEE ALSO Child Abuse Sourcebook, 2nd Edition

Drug Abuse Sourcebook, 3rd Edition

Basic Consumer Health Information about the Abuse of Cocaine, Club Drugs, Hallucinogens, Heroin, Inhalants, Marijuana, and Other Illicit Substances, Prescription Medications, and Over-the-Counter Medicines

Along with Facts about Addiction and Related Health Effects, Drug Abuse Treatment and Recovery, Drug Testing, Prevention Programs, Glossaries of Drug-Related Terms, and Directories of Resources for More Information

Edited by Joyce Brennfleck Shannon. 600 pages. 2010. 978-0-7808-1079-2.

SEE ALSO Alcoholism Sourcebook, 3rd Edition

Ear, Nose, and Throat Disorders Sourcebook, 2nd Edition

Basic Consumer Health Information about Disorders of the Ears, Hearing Loss, Vestibular Disorders, Nasal and Sinus Problems, Throat and Vocal Cord Disorders, and Otolaryngologic Cancers, Including Facts about Ear Infections and Injuries, Genetic and Congenital Deafness, Sensorineural Hearing Disorders, Tinnitus, Vertigo, Ménière Disease, Rhinitis, Sinusitis, Snoring, Sore Throats, Hoarseness, and More

Along with Reports on Current Research Initiatives, a Glossary of Related Medical Terms, and a Directory of Sources for Further Help and Information

Edited by Sandra J. Judd. 631 pages. 2007. 978-0-7808-0872-0.

"A resource book for the general public that provides comprehensive coverage of basic up-to-date medical information about the causes, symptoms, diagnosis, and treatment of diseases and disorders that affect the ears, nose, sinuses, throat, and voice... The majority of information is presented in question and answer format, much like questions a patient might ask of a health care provider. An extensive index facilitates the reader's ability to easily access information on any specific topic."
—*Journal of Dental Hygiene, Oct '07*

"A handy compilation of information on common and some not so common ailments of the ears, nose, and throat."
—*Doody's Review Service, 2007*

■

Eating Disorders Sourcebook, 2nd Edition
Basic Consumer Health Information about Anorexia Nervosa, Bulimia, Binge Eating, Compulsive Exercise, Female Athlete Triad, and Other Eating Disorders, Including Facts about Body Image and Other Cultural and Age-Related Risk Factors, Prevention Efforts, Adverse Health Effects, Treatment Options, and the Recovery Process

Along with Guidelines for Healthy Weight Control, a Glossary, and Directories of Additional Resources

Edited by Joyce Brennfleck Shannon. 557 pages. 2007. 978-0-7808-0948-2.

"Recommended for the reference collection of large public libraries."
—*American Reference Books Annual, 2008*

"A basic health reference any health or general library needs."
—*Internet Bookwatch, Jun '07*

SEE ALSO Diet and Nutrition Sourcebook, 3rd Edition, Mental Health Disorders Sourcebook, 4th Edition

■

Emergency Medical Services Sourcebook
Basic Consumer Health Information about Preventing, Preparing for, and Managing Emergency Situations, When and Who to Call for Help, What to Expect in the Emergency Room, the Emergency Medical Team,

Patient Issues, and Current Topics in Emergency Medicine

Along with Statistical Data, a Glossary, and Sources of Additional Help and Information

Edited by Jenni Lynn Colson. 472 pages. 2002. 978-0-7808-0420-3.

"Handy and convenient for home, public, school, and college libraries. Recommended."
—*CHOICE, Apr '03*

"This reference can provide the consumer with answers to most questions about emergency care in the United States, or it will direct them to a resource where the answer can be found."
—*American Reference Books Annual, 2003*

SEE ALSO Injury and Trauma Sourcebook

■

Endocrine and Metabolic Disorders Sourcebook, 2nd Edition
Basic Consumer Health Information about Hormonal and Metabolic Disorders that Affect the Body's Growth, Development, and Functioning, Including Disorders of the Pancreas, Ovaries and Testes, and Pituitary, Thyroid, Parathyroid, and Adrenal Glands, with Facts about Growth Disorders, Addison Disease, Cushing Syndrome, Conn Syndrome, Diabetic Disorders, Multiple Endocrine Neoplasia, Inborn Errors of Metabolism, and More

Along with Information about Endocrine Functioning, Diagnostic and Screening Tests, a Glossary of Related Terms, and Directories of Additional Resources

Edited by Joyce Brennfleck Shannon. 597 pages. 2007. 978-0-7808-0952-9.

SEE ALSO Diabetes Sourcebook, 4th Edition

■

Environmental Health Sourcebook, 3rd Edition
Basic Consumer Health Information about the Environment and Its Effects on Human Health, Including Facts about Air, Water, and Soil Contamination, Hazardous Chemicals, Foodborne Hazards and Illnesses, Household Hazards Such as Radon, Mold, and Carbon Monoxide, Consumer Hazards from Toxic Products and Imported Goods, and Disorders

591

Linked to Environmental Causes, Including Chemical Sensitivity, Cancer, Allergies, and Asthma

Along with Information about the Impact of Environmental Hazards on Specific Populations, a Glossary of Related Terms, and Resources for Additional Help and Information.

Edited by Laura Larsen. 600 pages. 2010. 978-0-7808-1078-5

Blindness, a Glossary of Related Terms, and Directories of Resources for More Help and Information

Edited by Amy L. Sutton. 646 pages. 2008. 978-0-7808-1000-6.

"A solid reference tool for eye care and a valuable addition to a collection."
—American Reference Books Annual, 2009

Ethnic Diseases Sourcebook

Basic Consumer Health Information for Ethnic and Racial Minority Groups in the United States, Including General Health Indicators and Behaviors, Ethnic Diseases, Genetic Testing, the Impact of Chronic Diseases, Women's Health, Mental Health Issues, and Preventive Health Care Services

Along with a Glossary and a Listing of Additional Resources

Edited by Joyce Brennfleck Shannon. 648 pages. 2001. 978-0-7808-0336-7.

"Not many books have been written on this topic to date, and the Ethnic Diseases Sourcebook is a strong addition to the list. It will be an important introductory resource for health consumers, students, health care personnel, and social scientists. It is recommended for public, academic, and large hospital libraries."
— American Reference Books Annual, 2002

"Will prove valuable to any library seeking to maintain a current, comprehensive reference collection of health resources... An excellent source of health information about genetic disorders which affect particular ethnic and racial minorities in the U.S."
—The Bookwatch, Aug '01

Eye Care Sourcebook, 3rd Edition

Basic Consumer Health Information about Eye Care and Eye Disorders, Including Facts about the Diagnosis, Prevention, and Treatment of Refractive Disorders, Cataracts, Glaucoma, Macular Degeneration, and Problems Affecting the Cornea, Retina, and Lacrimal Glands

Along with Advice about Preventing Eye Injuries and Tips for Living with Low Vision or

Family Planning Sourcebook

Basic Consumer Health Information about Planning for Pregnancy and Contraception, Including Traditional Methods, Barrier Methods, Hormonal Methods, Permanent Methods, Future Methods, Emergency Contraception, and Birth Control Choices for Women at Each Stage of Life

Along with Statistics, a Glossary, and Sources of Additional Information

Edited by Amy Marcaccio Keyzer. 503 pages. 2001. 978-0-7808-0379-4.

"Recommended for public, health, and undergraduate libraries as part of the circulating collection."
—E-Streams, Mar '02

"Will prove valuable to any library seeking to maintain a current, comprehensive reference collection of health resources... Excellent reference."
—The Bookwatch, Aug '01

SEE ALSO Pregnancy and Birth Sourcebook, 3rd Edition

Fitness and Exercise Sourcebook, 3rd Edition

Basic Consumer Health Information about the Physical and Mental Benefits of Fitness, Including Cardiorespiratory Endurance, Muscular Strength, Muscular Endurance, and Flexibility, with Facts about Sports Nutrition and Exercise-Related Injuries and Tips about Physical Activity and Exercises for People of All Ages and for People with Health Concerns

Along with Advice on Selecting and Using Exercise Equipment, Maintaining Exercise Motivation, a Glossary of Related Terms, and a Directory of Resources for More Help and Information

Edited by Amy L. Sutton. 635 pages. 2007. 978-0-7808-0946-8.

"Updates the consumer information on the physical and mental benefits of physical activity throughout the lifespan offered in earlier editions... Recommended. All readers; all levels."

—*CHOICE, Oct '07*

"An exceptionally well-rounded coverage perfect for any concerned about developing and understanding a fitness program."

—*California Bookwatch, Jun '07*

SEE ALSO Sports Injuries Sourcebook, 3rd Edition

Food Safety Sourcebook

Basic Consumer Health Information about the Safe Handling of Meat, Poultry, Seafood, Eggs, Fruit Juices, and Other Food Items, and Facts about Pesticides, Drinking Water, Food Safety Overseas, and the Onset, Duration, and Symptoms of Foodborne Illnesses, Including Types of Pathogenic Bacteria, Parasitic Protozoa, Worms, Viruses, and Natural Toxins

Along with the Role of the Consumer, the Food Handler, and the Government in Food Safety, a Glossary, and Resources for Additional Help and Information

Edited by Dawn D. Matthews. 327 pages. 1999. 978-0-7808-0326-8.

"Recommended reference source."

—*Booklist, May '00*

"This book takes the complex issues of food safety and foodborne pathogens and presents them in an easily understood manner. [It does] an excellent job of covering a large and often confusing topic."

— *American Reference Books Annual, 2000*

Forensic Medicine Sourcebook

Basic Consumer Information for the Layperson about Forensic Medicine, Including Crime Scene Investigation, Evidence Collection and Analysis, Expert Testimony, Computer-Aided Criminal Identification, Digital Imaging in the Courtroom, DNA Profiling, Accident Reconstruction, Autopsies, Ballistics, Drugs and Explosives Detection, Latent Fingerprints,

Product Tampering, and Questioned Document Examination

Along with Statistical Data, a Glossary of Forensics Terminology, and Listings of Sources for Further Help and Information

Edited by Annemarie S. Muth. 574 pages. 1999. 978-0-7808-0232-2.

"Given the expected widespread interest in its content and its easy to read style, this book is recommended for most public and all college and university libraries."

—*E-Streams, Feb '01*

"A wealth of information, useful statistics, references are up-to-date and extremely complete. This wonderful collection of data will help students who are interested in a career in any type of forensic field. It is a great resource for attorneys who need information about types of expert witnesses needed in a particular case. It also offers useful information for fiction and nonfiction writers whose work involves a crime. A fascinating compilation. All levels."

—*CHOICE, Jan '00*

"There are several items that make this book attractive to consumers who are seeking certain forensic data... This is a useful current source for those seeking general forensic medical answers."

—*American Reference Books Annual, 2000*

Gastrointestinal Diseases and Disorders Sourcebook, 2nd Edition

Basic Consumer Health Information about the Upper and Lower Gastrointestinal (GI) Tract, Including the Esophagus, Stomach, Intestines, Rectum, Liver, and Pancreas, with Facts about Gastroesophageal Reflux Disease, Gastritis, Hernias, Ulcers, Celiac Disease, Diverticulitis, Irritable Bowel Syndrome, Hemorrhoids, Gastrointestinal Cancers, and Other Diseases and Disorders Related to the Digestive Process

Along with Information about Commonly Used Diagnostic and Surgical Procedures, Statistics, Reports on Current Research Initiatives and Clinical Trials, a Glossary, and Resources for Additional Help and Information

Edited by Sandra J. Judd. 654 pages. 2006. 978-0-7808-0798-3.

"The text is designed for the general reader seeking information on prevention, disease warning signs, diagnostic and therapeutic questions... It is an excellent resource for the general reader to conveniently locate credible, coordinated and indexed information... The sourcebook will prove very helpful for patients, caregivers and should be available in every physician waiting room."

—*Doody's Review Service, 2006*

SEE ALSO *Diet and Nutrition Sourcebook, 3rd Edition, Digestive Diseases and Disorders Sourcebook*

Genetic Disorders Sourcebook, 4th Edition

Basic Consumer Health Information about Hereditary Diseases and Disorders, Including Facts about the Human Genome, Genetic Inheritance Patterns, Disorders Associated with Specific Genes, Such as Sickle Cell Disease, Hemophilia, and Cystic Fibrosis, Chromosome Disorders, Such as Down Syndrome, Fragile X Syndrome, and Turner Syndrome, and Complex Diseases and Disorders Resulting from the Interaction of Environmental and Genetic Factors, Such as Allergies, Cancer, and Obesity

Along with Facts about Genetic Testing, Suggestions for Parents of Children with Special Needs, Reports on Current Research Initiatives, a Glossary of Genetic Terminology, and Resources for Additional Help and Information

Edited by Sandra J. Judd. 600 pages. 2010. 978-0-7808-1076-1.

Head Trauma Sourcebook

Basic Information for the Layperson about Open-Head and Closed-Head Injuries, Treatment Advances, Recovery, and Rehabilitation

Along with Reports on Current Research Initiatives

Edited by Karen Bellenir. 414 pages. 1997. 978-0-7808-0208-7.

Headache Sourcebook

Basic Consumer Health Information about Migraine, Tension, Cluster, Rebound and Other Types of Headaches, with Facts about the Cause and Prevention of Headaches, the Effects of Stress and the Environment, Headaches during Pregnancy and Menopause, and Childhood Headaches

Along with a Glossary and Other Resources for Additional Help and Information

Edited by Dawn D. Matthews. 342 pages. 2002. 978-0-7808-0337-4.

"Highly recommended for academic and medical reference collections."

—*Library Bookwatch, Sep '02*

SEE ALSO *Pain Sourcebook, 3rd Edition*

Healthy Aging Sourcebook

Basic Consumer Health Information about Maintaining Health through the Aging Process, Including Advice on Nutrition, Exercise, and Sleep, Help in Making Decisions about Midlife Issues and Retirement, and Guidance Concerning Practical and Informed Choices in Health Consumerism

Along with Data Concerning the Theories of Aging, Different Experiences in Aging by Minority Groups, and Facts about Aging Now and Aging in the Future; and Featuring a Glossary, a Guide to Consumer Help, Additional Suggested Reading, and Practical Resource Directory

Edited by Jenifer Swanson. 537 pages. 1999. 978-0-7808-0390-9.

"Recommended reference source."

—*Booklist, Feb '00*

SEE ALSO *Adult Health Sourcebook, Physical and Mental Issues in Aging Sourcebook*

Healthy Children Sourcebook

Basic Consumer Health Information about the Physical and Mental Development of Children between the Ages of 3 and 12, Including Routine Health Care, Preventative Health Services, Safety and First Aid, Healthy Sleep, Dental Care, Nutrition, and Fitness, and Featuring Parenting Tips on Such Topics as Bedwetting, Choosing Day Care, Monitoring TV and Other Media, and Establishing a Foundation for Substance Abuse Prevention

Along with a Glossary of Commonly Used Pediatric Terms and Resources for Additional Help and Information.

Edited by Chad T. Kimball. 624 pages. 2003. 978-0-7808-0247-6.

"Should be required reading for parents and teachers."

—*E-Streams, Jun '04*

"It is hard to imagine that any other single resource exists that would provide such a comprehensive guide of timely information on health promotion and disease prevention for children aged 3 to 12."

—*American Reference Books Annual, 2004*

"This easy-to-read volume is a tremendous resource."

—*AORN Journal, May '05*

SEE ALSO *Childhood Diseases and Disorders Sourcebook, 2nd Edition*

Healthy Heart Sourcebook for Women

Basic Consumer Health Information about Cardiac Issues Specific to Women, Including Facts about Major Risk Factors and Prevention, Treatment and Control Strategies, and Important Dietary Issues

Along with a Special Section Regarding the Pros and Cons of Hormone Replacement Therapy and Its Impact on Heart Health, and Additional Help, Including Recipes, a Glossary, and a Directory of Resources

Edited by Dawn D. Matthews. 321 pages. 2000. 978-0-7808-0329-9.

"A good reference source and recommended for all public, academic, medical, and hospital libraries."

—*Medical Reference Services Quarterly, Summer '01*

"Contains very important information about coronary artery disease that all women should know. The information is current and presented in an easy-to-read format. The book will make a good addition to any library."

—*American Medical Writers Association Journal, Summer '00*

SEE ALSO *Cardiovascular Diseases and Disorders Sourcebook, 4th Edition, Women's Health Concerns Sourcebook, 3rd Edition*

Hepatitis Sourcebook

Basic Consumer Health Information about Hepatitis A, Hepatitis B, Hepatitis C, and Other Forms of Hepatitis, Including Autoimmune Hepatitis, Alcoholic Hepatitis, Nonalcoholic Steatohepatitis, and Toxic Hepatitis, with Facts about Risk Factors, Screening Methods, Diagnostic Tests, and Treatment Options

Along with Information on Liver Health, Tips for People Living with Chronic Hepatitis, Reports on Current Research Initiatives, a Glossary of Terms Related to Hepatitis, and a Directory of Sources for Further Help and Information

Edited by Sandra J. Judd. 570 pages. 2006. 978-0-7808-0749-5.

"The breadth of information found in this one book would not be readily found in another source. Highly recommended."

—*American Reference Books Annual, 2006*

SEE ALSO *Contagious Diseases Sourcebook, 2nd Edition*

Household Safety Sourcebook

Basic Consumer Health Information about Household Safety, Including Information about Poisons, Chemicals, Fire, and Water Hazards in the Home

Along with Advice about the Safe Use of Home Maintenance Equipment, Choosing Toys and Nursery Furniture, Holiday and Recreation Safety, a Glossary, and Resources for Further Help and Information

Edited by Dawn D. Matthews. 587 pages. 2002. 978-0-7808-0338-1.

"As a sourcebook on household safety this book meets its mark. It is encyclopedic in scope and covers a wide range of safety issues that are commonly seen in the home."

—*E-Streams, Jul '02*

Hypertension Sourcebook

Basic Consumer Health Information about the Causes, Diagnosis, and Treatment of High Blood Pressure, with Facts about Consequences, Complications, and Co-Occurring Disorders, Such as Coronary Heart Disease, Diabetes, Stroke, Kidney Disease, and Hypertensive Retinopathy, and Issues in Blood Pressure

Control, Including Dietary Choices, Stress Management, and Medications

Along with Reports on Current Research Initiatives and Clinical Trials, a Glossary, and Resources for Additional Help and Information

Edited by Dawn D. Matthews and Karen Bellenir. 588 pages. 2004. 978-0-7808-0674-0.

"Academic, public, and medical libraries will want to add the Hypertension Sourcebook to their collections."

—E-Streams, Aug '05

"The strength of this source is the wide range of information given about hypertension."

—American Reference Books Annual, 2005

SEE ALSO Stroke Sourcebook, 2nd Edition

▓

Immune System Disorders Sourcebook, 2nd Edition

Basic Consumer Health Information about Disorders of the Immune System, Including Immune System Function and Response, Diagnosis of Immune Disorders, Information about Inherited Immune Disease, Acquired Immune Disease, and Autoimmune Diseases, Including Primary Immune Deficiency, Acquired Immunodeficiency Syndrome (AIDS), Lupus, Multiple Sclerosis, Type 1 Diabetes, Rheumatoid Arthritis, and Graves' Disease

Along with Treatments, Tips for Coping with Immune Disorders, a Glossary, and a Directory of Additional Resources

Edited by Joyce Brennfleck Shannon. 643 pages. 2005. 978-0-7808-0748-8.

"Highly recommended for academic and public libraries."

—American Reference Books Annual, 2006

"The updated second edition is a 'must' for any consumer health library seeking a solid resource covering the treatments, symptoms, and options for immune disorder sufferers... An excellent guide."

—MBR Bookwatch, Jan '06

SEE ALSO AIDS Sourcebook, 4th Edition, Arthritis Sourcebook, 3rd Edition

▓

Infant and Toddler Health Sourcebook

Basic Consumer Health Information about the Physical and Mental Development of Newborns, Infants, and Toddlers, Including Neonatal Concerns, Nutrition Recommendations, Immunization Schedules, Common Pediatric Disorders, Assessments and Milestones, Safety Tips, and Advice for Parents and Other Caregivers

Along with a Glossary of Terms and Resource Listings for Additional Help

Edited by Jenifer Swanson. 570 pages. 2000. 978-0-7808-0246-9.

"As a reference for the general public, this would be useful in any library."

—E-Streams, May '01

"Recommended reference source."

—Booklist, Feb '01

▓

Infectious Diseases Sourcebook

Basic Consumer Health Information about Non-Contagious Bacterial, Viral, Prion, Fungal, and Parasitic Diseases Spread by Food and Water, Insects and Animals, or Environmental Contact, Including Botulism, E. Coli, Encephalitis, Legionnaires' Disease, Lyme Disease, Malaria, Plague, Rabies, Salmonella, Tetanus, and Others, and Facts about Newly Emerging Diseases, Such as Hantavirus, Mad Cow Disease, Monkeypox, and West Nile Virus

Along with Information about Preventing Disease Transmission, the Threat of Bioterrorism, and Current Research Initiatives, with a Glossary and Directory of Resources for More Information

Edited by Karen Bellenir. 610 pages. 2004. 978-0-7808-0675-7.

"This reference continues the excellent tradition of the Health Reference Series in consolidating a wealth of information on a selected topic into a format that is easy to use and accessible to the general public."

—American Reference Books Annual, 2005

"Recommended for public and academic libraries."

—E-Streams, Jan '05

SEE ALSO Environmental Health Sourcebook, 3rd Edition

Injury and Trauma Sourcebook

Basic Consumer Health Information about the Impact of Injury, the Diagnosis and Treatment of Common and Traumatic Injuries, Emergency Care, and Specific Injuries Related to Home, Community, Workplace, Transportation, and Recreation

Along with Guidelines for Injury Prevention, a Glossary, and a Directory of Additional Resources

Edited by Joyce Brennfleck Shannon. 675 pages. 2002. 978-0-7808-0421-0.

"Practitioners should be aware of guides such as this in order to facilitate their use by patients and their families."
—*Doody's Health Sciences Book Review Journal, Sep-Oct '02*

"Recommended reference source."
—*Booklist, Sep '02*

"Highly recommended for academic and medical reference collections."
—*Library Bookwatch, Sep '02*

SEE ALSO *Emergency Medical Services Sourcebook, Sports Injuries Sourcebook, 3rd Edition*

Learning Disabilities Sourcebook, 3rd Edition

Basic Consumer Health Information about Dyslexia, Auditory and Visual Processing Disorders, Communication Disorders, Dyscalculia, Dysgraphia, and Other Conditions That Impede Learning, Including Attention Deficit/ Hyperactivity Disorder, Autism Spectrum Disorders, Hearing and Visual Impairments, Chromosome-Based Disorders, and Brain Injury

Along with Facts about Brain Function, Assessment, Therapy and Remediation, Accommodations, Assistive Technology, Legal Protections, and Tips about Family Life, School Transitions, and Employment Strategies, a Glossary of Related Terms, and Directories of Additional Resources

Edited by Joyce Brennfleck Shannon. 613 pages. 2009. 978-0-7808-1039-6.

"Intended to be a starting point for people who need to know about learning disabilities. Each chapter on a specific disability includes readable,

well-organized descriptions... The book is well indexed and a glossary is included. Chapters on organizations and helpful websites will aid the reader who needs more information."
—*American Reference Books Annual, 2009*

"This book provides the necessary information to better understand learning disabilities and work with children who have them... It would be difficult to find another book that so comprehensively explains learning disabilities without becoming incomprehensible to the average parent who needs this information."
—*Doody's Review Service, 2009*

SEE ALSO *Attention Deficit Disorder Sourcebook, Autism and Pervasive Developmental Disorders Sourcebook*

Leukemia Sourcebook

Basic Consumer Health Information about Adult and Childhood Leukemias, Including Acute Lymphocytic Leukemia (ALL), Chronic Lymphocytic Leukemia (CLL), Acute Myelogenous Leukemia (AML), Chronic Myelogenous Leukemia (CML), and Hairy Cell Leukemia, and Treatments Such as Chemotherapy, Radiation Therapy, Peripheral Blood Stem Cell and Marrow Transplantation, and Immunotherapy

Along with Tips for Life During and After Treatment, a Glossary, and Directories of Additional Resources

Edited by Joyce Brennfleck Shannon. 564 pages. 2003. 978-0-7808-0627-6.

"Unlike other medical books for the layperson... the language does not talk down to the reader... This volume is highly recommended for all libraries."
—*American Reference Books Annual, 2004*

"A fine title which ranges from diagnosis to alternative treatments, staging, and tips for life during and after diagnosis."
—*The Bookwatch, Dec '03*

SEE ALSO *Blood & Circulatory Disorders Sourcebook, 3rd Edition, Cancer Sourcebook, 5th Edition*

Liver Disorders Sourcebook

Basic Consumer Health Information about the Liver and How It Works; Liver Diseases, Including Cancer, Cirrhosis, Hepatitis, and

Toxic and Drug Related Diseases; Tips for Maintaining a Healthy Liver; Laboratory Tests, Radiology Tests, and Facts about Liver Transplantation

Along with a Section on Support Groups, a Glossary, and Resource Listings

Edited by Joyce Brennfleck Shannon. 580 pages. 2000. 978-0-7808-0383-1.

"This title is recommended for health sciences and public libraries with consumer health collections."

—E-Streams, Oct '00

"Recommended reference source."

—Booklist, Jun '00

SEE ALSO Gastrointestinal Diseases and Disorders Sourcebook, 2nd Edition, Hepatitis Sourcebook

Lung Disorders Sourcebook

Basic Consumer Health Information about Emphysema, Pneumonia, Tuberculosis, Asthma, Cystic Fibrosis, and Other Lung Disorders, Including Facts about Diagnostic Procedures, Treatment Strategies, Disease Prevention Efforts, and Such Risk Factors as Smoking, Air Pollution, and Exposure to Asbestos, Radon, and Other Agents

Along with a Glossary and Resources for Additional Help and Information

Edited by Dawn D. Matthews. 657 pages. 2002. 978-0-7808-0339-8.

"Highly recommended for academic and medical reference collections."

—Library Bookwatch, Sep '02

SEE ALSO Asthma Sourcebook, 2nd Edition, Respiratory Disorders Sourcebook, 2nd Edition

Medical Tests Sourcebook, 3rd Edition

Basic Consumer Health Information about X-Rays, Blood Tests, Stool and Urine Tests, Biopsies, Mammography, Endoscopic Procedures, Ultrasound Exams, Computed Tomography, Magnetic Resonance Imaging (MRI), Nuclear Medicine, Genetic Testing, Home-Use Tests, and More

Along with Facts about Preventive Care and Screening Test Guidelines, Screening and

Assessment Tests Associated with Such Specific Concerns as Cancer, Heart Disease, Allergies, Diabetes, Thyroid Disfunction, and Infertility, a Glossary of Related Terms, and a Directory of Resources for Additional Help and Information

Edited by Karen Bellenir. 627 pages. 2008. 978-0-7808-1040-2

"This volume has a wide scope that makes it useful... Can be a valuable reference guide."

—American Reference Books Annual, 2009

"Would be a valuable contribution to any consumer health or public library."

—Doody's Book Review Service, 2009

Men's Health Concerns Sourcebook, 3rd Edition

Basic Consumer Health Information about Wellness in Men and Gender-Related Differences in Health, With Facts about Heart Disease, Cancer, Traumatic Injury, and Other Leading Causes of Death in Men, Reproductive Concerns, Sexual Dysfunction, Disorders of the Prostate, Penis, and Testes, Sex-Linked Genetic Disorders, and Other Medical and Mental Concerns of Men

Along with Statistical Data, a Glossary of Related Terms, and a Directory of Resources for Additional Information

Edited by Sandra J. Judd. 632 pages. 2009. 978-0-7808-1033-4.

"A good addition to any reference shelf in academic, consumer health, or hospital libraries."

—ARBAOnline, Oct '09

SEE ALSO Prostate and Urological Disorders Sourcebook

Mental Health Disorders Sourcebook, 4th Edition

Basic Consumer Health Information about the Causes and Symptoms of Mental Health Problems, Including Depression, Bipolar Disorder, Anxiety Disorders, Posttraumatic Stress Disorder, Obsessive-Compulsive Disorder, Eating Disorders, Addictions, and Personality and Psychotic Disorders

Along with Information about Medications and Treatments, Mental Health Concerns in

Children, Adolescents, and Adults, Tips on Living with Mental Health Disorders, a Glossary of Related Terms, and a Directory of Resources for Additional Help and Information

Edited by Amy L. Sutton. 680 pages. 2009. 978-0-7808-1041-9.

"Mental health concerns are presented in everyday language and intended for patients and their families as well as the general public... This resource is comprehensive and up to date... The easy-to-understand writing style helps to facilitate assimilation of needed facts and specifics on often challenging topics."
—*ARBAOnline*, Oct '09

"No health collection should be without this resource, which will reach into many a general lending library as well."
—*Internet Bookwatch*, Oct '09

SEE ALSO Depression Sourcebook, 2nd Edition, Stress-Related Disorders Sourcebook, 2nd Edition

Mental Retardation Sourcebook

Basic Consumer Health Information about Mental Retardation and Its Causes, Including Down Syndrome, Fetal Alcohol Syndrome, Fragile X Syndrome, Genetic Conditions, Injury, and Environmental Sources

Along with Preventive Strategies, Parenting Issues, Educational Implications, Health Care Needs, Employment and Economic Matters, Legal Issues, a Glossary, and a Resource Listing for Additional Help and Information

Edited by Joyce Brennfleck Shannon. 627 pages. 2000. 978-0-7808-0377-0.

"Public libraries will find the book useful for reference and as a beginning research point for students, parents, and caregivers."
—*American Reference Books Annual*, 2001

"The strength of this work is that it compiles many basic fact sheets and addresses for further information in one volume. It is intended and suitable for the general public."
—*E-Streams*, Nov '00

"An invaluable overview."
—*Reviewer's Bookwatch*, Jul '00

Movement Disorders Sourcebook, 2nd Edition

Basic Consumer Health Information about the Symptoms and Causes of Movement Disorders, Including Parkinson Disease, Amyotrophic Lateral Sclerosis, Cerebral Palsy, Muscular Dystrophy, Multiple Sclerosis, Myasthenia, Myoclonus, Spina Bifida, Dystonia, Essential Tremor, Choreatic Disorders, Huntington Disease, Tourette Syndrome, and Other Disorders That Cause Slowed, Absent, or Excessive Movements

Along with Information about Surgical and Nonsurgical Interventions, Physical Therapies, Strategies for Independent Living, a Glossary of Related Terms, and a Directory of Resources for Additional Help and Information

Edited by Amy L. Sutton. 618 pages. 2009. 978-0-7808-1034-1.

"The second updated edition of Movement Disorders Sourcebook is a winner, providing the latest research and health findings on all kinds of movement disorders in children and adults... a top pick for any health or general lending library's health reference collection."
—*California Bookwatch*, Aug '09

SEE ALSO Muscular Dystrophy Sourcebook

Multiple Sclerosis Sourcebook

Basic Consumer Health Information about Multiple Sclerosis (MS) and Its Effects on Mobility, Vision, Bladder Function, Speech, Swallowing, and Cognition, Including Facts about Risk Factors, Causes, Diagnostic Procedures, Pain Management, Drug Treatments, and Physical and Occupational Therapies

Along with Guidelines for Nutrition and Exercise, Tips on Choosing Assistive Equipment, Information about Disability, Work, Financial, and Legal Issues, a Glossary of Related Terms, and a Directory of Additional Resources

Edited by Joyce Brennfleck Shannon. 553 pages. 2007. 978-0-7808-0998-7.

Muscular Dystrophy Sourcebook

Basic Consumer Health Information about Congenital, Childhood-Onset, and Adult-Onset

Forms of Muscular Dystrophy, Such as Duchenne, Becker, Emery-Dreifuss, Distal, Limb-Girdle, Facioscapulohumeral (FSHD), Myotonic, and Ophthalmoplegic Muscular Dystrophies, Including Facts about Diagnostic Tests, Medical and Physical Therapies, Management of Co-Occurring Conditions, and Parenting Guidelines

Along with Practical Tips for Home Care, a Glossary, and Directories of Additional Resources

Edited by Joyce Brennfleck Shannon. 552 pages. 2004. 978-0-7808-0676-4.

"This book is highly recommended for public and academic libraries as well as health care offices that support the information needs of patients and their families."
—E-Streams, Apr '05

"Excellent reference."
—The Bookwatch, Jan '05

SEE ALSO Movement Disorders Sourcebook, 2nd Edition

Obesity Sourcebook

Basic Consumer Health Information about Diseases and Other Problems Associated with Obesity, and Including Facts about Risk Factors, Prevention Issues, and Management Approaches

Along with Statistical and Demographic Data, Information about Special Populations, Research Updates, a Glossary, and Source Listings for Further Help and Information

Edited by Wilma Caldwell and Chad T. Kimball. 360 pages. 2001. 978-0-7808-0333-6.

"The book synthesizes the reliable medical literature on obesity into one easy-to-read and useful resource for the general public."
—American Reference Books Annual, 2002

"Well suited for the health reference collection of a public library or an academic health science library that serves the general population."
—E-Streams, Sep '01

Osteoporosis Sourcebook

Basic Consumer Health Information about Primary and Secondary Osteoporosis and Juvenile Osteoporosis and Related Conditions, Including Fibrous Dysplasia, Gaucher Disease, Hyperthyroidism, Hypophosphatasia,

Myeloma, Osteopetrosis, Osteogenesis Imperfecta, and Paget's Disease

Along with Information about Risk Factors, Treatments, Traditional and Non-Traditional Pain Management, a Glossary of Related Terms, and a Directory of Resources

Edited by Allan R. Cook. 568 pages. 2001. 978-0-7808-0239-1.

"This resource is recommended as a great reference source for public, health, and academic libraries, and is another triumph for the editors of Omnigraphics."
—American Reference Books Annual, 2002

"Will prove valuable to any library seeking to maintain a current, comprehensive reference collection of health resources... From prevention to treatment and associated conditions, this provides an excellent survey."
—The Bookwatch, Aug '01

SEE ALSO Healthy Aging Sourcebook, Women's Health Concerns Sourcebook, 3rd Edition

Pain Sourcebook, 3rd Edition

Basic Consumer Health Information about Acute and Chronic Pain, Including Nerve Pain, Bone Pain, Muscle Pain, Cancer Pain, and Disorders Characterized by Pain, Such as Arthritis, Temporomandibular Muscle and Joint (TMJ) Disorder, Carpal Tunnel Syndrome, Headaches, Heartburn, Sciatica, and Shingles, and Facts about Diagnostic Tests and Treatment Options for Pain, Including Over-the-Counter and Prescription Drugs, Physical Rehabilitation, Injection and Infusion Therapies, Implantable Technologies, and Complementary Medicine

Along with Tips for Living with Pain, a Glossary of Related Terms, and a Directory of Additional Resources

Edited by Joyce Brennfleck Shannon. 644 pages. 2008. 978-0-7808-1006-8.

"Excellent for ready-reference users and can be used for beginning students in health fields... appropriate for the consumer health collection in both public and academic libraries."
—American Reference Books Annual, 2009

SEE ALSO Arthritis Sourcebook, 3rd Edition; Back and Neck Sourcebook, 2nd Edition;

Headache Sourcebook; Sports Injuries Sourcebook, 3rd Edition

Pediatric Cancer Sourcebook

Basic Consumer Health Information about Leukemias, Brain Tumors, Sarcomas, Lymphomas, and Other Cancers in Infants, Children, and Adolescents, Including Descriptions of Cancers, Treatments, and Coping Strategies

Along with Suggestions for Parents, Caregivers, and Concerned Relatives, a Glossary of Cancer Terms, and Resource Listings

Edited by Edward J. Prucha. 575 pages. 1999. 978-0-7808-0245-2.

"An excellent source of information. Recommended for public, hospital, and health science libraries with consumer health collections."
—*E-Streams, Jun '00*

"A valuable addition to all libraries specializing in health services and many public libraries."
—*American Reference Books Annual, 2000*

SEE ALSO *Childhood Diseases and Disorders Sourcebook, 2nd Edition, Healthy Children Sourcebook*

Physical and Mental Issues in Aging Sourcebook

Basic Consumer Health Information on Physical and Mental Disorders Associated with the Aging Process, Including Concerns about Cardiovascular Disease, Pulmonary Disease, Oral Health, Digestive Disorders, Musculoskeletal and Skin Disorders, Metabolic Changes, Sexual and Reproductive Issues, and Changes in Vision, Hearing, and Other Senses

Along with Data about Longevity and Causes of Death, Information on Acute and Chronic Pain, Descriptions of Mental Concerns, a Glossary of Terms, and Resource Listings for Additional Help

Edited by Jenifer Swanson. 660 pages. 1999. 978-0-7808-0233-9.

"This is a treasure of health information for the layperson."
—*CHOICE Health Sciences Supplement, May '00*

"Recommended for public libraries."
—*American Reference Books Annual, 2000*

SEE ALSO *Healthy Aging Sourcebook*

Podiatry Sourcebook, 2nd Edition

Basic Consumer Health Information about Disorders, Diseases, and Deformities that Affect the Foot and Ankle, Including Sprains, Corns, Calluses, Bunions, Plantar Warts, Plantar Fasciitis, Neuromas, Clubfoot, Flat Feet, Achilles Tendonitis, and Much More

Along with Information about Selecting a Foot Care Specialist, Foot Fitness, Shoes and Socks, Diagnostic Tests and Corrective Procedures, Financial Assistance for Corrective Devices, a Glossary of Related Terms, and a Directory of Resources for Additional Help and Information

Edited by Ivy L. Alexander. 516 pages. 2007. 978-0-7808-0944-4.

"An excellent resource... Although there have been various types of 'foot books' published in the past, none are as comprehensive as this one. 5 Stars (out of 5)!"
—*Doody's Review Service, 2007*

"Perfect for both health libraries and general-interest lending collections."
—*Internet Bookwatch, Jul '07*

Pregnancy and Birth Sourcebook, 3rd Edition

Basic Consumer Health Information about Pregnancy and Fetal Development, Including Facts about Fertility and Conception, Physical and Emotional Changes during Pregnancy, Prenatal Care and Diagnostic Tests, High-Risk Pregnancies and Complications, Labor, Delivery, and the Postpartum Period

Along with Tips on Maintaining Health and Wellness during Pregnancy and Caring for Newborn Infants, a Glossary of Related Terms, and Directories of Resources for Additional Help and Information

Edited by Amy L. Sutton. 645 pages. 2009. 978-0-7808-1074-7.

SEE ALSO *Breastfeeding Sourcebook, Congenital Disorders Sourcebook, 2nd Edition, Family Planning Sourcebook, Women's Health Concerns Sourcebook, 3rd Edition*

601

Prostate and Urological Disorders Sourcebook

Basic Consumer Health Information about Urogenital and Sexual Disorders in Men, Including Prostate and Other Andrological Cancers, Prostatitis, Benign Prostatic Hyperplasia, Testicular and Penile Trauma, Cryptorchidism, Peyronie Disease, Erectile Dysfunction, and Male Factor Infertility, and Facts about Commonly Used Tests and Procedures, Such as Prostatectomy, Vasectomy, Vasectomy Reversal, Penile Implants, and Semen Analysis

Along with a Glossary of Andrological Terms and a Directory of Resources for Additional Information

Edited by Karen Bellenir. 604 pages. 2006. 978-0-7808-0797-6.

"Certain to be a popular pick among library reference holdings... No prior knowledge is assumed for any of the conditions or terms herein, making it a most accessible general-interest reference."
—*California Bookwatch, Apr '06*

SEE ALSO *Men's Health Concerns Sourcebook, 3rd Edition, Urinary Tract and Kidney Diseases and Disorders Sourcebook, 2nd Edition*

Prostate Cancer Sourcebook

Basic Consumer Health Information about Prostate Cancer, Including Information about the Associated Risk Factors, Detection, Diagnosis, and Treatment of Prostate Cancer

Along with Information on Non-Malignant Prostate Conditions, and Featuring a Section Listing Support and Treatment Centers and a Glossary of Related Terms

Edited by Dawn D. Matthews. 340 pages. 2001. 978-0-7808-0324-4.

"Recommended reference source."
—*Booklist, Jan '02*

"A valuable resource for health care consumers seeking information on the subject... All text is written in a clear, easy-to-understand language that avoids technical jargon. Any library that collects consumer health resources would strengthen their collection with the addition of the Prostate Cancer Sourcebook."
—*American Reference Books Annual, 2002*

SEE ALSO *Cancer Sourcebook, 5th Edition, Men's Health Concerns Sourcebook, 3rd Edition*

Rehabilitation Sourcebook

Basic Consumer Health Information about Rehabilitation for People Recovering from Heart Surgery, Spinal Cord Injury, Stroke, Orthopedic Impairments, Amputation, Pulmonary Impairments, Traumatic Injury, and More, Including Physical Therapy, Occupational Therapy, Speech/Language Therapy, Massage Therapy, Dance Therapy, Art Therapy, and Recreational Therapy

Along with Information on Assistive and Adaptive Devices, a Glossary, and Resources for Additional Help and Information

Edited by Dawn D. Matthews. 519 pages. 2000. 978-0-7808-0236-0.

"This is an excellent resource for public library reference and health collections."
—*American Reference Books Annual, 2001*

"Recommended reference source."
—*Booklist, May '00*

Respiratory Disorders Sourcebook, 2nd Edition

Basic Consumer Health Information about Infectious, Inflammatory, and Chronic Conditions Affecting the Lungs and Respiratory System, Including Pneumonia, Bronchitis, Influenza, Tuberculosis, Sarcoidosis, Asthma, Cystic Fibrosis, Chronic Obstructive Pulmonary Disease, Lung Abscesses, Pulmonary Embolism, Occupational Lung Diseases, and Other Bacterial, Viral, and Fungal Infections

Along with Facts about the Structure and Function of the Lungs and Airways, Methods of Diagnosing Respiratory Disorders, and Treatment and Rehabilitation Options, a Glossary of Related Terms, and a Directory of Resources for Additional Help and Information

Edited by Sandra L. Judd. 638 pages. 2008. 978-0-7808-1007-5.

"An excellent book for patients, their families, or for those who are just curious about respiratory disease. Public libraries and physician offices would find this a valuable resource as well. 4 Stars! (out of 5)"
—*Doody's Review Service, 2009*

"A great addition for public and school libraries because it provides concise health information... readers can start with this reference source and get satisfactory answers before proceeding to other medical reference tools for

602

more in depth information... A good guide for health education on lung disorders."
—*American Reference Books Annual*, 2009

SEE ALSO *Asthma Sourcebook, 2nd Edition, Lung Disorders Sourcebook*

Sexually Transmitted Diseases Sourcebook, 4th Edition

Basic Consumer Health Information about Chlamydial Infections, Gonorrhea, Hepatitis, Herpes, HIV/AIDS, Human Papillomavirus, Pubic Lice, Scabies, Syphilis, Trichomoniasis, Vaginal Infections, and Other Sexually Transmitted Diseases, Including Facts about Risk Factors, Symptoms, Diagnosis, Treatment, and the Prevention of Sexually Transmitted Infections

Along with Updates on Current Research Initiatives, a Glossary of Related Terms, and Resources for Additional Help and Information

Edited by Laura Larsen. 623 pages. 2009. 978-0-7808-1073-0.

"Extremely beneficial... The question-and-answer format along with the index and table of contents make this well-organized resource extremely easy to reference, read, and comprehend... an invaluable medical reference source for lay readers, and a highly appropriate addition for public library collections, health clinics, and any library with a consumer health collection"
—*ARBAOnline*, Oct '09

SEE ALSO *AIDS Sourcebook, 4th Edition, Contagious Diseases Sourcebook, 2nd Edition, Men's Health Concerns Sourcebook, 3rd Edition, Women's Health Concerns Sourcebook, 3rd Edition*

Sleep Disorders Sourcebook, 3rd Edition

Basic Consumer Health Information about Sleep Disorders, Including Insomnia, Sleep Apnea and Snoring, Jet Lag and Other Circadian Rhythm Disorders, Narcolepsy, and Parasomnias, Such as Sleep Walking and Sleep Talking, and Featuring Facts about Other Health Problems that Affect Sleep, Why Sleep Is Necessary, How Much Sleep Is Needed, the Physical and Mental Effects of Sleep Deprivation, and Pediatric Sleep Issues

Along with Tips for Diagnosing and Treating Sleep Disorders, a Glossary of Related Terms, and a List of Resources for Additional Help and Information

Edited by Sandra J. Judd. 600 pages. 2010. 978-0-7808-1084-6.

Smoking Concerns Sourcebook

Basic Consumer Health Information about Nicotine Addiction and Smoking Cessation, Featuring Facts about the Health Effects of Tobacco Use, Including Lung and Other Cancers, Heart Disease, Stroke, and Respiratory Disorders, Such as Emphysema and Chronic Bronchitis

Along with Information about Smoking Prevention Programs, Suggestions for Achieving and Maintaining a Smoke-Free Lifestyle, Statistics about Tobacco Use, Reports on Current Research Initiatives, a Glossary of Related Terms, and Directories of Resources for Additional Help and Information

Edited by Karen Bellenir. 595 pages. 2004. 978-0-7808-0323-7.

"Provides everything needed for the student or general reader seeking practical details on the effects of tobacco use."
—*The Bookwatch*, Mar '05

"Public libraries and consumer health care libraries will find this work useful."
—*American Reference Books Annual*, 2005

SEE ALSO *Respiratory Disorders Sourcebook, 2nd Edition*

Sports Injuries Sourcebook, 3rd Edition

Basic Consumer Health Information about Sprains and Strains, Fractures, Growth Plate Injuries, Overtraining Injuries, and Injuries to the Head, Face, Shoulders, Elbows, Hands, Spinal Column, Knees, Ankles, and Feet, and with Facts about Heat-Related Illness, Steroids and Sport Supplements, Protective Equipment, Diagnostic Procedures, Treatment Options, and Rehabilitation

Along with a Glossary of Related Terms and a Directory of Resources for Additional Help and Information

Edited by Sandra J. Judd. 623 pages. 2007. 978-0-7808-0949-9.

SEE ALSO *Fitness and Exercise Sourcebook, 3rd Edition, Podiatry Sourcebook, 2nd Edition*

Stress-Related Disorders Sourcebook, 2nd Edition

Basic Consumer Health Information about Stress and Stress-Related Disorders, Including Types of Stress, Sources of Acute and Chronic Stress, the Impact of Stress on the Body's Systems, and Mental and Emotional Health Problems Associated with Stress, Such as Depression, Anxiety Disorders, Substance Abuse, Posttraumatic Stress Disorder, and Suicide

Along with Advice about Getting Help for Stress-Related Disorders, Information about Stress Management Techniques, a Glossary of Stress-Related Terms, and a Directory of Resources for Additional Help and Information

Edited by Amy L. Sutton. 608 pages. 2007. 978-0-7808-0996-3.

"Accessible to the lay reader. Highly recommended for medical and psychiatric collections."
—*Library Journal, Mar '08*

"Well-written for a general readership, the 2nd Edition of Stress-Related Disorders Sourcebook is a useful addition to the health reference literature."
—*American Reference Books Annual, 2008*

SEE ALSO *Mental Health Disorders Sourcebook, 4th Edition*

Stroke Sourcebook, 2nd Edition

Basic Consumer Health Information about Stroke, Including Ischemic, Hemorrhagic, and Mini Strokes, as Well as Risk Factors, Prevention Guidelines, Diagnostic Tests, Medications and Surgical Treatments, and Complications of Stroke

Along with Rehabilitation Techniques and Innovations, Tips on Staying Healthy and Maintaining Independence after Stroke, a Glossary of Related Terms, and a Directory of Resources for Stroke Survivors and Their Families

Edited by Amy L. Sutton. 626 pages. 2008. 978-0-7808-1035-8.

"An encyclopedic handbook on stroke that is written in a language the layperson can understand... This is one of the most helpful, readable books on stroke. This volume is highly recommended and should be in every medical, hospital and public library; in addition, every family practitioner should have a copy in his or her office."
—*American Reference Books Annual, 2009*

SEE ALSO *Brain Disorders Sourcebook, 3rd Edition, Hypertension Sourcebook*

Surgery Sourcebook, 2nd Edition

Basic Consumer Health Information about Common Inpatient and Outpatient Surgeries, Including Critical Care and Trauma, Gastrointestinal, Gynecologic and Obstetric, Cardiac and Vascular, Neurologic, Ophthalmologic, Orthopedic, Reconstructive and Cosmetic, and Other Major and Minor Surgeries

Along with Information about Anesthesia and Pain Relief Options, Risks and Complications, Postoperative Recovery Concerns, and Innovative Surgical Techniques and Tools, a Glossary of Related Terms, and a Directory of Additional Resources

Edited by Amy L. Sutton. 645 pages. 2008. 978-0-7808-1004-4.

"Large public libraries and medical libraries would benefit from this material in their reference collections."
—*American Reference Books Annual, 2009*

SEE ALSO *Cosmetic and Reconstructive Surgery Sourcebook, 2nd Edition*

Thyroid Disorders Sourcebook

Basic Consumer Health Information about Disorders of the Thyroid and Parathyroid Glands, Including Hypothyroidism, Hyperthyroidism, Graves Disease, Hashimoto Thyroiditis, Thyroid Cancer, and Parathyroid Disorders, Featuring Facts about Symptoms, Risk Factors, Tests, and Treatments

Along with Information about the Effects of Thyroid Imbalance on Other Body Systems, Environmental Factors That Affect the Thyroid Gland, a Glossary, and a Directory of Additional Resources

Edited by Joyce Brennfleck Shannon. 573 pages. 2005. 978-0-7808-0745-7.

"Recommended for consumer health collections."
—*American Reference Books Annual, 2006*

"Highly recommended pick for Basic Consumer health reference holdings at all levels."
—*The Bookwatch, Aug '05*

SEE ALSO *Endocrine and Metabolic Disorders Sourcebook, 2nd Edition*

Transplantation Sourcebook

Basic Consumer Health Information about Organ and Tissue Transplantation, Including Physical and Financial Preparations, Procedures and Issues Relating to Specific Solid Organ and Tissue Transplants, Rehabilitation, Pediatric Transplant Information, the Future of Transplantation, and Organ and Tissue Donation

Along with a Glossary and Listings of Additional Resources

Edited by Joyce Brennfleck Shannon. 610 pages. 2002. 978-0-7808-0322-0.

"Recommended for libraries with an interest in offering consumer health information."
—*E-Streams, Jul '02*

"This is a unique and valuable resource for patients facing transplantation and their families."
—*Doody's Review Service, Jun '02*

Traveler's Health Sourcebook

Basic Consumer Health Information for Travelers, Including Physical and Medical Preparations, Transportation Health and Safety, Essential Information about Food and Water, Sun Exposure, Insect and Snake Bites, Camping and Wilderness Medicine, and Travel with Physical or Medical Disabilities

Along with International Travel Tips, Vaccination Recommendations, Geographical Health Issues, Disease Risks, a Glossary, and a Listing of Additional Resources

Edited by Joyce Brennfleck Shannon. 619 pages. 2000. 978-0-7808-0384-8.

"Recommended reference source."
—*Booklist, Feb '01*

"This book is recommended for any public library, any travel collection, and especially any collection for the physically disabled."
—*American Reference Books Annual, 2001*

SEE ALSO *Worldwide Health Sourcebook*

Urinary Tract and Kidney Diseases and Disorders Sourcebook, 2nd Edition

Basic Consumer Health Information about the Urinary System, Including the Bladder, Urethra, Ureters, and Kidneys, with Facts about Urinary Tract Infections, Incontinence, Congenital Disorders, Kidney Stones, Cancers of the Urinary Tract and Kidneys, Kidney Failure, Dialysis, and Kidney Transplantation

Along with Statistical and Demographic Information, Reports on Current Research in Kidney and Urologic Health, a Summary of Commonly Used Diagnostic Tests, a Glossary of Related Terms, and a Directory of Resources for Additional Help and Information

Edited by Ivy L. Alexander. 621 pages. 2005. 978-0-7808-0750-1.

"A good choice for a consumer health information library or for a medical library needing information to refer to their patients."
—*American Reference Books Annual, 2006*

SEE ALSO *Prostate and Urological Disorders Sourcebook*

Vegetarian Sourcebook

Basic Consumer Health Information about Vegetarian Diets, Lifestyle, and Philosophy, Including Definitions of Vegetarianism and Veganism, Tips about Adopting Vegetarianism, Creating a Vegetarian Pantry, and Meeting Nutritional Needs of Vegetarians, with Facts Regarding Vegetarianism's Effect on Pregnant and Lactating Women, Children, Athletes, and Senior Citizens

Along with a Glossary of Commonly Used Vegetarian Terms and Resources for Additional Help and Information

Edited by Chad T. Kimball. 337 pages. 2002. 978-0-7808-0439-5.

"Organizes into one concise volume the answers to the most common questions concerning vegetarian diets and lifestyles. This title is recommended for public and secondary school libraries."

—E-Streams, Apr '03

"Invaluable reference for public and school library collections alike."
—Library Bookwatch, Apr '03

"The articles in this volume are easy to read and come from authoritative sources. The book does not necessarily support the vegetarian diet but instead provides the pros and cons of this important decision... Recommended for public libraries and consumer health libraries."
—American Reference Books Annual, 2003

SEE ALSO *Diet and Nutrition Sourcebook, 3rd Edition*

Women's Health Concerns Sourcebook, 3rd Edition

Basic Consumer Health Information about Issues and Trends in Women's Health and Health Conditions of Special Concern to Women, Including Endometriosis, Uterine Fibroids, Menstrual Irregularities, Menopause, Sexual Dysfunction, Infertility, Cancer in Women, and Other Such Chronic Disorders as Lupus, Fibromyalgia, and Thyroid Disease

Along with Statistical Data, Tips for Maintaining Wellness, a Glossary, and a Directory of Resources for Further Help and Information

Edited by Sandra J. Judd. 679 pages. 2009. 978-0-7808-1036-5.

"This useful resource provides information about a wide range of topics that will help women understand their bodies, prevent or treat disease, and maintain health... A detailed index helps readers locate information. This is a useful addition to public and consumer health library collections"
—ARBAOnline, Jun '09

SEE ALSO *Breast Cancer Sourcebook, 3rd Edition, Cancer Sourcebook for Women, 4th Edition, Healthy Heart Sourcebook for Women*

Workplace Health and Safety Sourcebook

Basic Consumer Health Information about Workplace Health and Safety, Including the Effect of Workplace Hazards on the Lungs,

Skin, Heart, Ears, Eyes, Brain, Reproductive Organs, Musculoskeletal System, and Other Organs and Body Parts

Along with Information about Occupational Cancer, Personal Protective Equipment, Toxic and Hazardous Chemicals, Child Labor, Stress, and Workplace Violence

Edited by Chad T. Kimball. 610 pages. 2000. 978-0-7808-0231-5.

"As a reference for the general public, this would be useful in any library."
—E-Streams, Jun '01

"Provides helpful information for primary care physicians and other caregivers interested in occupational medicine... General readers; professionals."
—CHOICE, May '01

Worldwide Health Sourcebook

Basic Information about Global Health Issues, Including Malnutrition, Reproductive Health, Disease Dispersion and Prevention, Emerging Diseases, Risky Health Behaviors, and the Leading Causes of Death

Along with Global Health Concerns for Children, Women, and the Elderly, Mental Health Issues, Research and Technology Advancements, and Economic, Environmental, and Political Health Implications, a Glossary, and a Resource Listing for Additional Help and Information

Edited by Joyce Brennfleck Shannon. 597 pages. 2001. 978-0-7808-0330-5.

"Named an Outstanding Academic Title."
—CHOICE, Jan '02

"Yet another handy but also unique compilation in the extensive Health Reference Series, this is a useful work because many of the international publications reprinted or excerpted are not readily available. Highly recommended."
—CHOICE, Nov '01

SEE ALSO *Traveler's Health Sourcebook*

Teen Health Series
Complete Catalog
List price $69 per volume. School and library price $62 per volume.

Abuse and Violence Information for Teens
Health Tips about the Causes and Consequences of Abusive and Violent Behavior
Including Facts about the Types of Abuse and Violence, the Warning Signs of Abusive and Violent Behavior, Health Concerns of Victims, and Getting Help and Staying Safe

Edited by Sandra Augustyn Lawton. 411 pages. 2008. 978-0-7808-1008-2.

"A useful resource for schools and organizations providing services to teens and may also be a starting point in research projects."
—*Reference and Research Book News, Aug '08*

"Violence is a serious problem for teens... This resource gives teens the information they need to face potential threats and get help—either for themselves or for their friends."
—*American Reference Books Annual, 2009*

Accident and Safety Information for Teens
Health Tips about Medical Emergencies, Traumatic Injuries, and Disaster Preparedness
Including Facts about Motor Vehicle Accidents, Burns, Poisoning, Firearms, Natural Disasters, National Security Threats, and More

Edited by Karen Bellenir. 420 pages. 2008. 978-0-7808-1046-4.

"Aimed at teenage audiences, this guide provides practical information for handling a comprehensive list of emergencies, from sport injuries and auto accidents to alcohol poisoning and natural disasters."
—*Library Journal, Apr 1, '09*

"Useful in the young adult collections of public libraries as well as high school libraries."
—*American Reference Books Annual, 2009*

SEE ALSO Sports Injuries Information for Teens, 2nd Edition

Alcohol Information for Teens, 2nd Edition
Health Tips about Alcohol and Alcoholism
Including Facts about Alcohol's Effects on the Body, Brain, and Behavior, the Consequences of Underage Drinking, Alcohol Abuse Prevention and Treatment, and Coping with Alcoholic Parents

Edited by Lisa Bakewell. 410 pages. 2009. 978-0-7808-1043-3.

"This handbook, written for a teenage audience, provides information on the causes, effects, and preventive measures related to alcohol abuse among teens... The chapters are quick to make a connection to their teenage reading audience. The prose is straightforward and the book lends itself to spot reading. It should be useful both for practical information and for research, and it is suitable for public and school libraries."
—*ARBAOnline, Jun '09*

SEE ALSO Drug Information for Teens, 2nd Edition

Allergy Information for Teens
Health Tips about Allergic Reactions Such as Anaphylaxis, Respiratory Problems, and Rashes
Including Facts about Identifying and Managing Allergies to Food, Pollen, Mold, Animals, Chemicals, Drugs, and Other Substances

Edited by Karen Bellenir. 410 pages. 2006. 978-0-7808-0799-0.

"This is a comprehensive, readable text on the subject of allergic diseases in teenagers. 5 Stars (out of 5)!"
—*Doody's Review Service, Jun '06*

"This authoritative and useful self-help title is a solid addition to YA collections, whether for personal interest or reports."
—*School Library Journal, Jul '06*

Asthma Information for Teens, 2nd Ed.
Health Tips about Managing Asthma and Related Concerns

Including Facts about Asthma Causes, Triggers and Symptoms, Diagnosis, and Treatment

Edited by Kim Wohlenhaus. 400 pages. 2010. 978-0-7808-1086-0.

Body Information for Teens

Health Tips about Maintaining Well-Being for a Lifetime

Including Facts about the Development and Functioning of the Body's Systems, Organs, and Structures and the Health Impact of Lifestyle Choices

Edited by Sandra Augustyn Lawton. 458 pages. 2007. 978-0-7808-0443-2.

Cancer Information for Teens, 2nd Edition

Health Tips about Cancer Awareness, Symptoms, Prevention, Diagnosis, and Treatment

Including Facts about Common Cancers Affecting Teens, Causes, Detection, Coping Strategies, Clinical Trials, Nutrition and Exercise, Cancer in Friends or Family, and More

Edited by Karen Bellenir and Lisa Bakewell. 445 pages. 2010. 978-0-7808-1085-3.

Complementary and Alternative Medicine Information for Teens

Health Tips about Non-Traditional and Non-Western Medical Practices

Including Information about Acupuncture, Chiropractic Medicine, Dietary and Herbal Supplements, Hypnosis, Massage Therapy, Prayer and Spirituality, Reflexology, Yoga, and More

Edited by Sandra Augustyn Lawton. 407 pages. 2007. 978-0-7808-0966-6.

"This volume covers CAM specifically for teenagers but of general use also. It should be a welcome addition to both public and academic libraries."
—*American Reference Books Annual, 2008*

"This volume provides a solid foundation for further investigation of the subject, making it useful for both public and high school libraries."
—*VOYA: Voice of Youth Advocates, Jun '07*

Diabetes Information for Teens

Health Tips about Managing Diabetes and Preventing Related Complications

Including Information about Insulin, Glucose Control, Healthy Eating, Physical Activity, and Learning to Live with Diabetes

Edited by Sandra Augustyn Lawton. 410 pages. 2006. 978-0-7808-0811-9.

"A comprehensive instructional guide for teens... some of the material may also be directed towards parents or teachers. 5 stars (out of 5)!"
—*Doody's Review Service, 2006*

"Students dealing with their own diabetes or that of a friend or family member or those writing reports on the topic will find this a valuable resource."
—*School Library Journal, Aug '06*

"This text is directed to the teen population and would be an excellent library resource for a health class or for the teacher as a reference for class preparation. It can, however, serve a much wider audience. The clinical educator on diabetes may find it valuable to educate the newly diagnosed client regardless of age. It also would be an excellent reference and education tool for a preventive medicine seminar on diabetes."
—*Physical Therapy, Mar '07*

Diet Information for Teens, 2nd Edition

Health Tips about Diet and Nutrition

Including Facts about Dietary Guidelines, Food Groups, Nutrients, Healthy Meals, Snacks, Weight Control, Medical Concerns Related to Diet, and More

Edited by Karen Bellenir. 432 pages. 2006. 978-0-7808-0820-1.

"A very quick and pleasant read in spite of the fact that it is very detailed in the information it gives... A book for anyone concerned about diet and nutrition."
—*American Reference Books Annual, 2007*

SEE ALSO *Eating Disorders Information for Teens, 2nd Edition*

Drug Information for Teens, 2nd Edition

Health Tips about the Physical and Mental Effects of Substance Abuse

Including Information about Marijuana, Inhalants, Club Drugs, Stimulants, Hallucinogens, Opiates, Prescription and Over-the-Counter Drugs, Herbal Products, Tobacco, Alcohol, and More

Edited by Sandra Augustyn Lawton. 468 pages. 2006. 978-0-7808-0862-1.

"As with earlier installments in Omnigraphics' Teen Health Series, Drug Information for Teens is designed specifically to meet the needs and interests of middle and high school students... Strongly recommended for both academic and public libraries."
—*American Reference Books Annual*, 2007

"Solid thoughtful advice is given about how to handle peer pressure, drug-related health concerns, and treatment strategies."
—*School Library Journal*, Dec '06

SEE ALSO *Alcohol Information for Teens, 2nd Edition, Tobacco Information for Teens, 2nd Edition*

Eating Disorders Information for Teens, 2nd Edition

Health Tips about Anorexia, Bulimia, Binge Eating, And Other Eating Disorders

Including Information about Risk Factors, Diagnosis and Treatment, Prevention, Related Health Concerns, and Other Issues

Edited by Sandra Augustyn Lawton. 377 pages. 2009. 978-0-7808-1044-0.

"This handy reference offers basic information and addresses specific disorders, consequences, prevention, diagnosis and treatment, healthy eating, and more. It is written in a conversational style that is easy to understand... Will provide plenty of facts for reports as well as browsing potential for students with an interest in the topic."
—*School Library Journal*, Jun '09

"Written in a straightforward style that will appeal to its teenage audience. The author does not play down the danger of living with an eating disorder and urges those struggling with this problem to seek professional help.

This work, as well as others in this series, will be a welcome addition to high school and undergraduate libraries."
—*American Reference Books Annual*, 2009

SEE ALSO *Diet Information for Teens, 2nd Edition*

Fitness Information for Teens, 2nd Edition

Health Tips about Exercise, Physical Well-Being, and Health Maintenance

Including Facts about Conditioning, Stretching, Strength Training, Body Shape and Body Image, Sports Nutrition, and Specific Activities for Athletes and Non-Athletes

Edited by Lisa Bakewell. 432 pages. 2009. 978-0-7808-1045-7.

"This no-nonsense guide packs a great deal into its pages... This is a helpful reference for basic diet and exercise information for health reports or personal use."
—*School Library Journal*, April 2009

"An excellent source for general information on why teens should be active, making time to exercise, the equipment people might need, various types of activities to try, how to maintain health and wellness, and how to avoid barriers to becoming healthier... This would still be an excellent addition to a public library ready-reference collection or a high school health library collection."
—*American Reference Books Annual*, 2009

"This easy to read, well-written, up-to-date overview of fitness for teenagers provides excellent wellness and exercise tips, information, and directions... It is a useful tool for them to obtain a base knowledge in fitness topics and different sports."
—*Doody's Review Service*, 2009

SEE ALSO *Diet Information for Teens, 2nd Edition, Sports Injuries Information for Teens, 2nd Edition*

Learning Disabilities Information for Teens

Health Tips about Academic Skills Disorders and Other Disabilities That Affect Learning

Including Information about Common Signs of Learning Disabilities, School Issues, Learning to Live with a Learning Disability, and Other Related Issues

Edited by Sandra Augustyn Lawton. 400 pages. 2006. 978-0-7808-0796-9.

"This book provides a wealth of information for any reader interested in the signs, causes, and consequences of learning disabilities, as well as related legal rights and educational interventions... Public and academic libraries should want this title for both students and general readers."

—*American Reference Books Annual, 2006*

▓

Mental Health Information for Teens, 3rd Edition
Health Tips about Mental Wellness and Mental Illness
Including Facts about Mental and Emotional Health, Depression and Other Mood Disorders, Anxiety Disorders, Behavior Disorders, Self-Injury, Psychosis, Schizophrenia, and More

Edited by Karen Bellenir. 400 pages. 2010. 978-0-7808-1087-7.

SEE ALSO *Stress Information for Teens, Suicide Information for Teens, 2nd Edition*

▓

Pregnancy Information for Teens
Health Tips about Teen Pregnancy and Teen Parenting
Including Facts about Prenatal Care, Pregnancy Complications, Labor and Delivery, Postpartum Care, Pregnancy-Related Lifestyle Concerns, and More

Edited by Sandra Augustyn Lawton. 434 pages. 2007. 978-0-7808-0984-0.

▓

Sexual Health Information for Teens, 2nd Edition
Health Tips about Sexual Development, Reproduction, Contraception, and Sexually Transmitted Infections
Including Facts about Puberty, Sexuality, Birth Control, Chlamydia, Gonorrhea, Herpes, Human Papillomavirus, Syphilis, and More

Edited by Sandra Augustyn Lawton. 430 pages. 2008. 978-0-7808-1010-5.

"This offering represents the most up-to-date information available on an array of topics including abstinence-only sexual education and pregnancy-prevention methods... The range of coverage—from puberty and anatomy to sexually transmitted diseases—is thorough and extensive. Each chapter includes a bibliographic citation, and the three back sections containing additional resources, further reading, and the index are all first-rate... This volume will be well used by students in need of the facts, whether for educational or personal reasons."

—*School Library Journal, Nov '08*

"Presents information related to the emotional, physical, and biological development of both males and females that occurs during puberty. It also strives to address some of the issues and questions that may arise... The text is easy to read and understand for young readers, with satisfactory definitions within the text to explain new terms."

—*American Reference Books Annual, 2009*

▓

Skin Health Information for Teens, 2nd Edition
Health Tips about Dermatological Concerns and Skin Cancer Risks
Including Facts about Acne, Warts, Hives, and Other Conditions and Lifestyle Choices, Such as Tanning, Tattooing, and Piercing, That Affect the Skin, Nails, Scalp, and Hair

Edited by Edited by Kim Wohlenhaus. 418 pages. 2009. 978-0-7808-1042-6.

"The material in this work will be easily understood by teenagers and young adults. The publisher has liberally used bulleted lists and sidebars to keep the reader's attention... A useful addition to school and public library collections."

—*ARBAOnline, Oct '09*

▓

Sleep Information for Teens
Health Tips about Adolescent Sleep Requirements, Sleep Disorders, and the Effects of Sleep Deprivation
Including Facts about Why People Need Sleep, Sleep Patterns, Circadian Rhythms, Dreaming, Insomnia, Sleep Apnea, Narcolepsy, and More

Edited by Karen Bellenir. 355 pages. 2008. 978-0-7808-1009-9.

"Clear, concise, and very readable and would be a good source of sleep information for anyone—not just teenagers. This work is highly recommended for medical libraries, public school libraries, and public libraries."
—*American Reference Books Annual, 2009*

SEE ALSO *Body Information for Teens*

Sports Injuries Information for Teens, 2nd Edition
Health Tips about Acute, Traumatic, and Chronic Injuries in Adolescent Athletes
Including Facts about Sprains, Fractures, and Overuse Injuries, Treatment, Rehabilitation, Sport-Specific Safety Guidelines, Fitness Suggestions, and More

Edited by Karen Bellenir. 429 pages. 2008. 978-0-7808-1011-2.

"An engaging selection of informative articles about the prevention and treatment of sports injuries... The value of this book is that the articles have been vetted and are often augmented with inserts of useful facts, definitions of technical terms, and quick tips. Sensitive topics like injuries to genitalia are discussed openly and responsibly. This revised edition contains updated articles and defines sport more broadly than the first edition."
—*School Library Journal, Nov '08*

"This work will be useful in the young adult collections of public libraries as well as high school libraries... A useful resource for student research."
—*American Reference Books Annual, 2009*

SEE ALSO *Accident and Safety Information for Teens*

Stress Information for Teens
Health Tips about the Mental and Physical Consequences of Stress
Including Information about the Different Kinds of Stress, Symptoms of Stress, Frequent Causes of Stress, Stress Management Techniques, and More

Edited by Sandra Augustyn Lawton. 392 pages. 2008. 978-0-7808-1012-9.

"Understanding what stress is, what causes it, how the body and the mind are impacted by it, and what teens can do are the general categories addressed here... The chapters are brief but informative, and the list of community-help organizations is exhaustive. Report writers will find information quickly and easily, as will those who have personal concerns. The print is clear and the format is readable, making this an accessible resource for struggling readers and researchers."
—*School Library Journal, Dec '08*

"The articles selected will specifically appeal to young adults and are designed to answer their most common questions."
— *American Reference Books Annual, 2009*

SEE ALSO *Mental Health Information for Teens, 3rd Edition*

Suicide Information for Teens, 2nd Edition
Health Tips about Suicide Causes and Prevention
Including Facts about Depression, Risk Factors, Getting Help, Survivor Support, and More

Edited by Kim Wohlenhaus. 400 pages. 2010. 978-0-7808-1088-4.

SEE ALSO *Mental Health Information for Teens, 3rd Edition*

Tobacco Information for Teens, 2nd Edition
Health Tips about the Hazards of Using Cigarettes, Smokeless Tobacco, and Other Nicotine Products
Including Facts about Nicotine Addiction, Nicotine Delivery Systems, Secondhand Smoke, Health Consequences of Tobacco Use, Related Cancers, Smoking Cessation, and Tobacco Use Statistics

Edited by Karen Bellenir. 400 pages. 2010. 978-0-7808-1153-9.

SEE ALSO **Drug Information for Teens, 2nd Edition**

Health Reference Series

Alcoholism Sourcebook, 3rd Edition

Allergies Sourcebook, 3rd Edition

Alzheimer Disease Sourcebook, 4th Edition

Arthritis Sourcebook, 3rd Edition

Asthma Sourcebook, 2nd Edition

Attention Deficit Disorder Sourcebook

Autism & Pervasive Developmental Disorders
Sourcebook

Back & Neck Sourcebook, 2nd Edition

Blood & Circulatory Disorders Sourcebook,
3rd Edition

Brain Disorders Sourcebook, 3rd Edition

Breast Cancer Sourcebook, 3rd Edition

Breastfeeding Sourcebook

Burns Sourcebook

Cancer Sourcebook for Women, 4th Edition

Cancer Sourcebook, 5th Edition

Cancer Survivorship Sourcebook

Cardiovascular Disorders Sourcebook,
4th Edition

Caregiving Sourcebook

Child Abuse Sourcebook

Childhood Diseases & Disorders Sourcebook,
2nd Edition

Colds, Flu & Other Common Ailments
Sourcebook

Communication Disorders Sourcebook

Complementary & Alternative Medicine
Sourcebook, 4th Edition

Congenital Disorders Sourcebook, 2nd Edition

Contagious Diseases Sourcebook

Cosmetic & Reconstructive Surgery
Sourcebook, 2nd Edition

Death & Dying Sourcebook, 2nd Edition

Dental Care & Oral Health Sourcebook,
3rd Edition

Depression Sourcebook, 2nd Edition

Dermatological Disorders Sourcebook,
2nd Edition

Diabetes Sourcebook, 4th Edition

Diet & Nutrition Sourcebook, 3rd Edition

Digestive Diseases & Disorder Sourcebook

Disabilities Sourcebook

Disease Management Sourcebook

Domestic Violence Sourcebook, 3rd Edition

Drug Abuse Sourcebook, 3rd Edition

Ear, Nose & Throat Disorders Sourcebook,
2nd Edition

Eating Disorders Sourcebook, 3rd Edition

Emergency Medical Services Sourcebook

Endocrine & Metabolic Disorders Sourcebook,
2nd Edition

Environmental Health Sourcebook, 3rd Edition

Ethnic Diseases Sourcebook

Eye Care Sourcebook, 3rd Edition

Family Planning Sourcebook

Fitness & Exercise Sourcebook, 4th Edition

Food Safety Sourcebook

Forensic Medicine Sourcebook

Gastrointestinal Diseases & Disorders
Sourcebook, 2nd Edition

Genetic Disorders Sourcebook, 3rd Edition

Head Trauma Sourcebook

Headache Sourcebook

Health Insurance Sourcebook

Healthy Aging Sourcebook

Healthy Children Sourcebook

Healthy Heart Sourcebook for Women

Hepatitis Sourcebook

Household Safety Sourcebook

Hypertension Sourcebook

Immune System Disorders Sourcebook,
2nd Edition

Infant & Toddler Health Sourcebook

Infectious Diseases Sourcebook

Injury & Trauma Sourcebook